Awakening and Sleep-Wake Cycle across Development

Advances in Consciousness Research

Advances in Consciousness Research provides a forum for scholars from different scientific disciplines and fields of knowledge who study consciousness in its multifaceted aspects. Thus the Series will include (but not be limited to) the various areas of cognitive science, including cognitive psychology, linguistics, brain science and philosophy. The orientation of the Series is toward developing new interdisciplinary and integrative approaches for the investigation, description and theory of consciousness, as well as the practical consequences of this research for the individual and society.

Series B: Research in progress. Experimental, descriptive and clinical research in consciousness.

Volume 38

Awakening and Sleep-Wake Cycle across Development
Edited by Piero Salzarulo and Gianluca Ficca

Awakening and Sleep-Wake Cycle across Development

Edited by

Piero Salzarulo
University of Florence

Gianluca Ficca
Second University of Naples

John Benjamins Publishing Company
Amsterdam / Philadelphia

TM The paper used in this publication meets the minimum requirements of American National Standard for Information Sciences – Permanence of Paper for Printed Library Materials, ANSI Z39.48-1984.

Library of Congress Cataloging-in-Publication Data

Awakening and sleep-wake cycle across development / edited by Piero Salzarulo, Gianluca Ficca.

p. cm. (Advances in Consciousness Research, ISSN 1381–589X ; v. 38)

Includes bibliographical references and index.

1. Sleep-wake cycle. 2. Developmental neurobiology. I. Salzarulo, Piero. II. Ficca, Gianluca. III. Series.

QP84.6.A935 2002
612.8'21--dc21 2002276248
ISBN 90 272 5158 4 (Eur.) / 1 58811 174 1 (US) (Pb; alk. paper)

John Benjamins Publishing Co. · P.O. Box 36224 · 1020 ME Amsterdam · The Netherlands
John Benjamins North America · P.O. Box 27519 · Philadelphia PA 19118-0519 · USA

Table of contents

3. Physiological and environmental influences on awakenings

4. Clinical contexts

Awakening

Which changes across development?

Piero Salzarulo
Department of Psychology, University of Florence

Sleep-wakefulness rhythm undergoes impressive changes across development: both sleep and wakefulness change not only in duration and temporal organization, but also in physiological and behavioural qualities. All these features have been extensively described in the last decades (for reviews see Salzarulo & Fagioli, 1999; Curzi & Challamel, 2000).The trend with development consists in the consolidation of sleep episodes of longer duration during the night and in the lengthening of wakefulness episodes during the day. Within this frame it is easily understandable that awakening is a crucial event. Nevertheless, contributions on this topic are relatively scarce. They come from different streams of investigation, sometimes with different terminologies. There are experimental researches on normal babies speaking about 'awakening', clinical approaches referring to 'night waking', and investigations about respiratory pathologies which often use the term 'arousal' (see for instance Groswasser et al. contribution, this volume).

It is important to examine the conceptual frame which underlies each of these domains; there are methodological and epistemological aspects which need to be underscored.

Experimental research showed frequency and age distribution in normal infants and was also intended to shed light on the processes which lead to awakening. Awakening was characterized by the appearance of behavioural manifestations of wakefulness (for a review see Hayes and Fagioli et al., this volume).

Night waking is a concept mainly used in pediatric and psychology practice which is related to an excessive frequency and, above all, duration of wakefulness during the night as a consequence of a single or of multiple awakenings. While the causes are multiple (see Messer & Richards, 1993 for a review), emphasis is put on practical approaches to solve this disturbing event for families.

A third approach comes mainly from the field of respiratory disturbances and uses a different term, 'arousal', which is often considered an 'equivalent' of awakening. Some authors, as Thach & Lijowska (1996), speak about 'full arousal' to indicate 'awakening'. In fact, this is an intriguing problem which deserves some comments and should be clarified. The term 'arousal', not only in the field of respiratory disturbances during development, often indicates a change in the depth of sleep, which resumes (in fact it never disappeared) after a short time interval measured in seconds (ASDA, 1992). These short time events have been interpreted as signs of physiological activation.To clarify the situation, a main research challenge could be to compare awakening features with arousal features, as far as the processes leading to and their consequences are concerned.

Besides the definition of the main features characterising each (arousal and awakening), the continuity between the two is of interest (a topic evoked also by Hayes and Ficca in this volume). Is the awakening the transformation of the arousal? Is arousal a necessary event preceding awakening? Thach & Lijowska (1996), for instance, consider sighs and 'trashing' (i.e. motor events), signs of 'arousal' necessarily preceding the 'full arousal' (i.e. 'awakening'). Chugh et al. (1996), speaking about the adult, are in favour of a continuum between arousal and awakening, whereas Scher et al. (1992), in studies on babies, pinpoint the marked difference between the mechanisms regulating the two. A further question: is arousal an expression of a temporary short instability of the CNS activity, while awakening is a 'true' change of state? Evidence could come also from the study of the developmental trends of both events: do arousal ad awakening share the same trends (i.e. change with age)? If not, this could be an additional argument to separate them.

It is important to remember that awakening is a transition between two different modes of CNS functionning (Wolff, 1984), facing each other: sleep state and wakefulness state. Time and modalities for passing the frontier (Garma, 1994) between these two blocks depend on several factors. First, the intrinsic features of each 'block' which are linked to maturation. Then, the ability of the brain to reconstruct a different mode of activity, which consists in the coordination of several physiological functions. The modalities of transition will be more or less smooth or abrupt, mainly on the basis of these capacities. The transition process should have its time course, which however is at present poorly known. A schematic sequence has been proposed recently by Thach and

Lijowska (1996), based on respiratory and motor events; a study taking into account the EEG activity level preceding spontaneous behavioural awakening in infants is currently being performed in our lab (Zampi et al., 2001).

Wakefulness is important for development (Salzarulo & Fagioli, 1995) and its characteristics change with age (Wolff, 1984). Thus, speaking about awakening, it seems important to take into account the kind of wakefulness which follows as a function of age. Waking up for doing what? Just move, look around or interact with objects, persons? There are possibilities which could be unavailable at the beginning of life, and become a 'choice' only later. Modalities and processes of transition between sleep and wakefulness could depend also from the repertoire of wakefulness that infants have at their disposal as expression of their maturational step (see Hopkins contribution, this volume).

In this book, in order to develop some of the topics mentioned above, we decided to include a set of papers by colleagues who made significant contributions in the field and who are involved in the study of the precocious development of behavioural and physiological components of sleep and wakefulness.

The book, mainly dealing with the issues discussed during a meeting held in Florence, April 14–15, 2000 (partially supported by University of Florence), is intended to present contributions from both experimental and clinical fields. Some of the papers refer to ongoing discussions within a working group (Wake up club) on a developing consensus about criteria to define awakening and arousal.

A first set of papers will raise methodological and theoretical problems dealing with awakening during development: in particular, the above mentioned confrontation "arousal vs awakening", which implies the construction and the agreement on criteria for defining each (see Hayes, Ficca and Ariagno contributions). Closely connected is the definition(s) of wakefulness(es) as a function of age, from its emergence to further qualitative and quantitative development (see Hopkins contribution).

A second group of papers will describe changes in awakening from preterm infants to school-age children (see Curzi et al.; Fagioli et al.; Bruni et al. papers). They include both systematic data collected up to now and suggestions on criteria as well as on models which could account for processes involved. In any case, they are a useful backgound for comparison with results obtained in clinical contexts.

Physiological and environmental factors influencing awakening will be considered in a third section. Interaction with temperature regulation is a topic of particular interest, since it raises the problem of the modalities of adaptation to external conditions and of mechanisms of biological regulation at early epochs of development (see Bach et al. paper). Obviously the family, and in particular the mother, has a role, also throughout parental practices, in modifying the frequency and possibly the characteristics of awakening. This kind of approach has been pursued in various social contexts (see Wulff & Siegmund; Scher; Sadeh; Giganti & Toselli contributions).

The fourth section concerns pathology and night waking. The frequency of arousals is greatly increased in some pathologies (see Gaultier; Vecchierini & Navelet; Groswasser et al. contributions; see also Curzi et al.). Interestingly, respiratory disturbances during sleep are accompanied by an increased frequency of arousals, but not of awakenings. This context represents a clear evidence of the usefulness to separate arousal from awakening.

In altered psychological relationships the excess of awakening, either real or claimed by the parents, represents a frequent and often distressing event (see Sadeh contribution), leading to what has been frequently reported in the literature as 'night waking' (see again Messer & Richards, 1993 for a review). Sadeh contribution opens a window on the sleep problems of infants and children. In future investigations it would be interesting to know which is the quality of wakefulness in those children and what kind of awakening they show, relative to children of the same age without sleep problems.

References

ASDA (1992). EEG arousals: scoring rules and examples. A preliminary report from the sleep disorders atlas task force of the American sleep disorders association. *Sleep*, 15, 174–184.

Chugh, Deepak K., Terri E. Weaver, & David F. Dinges (1996). Neurobehavioral consequences of arousals. *Sleep*, 19, S198–S201.

Curzi-Dascalova, Lilia, & Marie-Joséphe Challamel (2000). Neurophysiological basis of sleep development. In Loughin G.M., J.L. Carrol & C.L. Marcus (Eds.), *Sleep and breathing in children. A developmental approach* (3–37). New York: Dekker.

Garma, Lucile (1994). *Clinique de l'insomnie*. Paris: P.U.F.

Messer, David, & Martin Richards (1993). The development of sleeping difficulties. In St James-Roberts I., G. Harris & D. Messer (Eds.), *Crying, feeding and sleeping* (150–173). London: Harvester.

Salzarulo, Piero, & Igino Fagioli (1995). Sleep for development or development for waking? Some speculations from a human perspective. *Behavioural Brain Research*, *69*, 23–29.

Salzarulo, Piero, & Igino Fagioli (1999). Changes of sleep states and physiological activities across the first year of life. In Kalverboer Alex, Maria Luisa Genta & Brian Hopkins (Eds.), *Current issues in developmental psychology. Biopsychological perspectives* (53–74). Dordrecht: Kluwer.

Scher, Mark, Doris A. Steppe, Ronald E. Dahl, Shoba Asthana & Robert D. Guthrie (1992). Comparison of EEG sleep measures in healthy full-term and preterm infants at matched conceptional ages. *Sleep*, *15*, 442–448.

Thach, Bradley T., & Anna Lijowska (1996). Arousal in infants. *Sleep*, *19*, S271–S273.

Wolff, Peter (1984). Discontinuous changes in human wakefulness around the end of the second month of life: a developmental perspective. In Prechtl, Heinz F.R. (Ed.), Continuity of Neural functions; from prenatal to postnatal life (144–158). Oxford: Blackwell.

Zampi, Chiara, Igino Fagioli & Piero Salzarulo (2001). Attività EEG precedente il risveglio nei primi quattro mesi di vita. Italian Society of Sleep Research, 6° Congress, Bologna, May, 11 and 12.

Development of wakefulness

Re-awakening a neglected topic

Brian Hopkins
Department of Psychology,
Lancaster University, UK

Introduction

In a short note, published almost 25 years ago, a leading sleep investigator pleaded for more research on wakefulness (Kleitman, 1977). In subsequent years, this plea has largely gone unheeded and especially with regard to the development of wakefulness. There are many reasons for such a neglect. One is simply that describing sleep and accounting for its mechanisms are more tractable issues than is the case for wakefulness, which brings with it additional considerations like attention and how it develops. Another stems from the lack of a theoretical framework that would provide testable hypotheses about the nature of wakefulness and the developmental changes that it undergoes. Yet, despite these problems, there is at least one general principle with which most sleep researchers agree and that mitigates against studying sleep to the exclusion of wakefulness. This is that the functions of sleep and wakefulness are inextricably related (Salzarulo & Fagioli, 1995) – a principle embodied in both earlier theories (e.g., Roffwarg et al., 1966) and more recent ones (e.g., Crick & Mitchinson, 1995) concerning the roles played by REM sleep.

The present contribution does not endeavour to delve into how sleep and wakefulness may co-develop. Rather, it concerns the more restricted topic of how wakefulness develops, both quantitatively and qualitatively. In doing so, however, it will be impossible to ignore entirely drawing parallels between the two conditions. Given these qualifications, the topics to be addressed include the following: wakefulness from prenatal to postnatal life, the relevance of the behavioural state concept in studying the development of wakefulness, and the developmental processes involved in the change from transient to sustained periods of wakefulness. The latter topic has important theoretical ramifications, which raise questions about the relevance of dynamical systems thinking for understanding such a developmental change in wakefulness. Before addressing these topics, we begin with some preliminary remarks on the nature of wakefulness that will be elaborated upon in subsequent sections.

Some comments on the nature of wakefulness

In keeping with Kleitman's (1977) entreaty for more research on wakefulness, he had previously made an apposite distinction: wakefulness of necessity as against wakefulness of choice (Kleitman, 1963). The former refers to waking that is triggered and maintained by physiologically induced feelings of discomfort such as those associated with hunger, bowel or bladder distension or changes in body temperature. The latter implies wakefulness that is actively sustained through goal-directed movements that achieve observable effects in the physical or social environment. Developmentally, the import of the distinction is that wakefulness of necessity gives way to one that is qualitatively different in that it is dependent on the emergence of behaviours subject to voluntary control some time during the first year after birth (Kleitman, 1963).

In order to grasp the activity-dependent nature of wakefulness of choice, it is useful to recount the way it has been defined by Wolff (1987):

> ... that disposition when the infant practises and refines acquired sensorimotor patterns, discovers new novelties in the environment, and invents new combinations among component elements that become a means for intellectual exploration and social communication (p. 54)

While this definition is redolent of Piaget's (1952) account of how circular reactions develop, it contains the ingredients for the derivation of a theoretical framework applicable to the development of wakefulness. We will return to this promissory note later on and also to the question of whether the necessity-choice distinction is a meaningful one to apply to the behaviour of young infants. For the time being, we note that, relative to sleep, little is known about the development of wakefulness, especially with regard to any qualitative changes it may undergo. What then is known about quantitative changes in the amount of wakefulness during early development?

Development of wakefulness: Quantitative changes

Based on serial ultrasound and cardiotachographic recordings, the human foetus appears to be primarily a somnambulant, but active, organism (i.e., one that manifests a predominance of REM-like sleep). Even at term age, the percentage of recording time (viz., 2 hours) that the foetus was judged to be awake had a median value of only about 7% (Nijhuis et al., 1982). The same appears to be the case for preterm infants matched for gestational age and who also show an increasing differentiation between sleep and wakefulness as term age is approached (Mirmiran, 1995).

These comparisons suggest that the developmental foundations for both sleep and wakefulness arise from environment-independent processes rooted in the genetic regulation of monoamine metabolism (Greenspan et al., 2001). Moreover, the brain activation theory originally proposed by Roffwarg et al. (1966) has led to speculation that the high level of REM-like sleep evident from the second half of human pregnancy may serve as a replacement for wakefulness, particularly with regard to promoting the development of the visual system (see Hobson, 1995). While providing an attractive way of accounting for a continuity between prenatal and postnatal life in the development of wakefulness, findings from animal studies do not lend unequivocal support to the theory (see Mirmiran, 1995). Is, however, the transition to the extrauterine environment at term age associated with a marked quantitative discontinuity in wakefulness? The short answer is 'yes'.

In a comprehensive study of neonatal functions immediately after birth, it was reported that fullterm newborns are mainly awake during the first six hours relative to time thereafter (Desmond et al., 1963). After the first postpartum day, other studies would lead one to expect the newborn to be awake (but not drowsy or crying) for about 10 to 15% of a range of observation times (e.g., see Berg et al., 1973; Prechtl, 1965). In a pioneering programme of longitudinal research involving 14 infants, Wolff (1987) found prolonged periods of wakefulness during the first 24 hours, regardless of the mode of delivery. During these periods, they were able to pursue a moving target with their eyes, but not in conjunction with head movements. Some 48 hours later, this ability was much less evident.

Why is wakefulness so prominent in the first few hours after birth? The explanation is undoubtedly complicated, but it must have something to do with stresses and strains imposed by birth that are perhaps common to both vaginal and Caesarean section deliveries. It is known that during delivery high levels of the hormones adrenaline and noradrenaline are released (Lagercrantz &

Slotkin, 1986). With their diffuse effects on the sympathetic nervous system, but in particular on brain stem nuclei such as the locus coeruleous, an excess of these hormones acting together might promote a sort of wakefulness of necessity while at the same time suppressing sleep. In addition, their actions may help to clear the lungs and to establish independent respiration.

How do the quantitative features of wakefulness subsequently develop? In brief, its overall duration increases gradually from 24% of observation time at 2 weeks to 64% by the end of the third month. Wolff (1987) also reported concomitant increases in individual periods of uninterrupted wakefulness, especially between the second and third month. By about 6 months, these periods of wakefulness without crying were maintained for upwards of 200 min. at a time. Another feature is a progressive allocation of wakefulness to the daylight hours with sleep being mainly reserved for the night-time. This achievement of a stable circadian sleep-wake rhythm also becomes evident around 2 to 3 months as revealed by both parental diaries (Hellbrugge et al., 1964) and laboratory-based observations (Coons & Guilleminault, 1982).

Is the duration of wakefulness susceptible to alteration after the newborn period? There are a number of ways in which this question can be answered. One is to compare the findings of a home-based study like that of Wolff (1987) with those obtained by Dittrichova and Lapàckova (1964) from observations of institutionalized infants. As reported by Wolff (1987), this comparison revealed increasing differences between the two groups of infants, particularly from 12 weeks onwards: at this age, those who were home-reared were on average awake for more than twice as long (about 60%) as their institutionalized counterparts (less than 30%), and even 3 months later the relative amount of wakefulness (about 45%) was still less than for the infants in Wolff's study at 12 weeks. Another example comes from a comparison between bottle- and breast-fed infants, and showing that the former were awake for longer and slept less (Wolff, 1987). By 3 months, these differences had disappeared. These findings should be set against those derived from infants with a tracheoaesphogeal fistula who were tube fed for 24 hours a day and who therefore did not suffer from discomfort due to hunger (Salzarulo et al., 1980). Nevertheless, they had intermittent periods of waking – a finding that speaks against the view that wakefulness during the first three months only occurs out of necessity. Finally, Wolff (1987) demonstrated that visually- and auditory-based interventions could prolong periods of wakefulness by more than 15 min. Once again, these interventions were really only effective up to 3 months of age.

To summarize so far, both the overall duration and length of uninterrupted periods of wakefulness more than doubles between birth and 3 months of age in healthy fullterm infants. Prior to this age, both expressions of wakefulness can be substantially altered by environmental influences, which suggests that waking does not yet possess the self-regulatory properties typical of sleep. It also implies that wakefulness without crying undergoes both quantitative and qualitative changes at around 3 months. As for crying, it follows a somewhat different developmental trend, chief among which is a peak in its duration at about 6 weeks of age (see Hopkins, 2000). Thus, the next question to be addressed is whether wakefulness without crying does indeed manifest qualitative changes some time around the third month after a fullterm birth. Asking this question necessitates consideration of the concept of behavioural state as applied to infants.

Development of wakefulness: Qualitative changes

Behavioural state is a "... temporally enduring constellation of values of indicator variables" (McCarley, 1980, p. 379). For infants, such variables include condition of the eyes, respiratory patterns and the absence or presence of general movements. Each state has been treated as a particular mode of nervous activity and not as conditions along some continuum of arousal (Prechtl, 1974). While depicted as being qualitatively different from each other and having their own (non-linear) input-output relationships, these claims are the most convincing for REM (active) and NREM (quiet) sleep. With regard to wakefulness, crying is distinguished from two other states, which are labelled by Wolff (1987) as 'alert inactive' and 'alert active'. As for drowsiness, it is regarded as a discrete state (Brazelton, 1984), a transitional state (Thoman, 1990) or as a transitional period between waking and sleep (Wolff, 1987).

Three points need to be emphasised about the classification of waking states. Firstly, unlike sleep states, they do not adequately cater for the increasing differentiation of behaviour in the awake infant beyond the first couple of months after birth. Wolff (1987) proposed the state of alert activity as one way of overcoming this problem. Secondly, the distinction between alert inactive and alert active states rests on rather arbitrary distinctions between levels of activity (Ashton, 1973). It relies as such on some implicit judgement, sharpened by the experience of extensively observing the spontaneous behaviour of young infants (Wolff, 1987). Thirdly, waking states like those for sleep, have to endure for an arbitrarily imposed period of time (e.g., 3 min.). While, in conjunction with some form of smoothing technique, this may enable the identification of stable sleep states, it is of questionable value when applied to those during wakefulness given that it is especially susceptible to environmental influences during the first few months of postnatal life.

Prenatally, two sleep and two wake states comparable to those in the newborn have been identified, with those for sleep complying with criteria for stability by 36 to 38 weeks gestational age (Nijhuis et al., 1982; Groome & Watson, 1992). At this age, both quiet wakefulness (State 3F) and active wakefulness (State 4F) were difficult to detect and only fleetingly present. As with the newborn, a state was considered to be present only if its parameters of the indicator variables changed together within a moving window of 3 min. and then remained the same for at least another 3 min. (see Figure 1).

The consequences of using such an arbitrary time window to denote a change from one state to another are three-fold. The first is that the foetus (or infant) is always in one state or another. Consequently, the potential functional

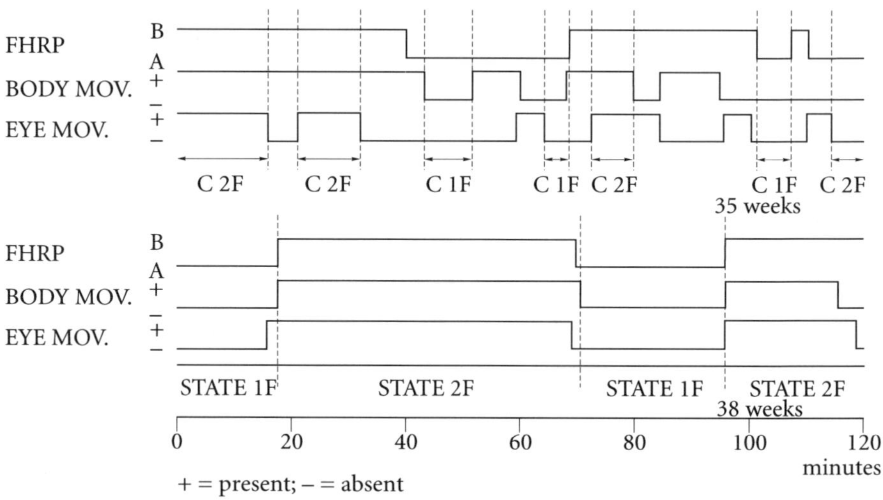

Figure 1. Changes in state parameters over 120 min at 35 weeks (upper profiles) and 38 weeks (lower profiles) gestational age. Parameters coincide (C) within a 3 min. moving window on a irregular basis indicating that sleep states 1F and 2F are not yet stable entities. By 38 weeks, stability of state has been achieved as shown by the three parameters always changing within 3 min. and then remaining unchanged for at least the same duration. Note that with the moving window technique, a foetus can only be in one state or another and that parameter fluctuations as well as transitional periods have been removed (Reproduced with permission from Nijhuis et al., 1984).
FHRP: Foetal heart pattern. A: heart rate stable within a narrow range. B: heart varies within a broader range than A. +/–: present/absent.

significance of fluctuations in indicator variables between states is ignored. Fluctuations (i.e., stochastic processes) in the state of a system have been portrayed as the 'motor' of change in both real time (i.e., seconds, minutes, hours) and ontogenetic time (i.e., weeks, months, years) by a number of authors (e.g., Kugler et al., 1982). Furthermore, if wake states have intrinsic durations of less than 3 min., then their presence will be infrequently detected.

Does crying have its origins in prenatal life? One possibility is that the pre-respiratory accompaniments of crying (e.g., facial movements) are established before birth such that they can be coordinated to form a 'cry face' (Hopkins, 2000). With the transition to the extrauterine environment and the ability to breathe independently, these non-vocal features of crying become linked to its vocal component. On this view, crying does not emerge *de novo* with the birth cry of the newborn, but in certain respects has a continuity in development between prenatal and postnatal life.

According to Wolff (1987), the postnatal development of waking states undergoes a striking qualitative change at around 2 to 3 months of age. During the newborn period, the alert active state is hardly present while some 2 months later its relative duration greatly exceeds that of alert inactivity (see Figure 2).

The defining feature of alert activity is the emergence of the ability to perform two or more actions simultaneously – a sort of dual-task performance

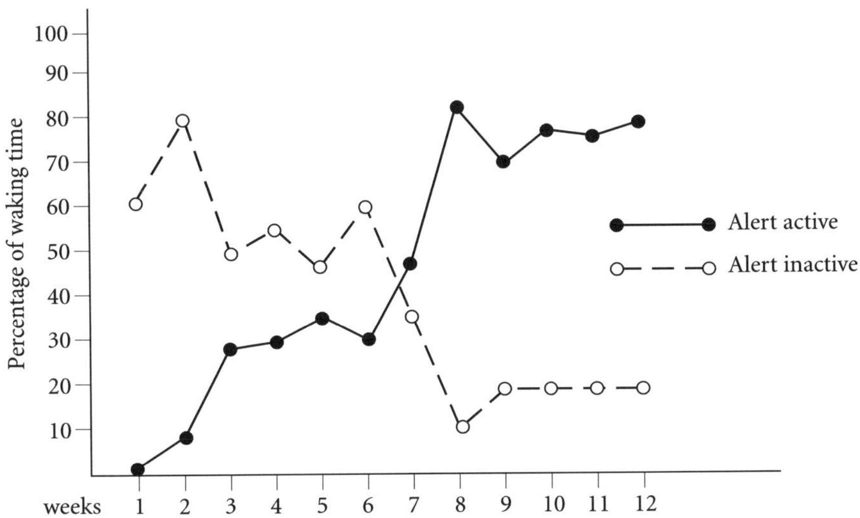

Figure 2. Presence of alert inactive and alert active states as percentage of waking time from 1 to 12 weeks (Reproduced with permission from Wolff, 1984).

liberated from 'stimulus boundedness'. Thus, for example, the infant can now grasp a foot while reaching for an object, engage in visual pursuit without having to inhibit other movements or abandon one action for another. Wakefulness of choice has become the *modus operandi* and is sustained not just by any interesting environmental event but through those events or effects engendered by the infant's self-initiated actions. In short, wakefulness has become self-regulatory or self-organizing and as such offers the possibility of new ways of combining actions (means) resulting in a marked expansion of possible outcomes (ends).

Crying also exhibits a change in quality some 2 to 3 months after birth with the appearance of 'interrupted fussing' (Hopkins & van Wulfften Palthe, 1987): rapid fluctuations between fussing and cooing during which the eyes remain

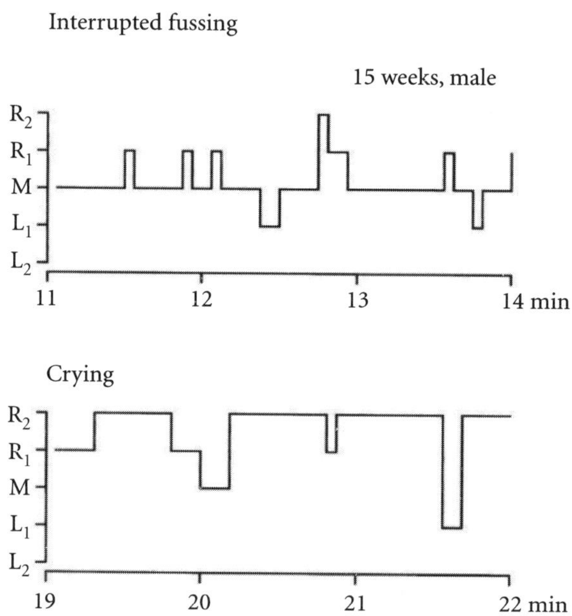

Figure 3. Typical example of head movements during interrupted fussing (eyes open) and crying (eyes closed) in the same infant at 15 weeks of age. Note that head movements during interrupted fussing shift relatively more frequently to the right (R) and left (L) from a midline (M) position. During crying, the head is mainly lateralized to the right.
R_1/L_1: head turned right /left up to 30° from midline.
R_2/L_2: head turned right/left more than 30° from midline.

open and the infant appears to be 'scanning' the immediate environment by means of coordinated head and eye movements (see Figure 3).

Occurring only when the infant is alone, it may constitute a form of 'vocal play' for exercising the articulatory and laryngeal mechanisms involved in speech acquisition or as a means of signalling a readiness to engage in social interactions. Subsequently, crying shows another qualitative change at about 6 months, but now when the infant is looking at the mother (see Gustafson & Green, 1991 who refer to it as elaborated crying).

'Alertness' as portrayed by Wolff (1987) seems to be synonymous in some respects with 'visual attention' as employed by others (e.g., Stechler & Latz, 1966). Acknowledging the shortcomings of using current classifications of wake states beyond the newborn period, further progress in understanding how wakefulness develops may accrue from incorporating recent models of (covert) attentional processes (e.g., see Posner et al., 1994) into the concept of behavioural state. A finding that moves us in this direction is that infants of about 6 weeks can enter periods of 'staring', lasting from about 10 to more than 80 sec. (Hopkins & van Wulfften Palthe, 1985). Absent after 3 months, the eyes are open but immobile while breathing and heart rate are irregular (see Figure 4), all of which go together with a loss of an active anti-gravity posture.

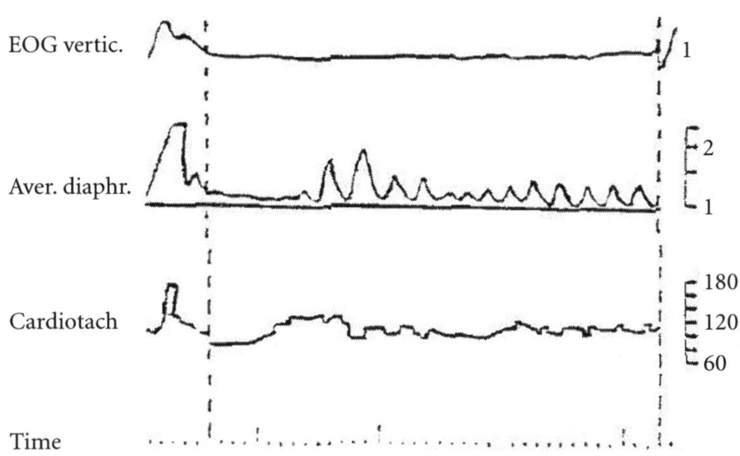

Figure 4. Recordings of eye movements (EOG vert.), respiration (Aver. diaphr.) and heart rate (Cardiotach.) during a period of staring lasting 37 sec. in an infant aged 6 weeks. Note the presence of a blink at the beginning and end of the period and the absence of eye movements during the period.

Phenomenologically at least, these periods appear to correspond with the 'sticky' attention reported for infants less than 2 months of age (e.g., see Atkinson et al., 1992). By this is meant an inability to disengage attention from its current focus. Some 2 months later, the infant is able to shift gaze both between and within visual arrays in an accurate, fast and reliable manner (see Johnson et al., 1991). Do such changes in covert attentional processes represent a qualitative shift in how wakefulness is organized? In principle, contemporary applications of dynamical systems thinking to ontogenetic development should provide an appropriate theoretical framework for tackling this sort of question.

On the developmental dynamics of wakefulness

In a nutshell, a dynamical systems approach attempts to capture the organizational principles governing transitions between stable states in complex, time-evolving systems (Hopkins & Butterworth, 1997). Space does not permit a detailed account of this approach and the reader is referred to Thelen and Smith (1994) and more recently to Hopkins (2001) for in-depth treatments. However, some indication of its relevance for studying the development of wakefulness can be conveyed through considering the meaning of self-organization and the distinction between order and control parameters.

Self-organization is a process by which new states spontaneously emerge in complex, open systems without any specification from the outside environment (Ball, 1999). The simplest form of self-organization is a non-equilibrium phase shift and which is flagged by fluctuations and a sudden jump, among other things, in the system's macroscopical behaviour prior to a change in state (see van der Maas & Hopkins, 1998). The system's global behaviour is captured by an order parameter or collective variable (i.e., the simplest descriptor of a high-dimensional complex system's behaviour in a stable state). A control parameter exerts constraints on the dynamics of the order parameter. However, when the control parameter is scaled up (or down) beyond some critical value, it may induce stochastic or even chaotic behaviour in the order parameter before it makes a sudden transition to a different state. A control parameter does not prescribe how an order parameter should change, but instead controls in the sense of leading the system through regions of instabilities between two stable states. An example of an order parameter is relative phase (i.e., the angular difference between the motions of two limbs that are approximately sinusoidal). Increasing the frequency of index finger flexions and extensions moving in anti-phase relative to each other results in an abrupt change to an in-phase mode following fluctuations and other markers of a non-equilibrium phase shift (Kelso, 1995). A relevant illustration of using relative phase in a developmental context can be found in a study of changes in EEG coherence between the ages of 1.5 and 16 years (Thatcher, 1998).

The distinction between order and control parameters warns us that a strict separation of qualitative from quantitative change is somewhat misleading. This is because a qualitative alteration in an order parameter can be triggered by a quantitative change of a control parameter beyond some critical value. Having said this, we are still confronted with the problem of identifying appropriate order and control parameters in studying the development of waking states. One potential order parameter could be the phase relationships between the respiratory movements of the diaphragm and intercostal muscles as recorded by surface EMG (see Prechtl et al., 1977). A control parameter might be derived from some continuously scaled measure of postural control given its intimate relationship to behavioural state in the young infant (see Casaer, 1979).

Ultimately, the goal of a dynamical systems approach should be that of appropriating the mathematical tools it offers to detect and model the nature of change in both real time and ontogenetic time during early development. An example of change along the first time scale involves modelling the dynamics of the transition from crying to an alert state as response to the administration of sucrose in 6 week-old infants (Barr et al., 1999). With regard to the second time scale, the development of wakefulness in general appears to adopt the hallmarks of a chaotic state by 2 months of age such that cyclical movements and visual attention become more strongly coupled (Robertson et al., 1993). This change may reflect the underlying dynamical regime (i.e., attractor state) that allows the infant to engage in 'doing two things at the same time' during Wolff's (1987) state of alert activity.

Concluding remarks

From its rather humble beginnings in prenatal life, wakefulness without crying becomes a defining feature of an infant's behaviour during daylight hours some 2 to 3 months after birth. Qualitatively, waking states have assumed some of the characteristics of sleep states by this age in that they have become more resistant to both internal and external sources of perturbation. The infant is now not just reactive, but also active as a consequence of improvements in perception and the control of movement and of the coupling between them.

Wakefulness has a new property, namely, that it is sustained by the infant's own actions, which have lost their obligatory character and assumed a voluntary-like appearance. It is perhaps this change in the quality of wakefulness that encapsulates the essence of the two-to-three month transformation in neural functions and which signifies a final break with a foetal behavioural repertoire. Wakefulness is now primed for the achievement of cognitive and social abilities that bear the stamp of executive functions.

This depiction of the early development of wakefulness glosses over two important hurdles to be crossed. One is the inadequacy of existing state classifications to cater for the substantive changes in the development of wakefulness occurring after 2 to 3 months of age. This problem is, for example, epitomized by the incursion of interrupted fussing into the development of crying at around the same age. As Wolff (1987) rightly points out, devising a taxonomy appropriate for classifying waking states beyond the newborn period is really not a satisfactory solution. Thus, adjusting state criteria to deal with the developmental differentiation of behaviour would give rise to an unmanageable list of age-specific indicator variables that then makes it impossible to carry out much needed longitudinal studies on the development of waking states.

The other, not unconnected, hurdle is the lack of a theoretical framework germane to studying infant waking states in both real and ontogenetic time. Following Wolff (1987), it was suggested that a dynamical systems approach to the development of wakefulness offers the scaffolding for constructing such a framework. With its emphasis on detecting and modelling stabilities and instabilities in time-evolving systems, it seems ideally suited for identifying transitions between states across both time scales. Moreover, it has the decided advantage of not requiring the imposition of arbitrary time limits on the duration of states as a transition to a new state will be signalled by hallmark changes in the behaviour of an appropriate order parameter. The problem then is to identify such an age-invariant descriptor (e.g., relative phase) together with those control parameters that induce it to re-organise in some way, and which probably differ from one age to the next (see Hopkins et al., 1993).

While the distinction between wakefulness of necessity and wakefulness of choice is helpful, it is too simplistic when applied to a developmental context. Rather than a change in wakefulness from one of necessity to one of choice, it is more likely that they co-develop, with the former having a less de-stabilising influence on the latter as the infant develops. One way of operationalizing the development of wakefulness of choice is contained in the suggestion of studying changes in covert attention during infancy. This suggestion rests on a deep-seated issue with implications for how we construe wakefulness, namely, consciousness.

Broadly speaking, consciousness can be defined as an awareness of one's surroundings and of one's thoughts and feelings. In the past, it was considered to be a scientifically impenetrable concept best suited to the arm-chair ruminations of philosophers. More recently, it has figured highly in the research agenda of the neurosciences due to the appearance of testable hypotheses based on new insights into brain functioning. Examples include Baars' (1997) theory of a global workspace and Crick's (1994) model of visual consciousness. Common to both is the supposition that one of the main functions of consciousness is to provide access to unconsciousness regions of the brain in order to activate, control and coordinate behaviour. This function is referred to access consciousness (AC), which is distinguished from phenomenal consciousness (PC).

AC is a form of direct control involving awareness and with its neural substrates residing in the frontal cortex (Block, 1996). In contrast, PC corresponds to selective attention and necessitates activity in the ventral pathway linking the striate cortex to prestriate areas and eventually to the infereotemporal cortex (see Milner & Goodale, 1995). From what is known about the prolonged functional development of the frontal cortex (Fuster, 1997), it would seem reasonable to propose PC as a necessary precursor for the emergence of the executive-like control ascribed to AC.

To return to Kleitman (1977), the rise of neuroscientific interest in what constitutes consciousness has begun to fulfil his request for better insights into the nature of wakefulness. How wakefulness relates to consciousness is a weighty topic for another time. However, an empirical approach to unravelling the functions of consciousness should serve to re-awaken interest in the development of wakefulness.

References

Ashton, R. (1973). The state variable in neonatal research: A review. *Merrill-Palmer Quarterly*, *19*, 3–20.

Atkinson, J., Hood, B., Wattam-Bell, J., & Braddick, O.J. (1992). Changes in infants' ability to switch visual attention in the first three months of life. *Perception*, *21*, 643–653.

Baars, B.J. (1997). *In the theater of consciousness: The workspace of the mind.* Oxford: Oxford University Press.

Ball, P. (1999). *The self-made tapestry: Pattern formation in nature.* Oxford: Oxford University Press.

Barr, R.G., Beek, P.J., & Calinoiu, N. (1999). Challenges to nonlinear modelling of infant emotion regulation in real and developmental time. In G.J.P. Savelsbergh, H.L.J. van der Maas, & P.L.C. van Geert (Eds.), *Non-linear developmental processes* (pp. 15–37). Amsterdam: Royal Netherlands Academy of Arts and Sciences.

Berg, W.K., Adkinson, C.D., & Strock, B.D. (1973). Duration and frequency of periods of alertness in neonates. *Developmental Psychology, 9*, 434.

Block, N. (1996). How can we find the neural correlate of consciousness? *Trends in Neurosciences, 19*, 456–459.

Brazelton, T.B. (1984). *Neonatal behavioral assessment scale* (2nd ed.). London: Heinemann Medical Books.

Casaer, P. (1979). *Postural behaviour in newborn infants.* London: Heinemann Medical Books.

Coons, S., & Guilleminault, C. (1982). Development of sleep-wake patterns and non-rapid eye movement sleep stages during the first six months of life in normal infants. *Pediatrics, 69*, 793–798.

Crick, F. (1994). *The astonishing hypothesis: The scientific search for the soul.* New York: Simon & Schuster.

Crick, F., & Mitchinson, G. (1995). REM sleep and neural nets. *Behavioural Brain Research, 69*, 147–155.

Desmond, M.M., Franklin, R.R., Vallbona, C., Hill, R.M., Plumb, R., Arnold, H., & Watts, J. (1963). The clinical behavior of the newly born. I. The term baby. *Journal of Pediatrics, 62*, 307–325.

Dittrichova, J., & Lapàckova, V. (1964). Development of the waking state in young infants. *Child Development, 35*, 365–370.

Fuster, J.M. (1997). *The prefrontal cortex: Anatomy, physiology, and neuropsychology of the frontal lobe* (3rd ed.). New York: Raven Press.

Greenspan, R.J., Tononi, G., Cirelli, C., & Shaw, P.J. (2001). Sleep and the fruit fly. *Trends in Neurosciences, 24*, 142–145.

Groome, L.J., & Watson, J.E. (1992). Assessment of in utero neurobehavioral development: I. Fetal behavioral states. *Journal of Maternal-Fetal Investigation, 2*, 183–194.

Gustafson, G., & Green, J. (1991). Developmental coordination of cry sounds with visual regard and gestures. *Infant Behavior and Development, 14*, 51–57.

Hellbrugge, T., Ehrengut-Lange, J., Stehr, K., & Rutenfranz, J. (1964). Circadian periodicity of physiological functions in different stages of infancy and childhood. *Annals of the New York Academy of Sciences, 117*, 361–373.

Hobson, J.A. (1995). *Sleep.* New York: Scientific American Library.

Hopkins, B. (2000). Development of crying in normal infants: Method, theory and some speculations. In R.G. Barr, B. Hopkins, & J.A. Green (Eds.), *Crying as a sign, a symptom, & a signal: Clinical, emotional and developmental aspects of infant and toddler crying* (pp. 176–209). London: MacKeith Press.

Hopkins, B. (2001). Understanding motor development: Insights from dynamical systems perspectives. In A.F. Kalverboer, & A. Gramsbergen (Eds.), *Handbook on brain and behaviour in human development* (pp. 591–620). Dordrecht: Kluwer.

Hopkins, Beek, P.J., & Kalverboer, A.F. (1993). Theoretical issues in the longitudinal study of motor development. In A.F. Kalverboer, B. Hopkins, & R. Geuze (Eds.), *Motor development in early and later childhood: Longitudinal approaches* (pp. 343–371). Cambridge: Cambridge University Press.

Hopkins, B., & Butterworth, G. (1997). Dynamical system approaches to the development of action. In G. Bremner, A. Slater, & G. Butterworth (Eds.), *Infant development: Recent advances* (pp. 75–100). Hove: Psychology Press.

Hopkins, B. & van Wulfften Palthe, T. (1985). Staring in infancy. *Early Human Development, 12*, 261–267.

Hopkins, B. & van Wulfften Palthe, T. (1987). The development of the crying state. *Developmental Psychobiology, 20*, 165–175.

Johnson, M.H., Posner, M.I., & Rothbart, M.K. (1991). The development of visual attention in infancy: Contingency learning, anticipation and disengagement. *Journal of Cognitive Neuroscience, 3*, 335–344.

Kelso, J.A.S. (1995). *Dynamic patterns: The self-organization of brain and behavior.* Cambridge, MA: MIT Press.

Kleitman, N. (1963). *Sleep and wakefulness* (2nd ed.). Chicago: University of Chicago Press.

Kleitman, N. (1977). Not only sleep-wakefulness as well!. *Waking and Sleeping, 1*, 121.

Kugler, P.N., Kelso, J.A.S., & Turvey, M.T. (1982). On coordination and control in naturally developing systems. In J.A.S. Kelso, & J.E. Clark (Eds.), *The development of movement coordination and control* (pp. 5–78). New York: Wiley.

Lagercrantz, H., & Slotkin, T.A. (1986). The 'stress' of being born. *Scientific American, 254*, 100–107.

McCarley, R.W. (1980). Mechanisms and models of behavioral state control. In Hobson, J.A., & Brazier, M.A.B. (Eds.), *The reticular formation revisited* (pp. 375–403). New York: Raven Press.

Milner, A.D., & Goodale, M.A. (1995). *The visual brain in action.* Oxford: Oxford University Press.

Mirmiran, M. (1995). The function of fetal/neonatal rapid eye movement sleep. *Behavioural Brain Research, 69*, 13–22.

Nijhuis, J.G., Prechtl, H.F.R., Martin, C.B., & Bots, R.S.G.M. (1982). Are there behavioural states in the human fetus? *Early Human Development, 6*, 177–195.

Nijhuis, J.G. Martin, C.B., & Prechtl, H.F.R. (1984). Behavioural states of the human fetus. In H.F.R Prechtl (Ed.), *Continuity of neural functions from prenatal to postnatal life* (pp. 65–78). Oxford: Blackwell.

Piaget, J. (1952).*The origins of intelligence in children.* New York: Norton.

Posner, M.I., Rothbart, M.K., & Thomas-Thrapp, L. (1994). Functions of orienting in early infancy. In P.J. Lang, R.F. Simons & M. Balabov (Eds.), *Attention and orienting: Sensory and motivational processes* (pp. 327–345). Mahwah, NJ: Erlbaum.

Prechtl, H.F.R. (1965). Problems of behavioral studies in the newborn infant. In D.S. Lehrman, R.A. Hinde & E. Shaw (Eds.), *Advances in the study of behavior* (pp. 75–98). New York: Academic Press.

Prechtl, H.F.R. (1974). The behavioural states of the newborn infant (a review). *Brain Research, 76*, 185–212.

Prechtl, H.F.R., Eykern, L.A. van, & O'Brien, M.J. (1977). Respiratory muscle EMG in newborns: A non-intrusive method. *Early Human Development, 1*, 265–283.

Robertson, S.S., Cohen, A.H., & Mayer-Kress, G. (1993). Behavioral chaos: Beyond the metaphor. In L.B. Smith & E. Thelen (Eds.), *A dynamic systems theory approach to development: Applications* (pp. 119–150). Cambridge, MA: MIT Press.

Roffwarg, H.P., Muzio, J.N., & Dement, W.C. (1966). Ontogenetic development of the human sleep-dream cycle. *Science, 152*, 604–619.

Salzarulo, P., & Fagioli, I. (1995). Sleep for development or development for waking? – some speculations from a human perspective. *Behavioural Brain Research, 69*, 23–27.

Salzarulo, P., Fagioli, I., Salomon, F., Ricour, C., Raimbault, G., Ambrosi, S., Cicchi, O., Duhamel, J.F., & Rigoard, M.T. (1980). Sleep patterns in infants under continuous feeding from birth. *Electroencephalography & Clinical Neurophysiology, 49*, 330–336.

Stechler, G., & Latz, E. (1966). Some observations on attention and arousal in the human infant. *Journal of the American Academy of Child Psychiatry, 5*, 517–525.

Thatcher, R.W. (1998). A predator-prey model of human cerebral development. In K.M. Newell, & P.C.M. Molenaar (Eds.), *Applications of nonlinear dynamics to developmental process modeling* (pp. 67–128). Mahwah, NJ: Erlbaum.

Thelen, E., & Smith, L.B. (1994). *A dynamic systems approach to the development of cognition and action*. Cambridge, MA: MIT Press.

Thoman, E.B. (1990). Sleeping and waking states in infants: A functional perspective. *Neuroscience Biobehavioral Review, 14*, 93–107.

van der Maas, H. L.J., & Hopkins, B. (1998). Dynamical systems theory: So what's new? *British Journal of Developmental Psychology, 16*, 1–13.

Wolff, P.H. (1984). Discontinuous changes in human wakefulness around the end of the second month of life: A developmental perspective. In H.F.R Prechtl (Ed.), *Continuity of neural functions from prenatal to postnatal life* (pp. 144–158). Oxford: Blackwell.

Wolff, P.H. (1987). *The development of behavioral states and the expression of emotions in early infancy: New proposals for investigation*. Chicago: University of Chicago Press.

Methodological issues in the study of arousals and awakenings during sleep in the human infant

Marie J. Hayes
Department of Psychology, University of Maine,
Orono, ME

The development of sleep and arousal systems in infancy is driven by the explosive growth of brain development from late fetal life through the first year (Salzarulo & Fagioli, 1995). Much research has focused on sleep processes with relatively little work specifically on waking and arousal mechanisms, even though this process undergoes dramatic change during infancy that: 1. reflects organisational/maturational processes in the development of the forebrain and associative neural networks within the neuraxis (Curzi-Dascalova, 1977; Fagioli & Salzarulo, 1982; Steriade, 1996); 2. represents the opening of consciousness and the development of infant psychology (Scher, 1991; Anders, 1994); 3. may be linked to important dysfunction in developing neural systems, e.g. SIDS (Sudden Infant Death Syndrome), ALTE (Apparent Life Threatening Event(s)), sleep apnea (obstructive, central or mixed); 4. developmental sleep disorders such as night-waking, etc. (Fleming et al., 1996; Haddad et al., 1979; Guilleminault et al., 1978); 5. may provide insight concerning the evolutionary role of awakenings and arousals across ages, species and ecological demands (Siegel, 1994; McKenna et al., 1990).

Emergence. Sometime after 28 weeks postconceptional age, motor movements and quiescence become temporally patterned and macrostructurally segregated. These on-off periods have the behavioural characteristics of active and quiet sleep although state integrity is often problematic and short-lived. The exact timing of emergent processes of sleep state organisation is still a matter of considerable debate (Prechtl, 1974; Scher, 1996; Stefanski et al., 1984;

Curzi-Dascalova, Peirano & Morel-Kahn, 1988; Curzi-Dascalova et al., 1985). Nonetheless, true waking state, as distinguished from sleep, is believed to emerge in the same period in the fetus and premature infant (Prechtl, 1974; Curzi-Dascalova, 1995; Stefanski et al., 1984; Visser et al., 1987; Parmelee et al., 1967).

The identification of waking as a distinct state has been pursued by monitoring autonomic, motility and/or EEG parameters both *in* and *ex utero* (Visser et al., 1987; Prechtl, 1982; Sterman & Hoppenbrouwer, 1971). Electrocortical and behavioural identification of waking state as early as 28 weeks has been made in the premature infant (Curzi-Dascalova, 1995). As a behavioural state, waking can be reliably distinguished from sleep in premature infants by 30 weeks PCA (Holditch-Davis, 1990; Myers et al., 1998). The controversy over coding criteria is fueled by the observation that characteristics of multiple states frequently co-exist in the early organisational phase.

The incidence and stability of waking increase dynamically in frequency, duration and circadian temporal patterning throughout infancy (Louis et al., 1997; Schulz et al., 1985; Salzarulo et al., 1979). Beginning in the full-term neonatal period, and continuing through the first year, sub–types of waking can be distinguished (e.g. cry/fuss, quiet alert, active alert, drowse, etc; (Wolff, 1959; Thoman, 1990; Prechtl, 1974)). The ability to sustain waking state which increases in the first postnatal year is a critical avenue of CNS stimulation, promoting experience-expectant plasticity in cognitive, sensory, motor and emotional development (Greenough & Black, 1992).

Arousal and childhood disease. Disorders of arousal or waking in the first year are believed to be comorbid with, and perhaps mediate, some developmental illnesses. For example, one proposed etiology for SIDS/ALTE (Sudden Infant Death Syndrome/Apparent Life Threatening Event) is suggested by the finding that arousal threshold and quiet sleep propensity are increased dramatically during prone position sleeping, a position in which most infants are found in SIDS/ALTE (AAP Task Force, 1992; Hoffman et al., 1988; Dwyer et al., 1995). Recent work suggests that contextual factors such as ambient temperature, nasal congestion, soft bedding and social sleeping may reduce or compound risk (McKenna et al., 1993; Bach et al., 1994; Chiodini & Thach, 1993). Infant factors such as cardiac Q–T interval abnormalities, prematurity, a history of respiratory distress syndrome; autonomic dysfunction or brainstem immaturity may also increase vulnerability (McKenna et al., 1993; Fleming et al., 1996; Schwartz et al., 1998). Nonetheless, there is strong suspicion that failure to arouse to an hypoxic stimulus is instrumental in SIDS mortality.

Another developmental syndrome associated with impaired arousal is sleep apnea characterized by frequent, sleep-disrupting arousals of short duration (Brouillette, Fernback & Hunt, 1982). These arousal events can be very difficult to distinguish from sleep because they are typically very brief, not associated with state change and have only some of the behavioural and electrocortical features of spontaneous arousal or awakening. One of the many stimuli capable of producing such brief arousals is activation of chemosensitive cells in the respiratory tract which respond to hypercarbic or hypoxic conditions during respiratory pauses of central, peripheral or mixed origin (Phillipson et al., 1978). The effects of chronic sleep apnea at all ages are chronic sleep fragmentation, night-time arousals and awakenings and day-time sleepiness (review: Berry & Gleason, 1997).

Universal standards to distinguish arousal events from sleep have been difficult to establish. One issue is the dynamic changes in waking and arousal during early development making comparison to the adult literature problematic. Curzi-Dascalova and Mirmiran (1996) have addressed this problem formally and suggest that new, developmentally appropriate standards must be established.

This paper will examine the methodological problems in the study of arousals and awakenings, especially the problem of determining what constitutes an arousal or awakening episode, what stimuli are believed to be involved, and what measures constitute the most sensitive or appropriate yardsticks for determining whether an arousal-related event or transition has occurred. It is generally acknowledged that waking/arousal can be divided into two types: 1. related to so-called "spontaneous" or unknown factors; and 2. those that are reactive to identifiable, extrinsic or intrinsic events.

Awakenings

Awakenings represent unambiguous transitions from sleep to waking. They are age-dependent and based on behavioural criteria. In the adult and child literature, awakenings and arousals are typically distinguished by duration (1–2 min are typical breakpoints to establish awakening; 3 seconds for an arousal). In adults, awakening is behaviourally defined when the individual engages in conscious behaviours that reflect awareness of their surroundings such as eyes open, talking, or positional and motor movements incompatible with sleep (sitting up, walking, etc.), unless there is a specific sleep disorder. On the other hand, arousals have also been defined in terms of electrocortical criteria only (Atlas Task Force, 1992).

In infants and fetuses the development of behaviourally quantifiable, sustained awakenings are controversial between 30–36 weeks PCA. Attempts to quantify premature infant sleep before 36 weeks PCA using EEG methods have been generally unsuccessful (Dreyfus-Brisac, 1975) presumably because of weak cortical signals at the skull due to CNS immaturity. Behavioural and autonomic criteria (respiration, heart rate variability) have been used with some success (Hayes et al., 1994; Myers, et al., 1998; Stefanski et al., 1984; Holditch-Davis, 1990), although Prechtl's group has contended that state is not sufficiently organised to code at these ages. Recent work has proposed that EEG can be used with traditional autonomic and behavioural measures in premature infants <36 weeks of age to discriminate sleep states but little has been discussed methodologically about waking state (Curzi-Dascalova, 1993; Scher et al., 1995).

Ethologically-based approach. Early waking processes in infants 30–35 week PCA can be reliably indexed by longterm videotaped recordings using behavioural criteria: open eyes, focused scanning eye movements and body movements; and duration requirements for definitions of awakenings. Infant studies have used various coding intervals and requirements for coding an awakening (1-min, Stefanski, et al; 1984; 10-sec, Holditch-Davis et al.; 2-min, Ficca et al., 1999; Kahn et al., 1993).

In our studies, approximately 10% of a night record can be identified as waking state in 30–35 week old infants when a 1.5 minute criterion is used for state stability (Hayes et al, 1999). Stefanski et al. (1984) found that 8–12% of the time during the day premature infants were awake; whereas, Gabriel et al. (1981) report 13% wake time when 96 hours were examined continuously. Using a 1-min criterion for behavioural state, Giganti et al. (2001) examined infants over 24 hour periods and detected a circadian pattern of sleep-wake distribution that was developmental: more wake time at preterm ages during the nocturnal phase which is reversed to daytime in full-term age infants. Hence, the patterning and circadian distribution of awakenings varies dramatically during the emergent phase. Salzarulo and colleagues have emphasized the methodology of continuous 24-hour evaluations of sleep-wake states during early development and the importance of circadian factors in the temporal distribution of states during infancy (Fagioli, Salomon & Salzarulo, 1981; Fagioli & Salzarulo, 1982; Fagioli, Bes & Salzarulo, 1988).

Methods of measuring awakenings during normative development. As described above, the developmental processes in the circadian distribution of postnatal awakenings and waking state (less in the night, more sustained waking periods in the day) have been described using primarily behavioural methods, although EEG has been be used for this purpose (Wolff, 1959; Prechtl, 1982; Kahn et al., 1993; Anders, Emde & Parmelee, 1971).

Real-time and time-lapse videography have been very useful in establishing awakening patterns across long observation periods (Anders, 1979; Fagioli & Salzarulo, 1982). Challamel's group showed that young infants experience significantly more awakenings (>1-min) and less sleep continuity than older infants, but this trend decreases with advancing age (Louis et al., 1997). Awakenings gradually express a strong diurnal rhythm, decreased daytime napping and increases in nocturnal sleep consolidation, a result that has been reported previously (Bruni et al., 1996; Anders & Keener, 1985).

Ficca, Fagioli, Giganti & Salzarulo (1999) examined awakenings between 1–54 weeks of age using EEG and observation methods. Awakenings during REM were the most common, but decreased with age. By 6 months of age, there was a decrease in the frequency of REM awakenings although the duration of wakefulness bouts remained stable. In younger infants, the durations of wakefulness out of QS were longer. This result suggests that REM/wake couplings decline with age as waking state becomes more organised. Also, the duration of waking and, hence, waking state stability, may be qualitatively different and more robust following QS episodes.

Parental report. One question in the awakening literature is whether sleep-disordered infants and children with night-waking and calling out reported by parents actually *wake up more often* than infants that do not signal to their parents. At these ages, nightwaking is often quantified based on parental reports usually of some proscribed period such as during the last week (Crowell et al., 1987; Scher, 1991). Nightwaking may be symptomatic of a greater difficulty returning to sleep following spontaneous, night-time awakenings. Anders (1979), using a videotaping procedure, has established that infants who call out during the night have the same number of awakenings as non-signalling infants. Not surprisingly, parents of nonsignallers promoted independent sleep onset skills. Hence, the issue of the developmental context of awakenings is important in addressing mechanism, in this case, vis à vis parent-infant night-time interactions. Infants who habitually returned to sleep in the parent's bed following night-feeding in infancy, are more likely to night-wake, parent-seek and engage in child-initiated co-sleeping in early childhood (Hayes et al., 1996).

Biologically-based child factors, such as regulatory problems (rhythmicity, hyperactivity, feeding difficulties etc.), illness or prematurity (Wolke, 1994); drug exposure (Dahl et al., 1995) and temperament are also involved in persistent night-waking and calling out in early childhood (Keener, Zeanah & Anders, 1988; Scher, 1991; Hayes et al., 2001). Environmental factors such as parent-child interactions (Sadeh & Anders, 1993); parental beliefs and culture (McKenna et al., 1990; Lozoff, 1984); and parental psychopathology interact dynamically with child factors over the course of individual developmental history to affect both night-waking and the temporal distribution of waking state (Gottlieb, 1996).

Importance of methodology. Objective (video-, acti- or electrographic) measures vs. subjective (parental report) measures have been compared and will continue to be in the resolution of the best methods to quantify sleep and waking state development. Actigraphic estimates of night-waking in sleep disordered children show an increased number of awakenings and shorter periods of continuous, consolidated sleep (Sadeh et al., 1991). If you accept that actigraphic measures are accurate indicators of wake time, sleep-disrupted children have quantitatively more waking episodes than non-sleep disordered children.

Wake vs. sleep which is quantified using piezoelectric actigraphy in infants and children is accomplished typically with a commercial actigraphic wrist device which is attached to the thigh or upper arm. Acceleromotor output is correlated with the forcefulness of movements and, when digitized, represents both the relative magnitude and duration of movements. The data are binned depending on the experimenter's interests and the device's limitations (typically, accelerations are averaged every 1-sec to 20-min).

Algorithms distinguishing awakenings from sleep have been developed for adults, the most accepted being Cole et al. (1992). Sadeh and colleagues (Sadeh, Hauri, Kripke & Lavie, 1995; Sadeh, Sharkey & Carskadon, 1994) have proposed a sleep-wake algorithm for children that is similar to Cole & Kripke's algorithm and is informed by Thoman's work on state determination in infants using a mattress-method (Thoman & Glazier, 1987). These actigraphic methods have been used to characterize normative sleep and waking patterns in the first year (Sadeh et al., 1995).

Thoman's method uses mattress piezoelectric actigraphy and her group has published extensively on infant state coding, not only for wake vs. sleep but also for AS and QS states in infants, in both human and animal species. EEG-actigraphic concordance estimates suggest that the actigraphy method is best used for sleep-wake state determination. Observed error rates vary from 5–15% for actigraphy-based state determination compared to EEG (Sadeh et al., 1994). Results in infants with the "static charge bed," another actigraphic method, combined respiratory and body movement signals. Positive predictive value in coding REM sleep was reported to be only 54–67% although waking (defined as 30-sec of movement during a 1-min epoch) was 94% (Erkinjuntii et al., 1990; Kirjavainen et al., 1996).

One fundamental issue in infant state coding using actigraphy is distinguishing phasic motor bursts during AS and wake state. Thoman's group has shown that actigraphy-based patterning between awake state and phasic motor activity in AS produces a different signal that can be distinguished analytically, at least in infants. QS is more easy to determine since it is characterized by low motor output and regular respirations (Thoman & Tynan, 1979).

There has been interest in using other physiological signals to code state in infants such as respiratory patterning (which is part of the mattress-based actigraphy signal) or cardiac variability and rhythmicity, measures which are strongly state-dependent in infants (Meyers et al., 1998; Schechtman et al., 1992; Curzi-Dascalova et al., 1981).

Is there continuity between arousals and awakenings?

Spontaneous awakenings and briefer, arousal-like events occur ubiquitously during sleep across all ages, and are a part of sleep that is both maturational *and* normative. The term spontaneous refers to events whose mechanisms are poorly understood. Spontaneous events resembling waking or arousals, whether defined behaviourally, actigraphically or electrocortically, are more prevalent in sleep-disordered adults and children, individuals with psychiatric (hyperactivity, depression, psychosis) or illness conditions and in normal sleepers during anxious periods.

Of course, distinguishing between spontaneous awakenings and arousals depends on the criteria used to define each category. Nonetheless, according to any criteria, it is known that transient arousals are more frequent; whereas, full awakenings are less common. These sleep discontinuities, if they can be called that, do not negatively impact sleep integrity in healthy individuals.

Age. For this first discussion, rates of spontaneous arousals and awakenings will be described from a developmental perspective. In healthy infants and children, age determines the number of spontaneous awakenings. By the end of the first year, nocturnal sleep continuity without sustained awakening or calling out is accomplished in most infants (Ficca et al., 1999; Louis et al. 1997). Interestingly, a substantial minority of infants begin to express nightwakings again toward the end of the first year and again in toddlerhood (Richman & Graham, 1971; Scher, 1991).

The achievement of comprehensive nocturnal sleep continuity and predominant circadian distribution of waking to the diurnal phase develops over most of childhood. The maturational process is gradual. Adult-like proportions and durations of sleep and wake states (Salzarulo et al., 2001); and the full complement of adult characteristics of sleep and wake processes (e.g. motor atonia during REM sleep) (Kohyama & Iwakama, 1990; Erkinjuntii et al., 1984); delta proportion and spindle activity (Feinberg, 1974; Guillaminault, 1978); levels and patterning of spontaneous movements (Hayes & Mitchell, 1998), etc. are not mature until puberty.

One year old and younger infants experience significantly more awakenings than older children. With age, both the rate of spontaneous awakenings and wake state duration show a strong diurnal rhythm as infants decrease daytime napping and increase nocturnal sleep consolidation (Louis et al., 1997; Bruni et al., 1996; Ficca et al., 1999). In premature infants/fetuses, such awakenings occur briefly and sporadically; often defined primarily by spontaneous movements and orientation responses (Stefanski et al., 1994; Giganti et al., 2001; Hayes et al, 1999).

Arousals. Although awakenings have been successfully defined behaviourally, arousals have most often been measured with electrographic techniques (i.e. a change to theta or alpha frequencies in central and occipital leads) or are movement defined (i.e. movements as pen deflections or videographically-verified movement bursts) (Mograss et al., 1994; Phillipson & Sullivan, 1978).

Brief arousal events occur more frequently during sleep at all ages in individuals with sleep apnea leading to the hypothesis that arousal events function to terminate apneic episodes (Berry & Gleason, 1997; Sullivan & Issa, 1985; Phillipson & Sullivan, 1978). One function of brief/transient arousals in apneic adults is believed to be the reestablishment of a patent airway during the motor circuit activation that is part of the response (Remmers et al., 1978). Individuals suffering from obstructive apnea have spontaneous arousals admixed with "respiratory reactive" arousals (Berthon-Jones & Sullivan, 1982). For this reason, it is necessary to carefully separate spontaneous from suspected reactive arousal and awakening events through baseline assessments during non-apneic periods, evaluation of the role of state and examination of apneic type (obstructive, central or mixed origin) (Brouillette et al., 1982).

The American Sleep Disorders Association (ASDA) has recently established clinical criteria when it became clear that transient or brief arousals were being coded in nonstandard ways and it was not known whether "clinical significant" arousals were being coded. The recommendation was to establish a criterion duration of 3 seconds for a true arousal event following at least 10-min of continuous sleep, although it was acknowledged that this duration was arbitrary. Electrocortical criteria required evidence of thalamocortical activation (>3-sec of alpha or theta activity). One source of confusion was the need to separate cortical EEG activation associated with arousal from an ongoing REM state desynchronization episode. This was resolved by examining current state. During REM, movement may or may not be overtly present *but* chin EMG activity was required in order to distinguish an arousal event from REM-related cortical activation (Atlas Task Force, 1992).

However, sleep and arousal in infants are fundamentally different from the adult (Bes et al., 1991). Curzi-Dascalova & Mirmiran (1996) address several problems with adult criteria for arousals in infant coding. First, infant EEG activity is often not in the requisite frequency bands required for adult arousal determination. Secondly, EEG pattern variations are frequent and change "spontaneously" (Eiselt et al., 1997). Finally, submental EMG in young infants is of low amplitude & difficult to record (Wuldebrand et al., 1995).

Another concern that will be discussed below is that, in infants, there are motor responses and autonomic responses without accompanying electrocortical changes. These events (termed subcortical arousals) are also seen in adults and may be more instrumental than electrocortical arousals in addressing motor patency during airway challenge (Berry & Gleeson, 1997). For example, far less than 100% of apneas are terminated by electrocortical arousals in both adults and developmental groups. Berry & Gleason (1997) speculate that, besides the possibility that arousals have no role in apnea termination, ASDA arousal criteria may be too restrictive, methods for detection may be insensitive and/or subcortical arousals may be instrumental for apnea termination.

Another issue is that arousal durations can be extraordinarily brief (e.g. 1-sec) in infants and do not necessarily disrupt ongoing sleep architecture (Mograss et al., 1994). McNamara et al. (1996) found that apneic infants had significantly more arousals following obstructive events during REM sleep using a 1-sec criterion duration, (combined with the adult criteria of an abrupt shift in EEG frequency and augmentation of submental EMG in AS), although the frequency of spontaneous arousals was not different from controls (McNamara et al., 1996). Hence, the features of arousals during development are often poorly described with the current adult criteria, especially the emphasis on electrocortical markers and minimal durations (Curzi-Dascalova & Mirmiran, 1996).

Position, arousals and awakenings in newborns. The naturalistic condition in which SIDS/ALTE infants are most frequently found is the prone position, leading to speculation that failure to awaken or adequately arouse in response to environmentally-mediated or intrinsic airway challenge (e.g. hypercapnia, hypoxia, esophageal reflux) may be due to the general finding that infants sleep more soundly in this position (Hoffman et al., 1988; Fleming & Blair, 1997). It should be noted that age may be an important factor in the risk to the infant and SIDS incidence is, in general, confined to the first six months of life, peaking at 3–4 months. Further, prone position in the premature improves lung function; decreases chest wall movement; increases breathing; decreases energy expenditure and improves oxygenation (Masterson et al., 1987).

Using a within-subjects, counterbalanced design, Kahn and colleagues found that infants sleeping in the prone position had fewer and shorter spontaneous arousals defined by electrocortical criteria as well as increased NREM sleep (Kahn et al., 1993, 1994). Meyers et al. (1998) examined prone premature infants and found that *spontaneous waking* (coded in 1-min bins according to Stefanski et al. (1984) with a 3-min smoothing criterion for state stability), was suppressed by 71% when premature infants were placed in the prone position. QS was also increased.

In a followup study from Kahn's group, prone-sleeping infants were found to have higher arousal thresholds to a white noise (Franco et al., 1997). *Reactive, polygraphic* arousals were coded according to the ASDA criteria *plus body movements for at least 3-sec. "Clinical awakening"* was defined by opening of the eyes and crying. No clinical awakenings occurred in the prone position, although only 3 infants of 22 awoke in the supine position. These results suggest that arousability defined electrographically was less efficient in the prone position, but the effects on awakening are less clear and perhaps, negligible.

Autonomic reactivity, such as cardiac and respiratory responsiveness to environmental noise or a tilt stimulus, are also damped when sleeping prone (Franco et al., 1996; Fifer et al., 1997) and in infants who succumb to SIDS (Schectman et al., 1991, 1992; Kahn et al., 1992). In the prone position, sympathovagal balance, specifically parasympathetic activity, is disrupted when heart rate was examined through power spectral procedures. In combination with gravitational challenge using the TILT stimulus, Galland et al. (1998) and Schechtman et al. (1988) found decreases in heart rate variablility in SIDS infants studied prospectively.

Interestingly, the social context of sleep, solitary vs. with the mother, has been found to increase the rate of spontaneous arousals and decrease NREM sleep, opposite effects to those found in prone, solitary sleepers. Social sleeping infants usually slept on the side or back and was associated with an increase in spontaneous, behaviourally defined "arousals" (i.e. awakenings in this context) and a decrease in electrocortically defined arousals than when sleeping alone (Mosko et al., 1997; McKenna, 1996). Duration, but not onset, of awakenings was augmented by maternal stimulation.

In this venue the SIDS risk literature cannot be comprehensively reviewed. It can be stated, however, that much research suggests that age, general health (autonomic function, respiratory disease, prenatal exposures, prematurity), body position during sleep, sensory cues (*extrinsic*: ambient temperature, hypercarbic/hypoxic environmental cues associated with CO2 rebreathing, social cues, noise; *intrinsic*: airway obstruction, bradycardia, chemo/mechanoreceptor threshold) and body position are important factors in both arousability in infants and perhaps in risk for SIDS (McKenna et al., 1993; Hoffman et al., 1988; Fleming et al., 1996; Bolton et al., 1993; Hunt, 1981).

Movement-based arousal measures. Electrocortical arousal standards have recently been compared to so-called subcortical or movement arousals based on the finding that the latter is more common and often more strongly correlated with apnea resolution or airway defense. The evolution of the study of movement/subcortical arousals in developmental populations has led to a reconsideration of behaviour as potentially the best measure for both spontaneous and reactive arousals.

Prone position affects arousal threshold independent of sleep state. Galland et al. (1998) found that the prone position decreases heart rate variability and arousability to a whole range of stimuli. In this study, arousal was coded as a graded continuous response according to behavioural criteria: 0, no movement; 0.5 startle; 1.0 gross head movements or eyes open (asleep again within 15–30"); 2.0 full awakening with eyes open. *Full awakening* was significantly less likely in QS (15%) compared to AS (54%). In the prone position, full awakening was significantly depressed in AS only when compared to the supine position. Importantly, the data show that movement arousals (e.g. 0.5, 1.0 scores) occurred more in the prone condition. The authors speculate that "movement" arousals, as defined in this study, may serve a protective function in that motor tone in the airway is restored during these events.

Brouillette and Thach (1999) used a modification of the ASDA arousal duration criterion: in their coding the minimum duration of an arousal was regarded as 1-sec. Historically, with EEG criteria, respiratory events rarely were terminated with an arousal; in this study, with movement-only criteria, they were. However, there was no difference in the incidence of movement-associated arousals across sleep state. They propose a role for motor activity that 1. has the properties of an arousal response; 2. precedes and increases the probability of a full awakening; and 3. may constitute a critically important airway defense mechanism.

Thoppil et al. (1991) examined spontaneous behavioural arousal on video with and without instrumentation. Movement-defined, transient arousals were only associated with EEG in one half of the cases. They maintained that movements are more sensitive to apnea termination than EEG arousal in premature infants and that most of the "squirming" episodes represent movements associated with behavioural arousal.

Wulbrand et al. (1995) examined obstructive apneas in premature infants and defined cardiorespiratory arousals as: presence of bradycardia, decrease in submental EMG, and decrease in the EMG of diaphragmatic muscles. They note that bradycardia always ceased at the termination of apnea in parallel with a gasp (short expiratory, deep inspiratory movements) without a change in EEG activity, sleep phase or other evidence of arousal.

Mograss, Ducharme and Broullette (1994) examined apnea and hypopneas in children from 2–11 years of age and defined movement arousals in the following way: 1. No EEG criteria; 2. duration 1-sec or longer; 3. any two parameters showing evidence of arousal (EEG, EMG (chin or arm), heart rate, distortion of respiratory signal); 4. duration of event must be > 15 seconds; and, 5. subject must be asleep for 10-sec for a second arousal. They also coded the arousals with videography to include three types: respiratory, technician-induced or spontaneous. The results showed that all arousals were less than 3 seconds. Spontaneous arousals were variable in duration and behavioural content, did not differ based on state and represented half of all arousals in these sleep-disordered children. Seventy-one percent of respiratory events resulted in movement arousals with no sleep state change and increased airway patency.

The most comprehensive analysis of movement arousals has been reported by Thach and colleagues (Lijowska et al., 1995; Thach, Wulbrand & McNamara, 1999) in which a highly stereotyped sequence of responses was found to follow airway challenges to a mixed hypercarbic and hypoxic environmental challenge using a cloth overlay in a prone or supine sleeping infant 2–8 months of age. Sleep state was determined by behavioural criteria using videography and infants were monitored with standard EEG, respiratory and heart rate measures. Carefully defined behavioural sequences could be observed consisting of a sigh, startle, thrashing, e.g. slow repeated movements, asymmetrical, head movements, etc, leading in some cases to EEG arousal and then full awakening. The movement response resulted in decreased inspired CO2 (Lijowska et al., 1995).

These studies share the conclusion that respiratory protective responses can be achieved in infants and children without the occurrence of an EEG change and other criteria of the ASDA task force. Further, there is some consensus that movement arousals (whose criteria differ from study to study) are better correlated with respiratory challenge, restore airway patency effectively and if not, probably lead to full awakening.

Spontaneous motility rhythms. What has not been addressed in this discussion is the relationship of movement arousals to environmental challenge and endogenous rhythms of motility that occur independent of state in fetuses and infants for at least the first 5 months postnatally (Robertson, 1982; Robertson, 1987). This cyclic process is ubiquitous in mammals (Corner, 1972; Narayanan et al., 1971), and has a periodicity of 1–3 minutes in humans, can be perturbed by environmental stimuli and results in a burst of gross body movement of relatively brief duration (<5 seconds). Scher (1996) reports "arousal" rates of 0.2 episodes per minute; Abu-Osba et al. (1991) have found 0.15 squirming episodes per minute. These events have the same periodicity as cyclic motility and arguable represent the same phenomenon. Hence, this fast cycle may allow the infant's nervous system to sample the environment and temporarily restore motor tone (and airway patency) well within the zone of asphyxiation.

McNamara (1996) has reported rates of spontaneous arousals in infants according to the 1-sec EEG criteria every 3–6 min in controls and 6–10 minutes in OSA infants. Lower levels of endogenous motility and increased apnea index has been found during 24 hour recordings in near miss infants (Coons & Guilleminault, 1985). Atypical patterns of spontaneous movements have recently been found in brain damaged infants (Prechtl, 1997). Hoppenbrouwers et al., (1982) found that spontaneous motility during AS and QS increased across the night at 2 to 3 months of age.

An independent source of movement cyclicity is determined by sleep state. AS motility bursts occur phasically between eye movements in infants during the first 9 months and beyond as motor atonia matures (Kohyama, 1997; Hayes & Mitchell, 1998; Aserinsky and Kleitman, 1955; Dement & Kleitman, 1957;

Glazier & Thoman, 1987). It should be mentioned that fast cyclic motility is enhanced in strength during AS in infants (Robertson, 1987).

Harper et al. (1978) found that SIDS infants exhibited less motility during AS specifically. It is proposed here that, typically, "spontaneous" subcortical/ movement arousals are part of the endogenous, cyclic motility phenomenon that may not be functioning normally in SIDS infants. Further, AS may create another opportunity for "protective" movements and were found to be depressed in SIDS infants. Importantly, apneic events have been found to be more common and of longer duration according to the respiratory distress index during AS further increasing the risk of asphyxiation in infants with lower movement rates.

Concluding remarks

Methodological concerns in the study of awakenings and arousal in infants have suffered from the lack of consensus on criteria for scoring, the philosophical bias for neurophysiological vs. behavioural indices and the dramatic developmental progression of waking state in the first year of life. Awakenings present clear behavioural distinction from sleep, often leading to state change. The probability of stable waking following awakening depends on the state from which the awakening arises.

The distinction between awakening and arousals has led to a debate concerning their common or uncommon etiology. Arousals have been studied mostly from the perspective of respiratory illness, specifically sleep apnea and SIDS. They have been defined electrocortically until very recently. Identifying the external or physiologic events that promote arousals and awakenings, disrupt sleep efficiency and promote daytime somnolence have been the primary goals of this research. Problems with electrocortical criteria for coding infant arousals is challenged by the need for more developmentally appropriate standards. The importance of adopting behavioural methodologies for measuring both spontaneous and reactive arousal events is argued. The finding that subcortical arousals are more common, can be stimulus-driven, precede electrocortical arousal by some seconds (but, most often are not succeeded by them), and can be studied with behavioural criteria alone suggests that the electrocortical approach to the study of awakening and arousal may be too narrow.

The extent to which spontaneous and reactive arousals and awakenings are discontinuous mechanistically is explored. A role for spontaneous motility cycles is proposed as an overlapping system that utilizes subcortical arousal substrates, is responsive to environmental input and periodically activates the subcortical movement system (that is, the ascending cholinergic arousal circuits, Steriade, 1996). This cycle is independent of state and is a unique feature of the infancy period that may play a role in protecting infants from adverse environmental or physiologic airway challenge.

In conclusion, the current state of methodological issues of awakening and arousal research clearly requires a renewed attention to behavioural measures as indispensable to advancing our knowledge and understanding of developing sleep and arousal systems.

References

AAP Task Force on Infant Positioning and SIDS (1992). Positioning in SIDS. *Pediatrics, 89,* 1120–1126.

Abu-Osba, Y.K. (1991). Treatment of persistent pulmonary hypertension of the newborn: update. *Archives of Disease in Childhood, 66,* 74–77.

American Sleep Disorders Association – The Atlas Task Force (1992). EEG arousals: Scoring rules and examples. *Sleep, 15,* 174–184.

Anders, Thomas F., R. Emde & Arthur H. Jr. Parmelee (1971). *A manual for standardized terminology, techniques and criteria for the scoring of states of sleep and wakefulness in newborn infants*: Los Angeles: Brain Information Service, School of Health Sciences, UCLA.

Anders, Thomas F. (1979). Night waking in infants during the first year of life. *Pediatrics, 63,* 860–864.

Anders, Thomas F., & M. Keener (1985). Developmental course of nighttime sleep-wake patterns in full-term and premature infants during the first year of life. I. *Sleep, 8,* 173–192.

Anders, Thomas F., (1994). Infant sleep, nighttime relationships and attachment. *Psychiatry, 57,* 11–21.

Aserinsky, E., & Nathaniel Kleitman (1955). A motility cycle in sleeping infants as manifested by ocular and gross bodily activity. *Journal of Applied Physiology, 8,* 11–18.

Berry, R.B., & K. Gleeson (1997). Respiratory arousal from sleep. *Sleep, 20,* 655–675.

Berthon-Jones, M., & C.E. Sullivan (1982). Ventilatory and arousal responses to hypoxia in sleeping humans. *American Review of Respiratory Disorders, 125,* 632–639.

Bes, Frederik, Hartmut Schulz, Yvonne Navelet & Piero Salzarulo (1991). The distribution of slow-wave sleep across the night: a comparison for infants, children, and adults. *Sleep, 14,* 5–12.

Bolton, D., B. Taylor, A. Campbell, B. Galland, B., & C. Cresswell (1993). Rebreathing expired gases from bedding: A cause of cot death? *Archives of Disease in Childhood, 69,* 187–190.

Booth, C.L., H.L. Leonard, S.P. Waite & Evelyn B. Thoman (1983). Sleep states and behaviors patterns in preterm and fullterm infants. *Neuropediatrics, 11,* 354–364.

Bowes, G., & E.A. Phillipson (1980). Arousal, ventilatory and airway responses to laryngeal stimulation following sleep fragmentation. *American Review of Respiratory Disorders, 121,* 316–320.

Brouillette, R.T., S.K. Fernback & C.E. Hunt (1982). Obstructive sleep apnea in infants and children. *Journal of Pediatrics, 100,* 31–40.

Bruni, Oliviero, S. Ottaviano, V. Guidetti, M. Romoli, M. Innocenzi, F. Cortesis & F. Giannotti (1996). The Sleep Disturbance Scale for Children (SDSC). Construction and validation of an instrument to evaluate sleep disturbances in childhood and adolescence. *Journal of Sleep Research, 5,* 251–261.

Chiodini, B.A., & Bradley T. Thach (1993). Impaired ventilation in infants sleeping face down: Potential significance for sudden infant death syndrome. *Journal of Pediatrics, 123,* 686–692.

Cole, R.J., Daniel F. Kripke, William D.F. Gruen, D.J. Mullaney & J.C. Gillin (1992). Automatic sleep-wake identification from wrist activity. *Sleep, 15,* 461–469.

Coons, Susan, & Christiane Guilleminault (1985). Motility and arousal in near miss sudden infant death syndrome. *Journal of Pediatrics, 107,* 728–732.

Crowell, J., M. Keener, N. Ginsburg & Thomas F. Anders (1987). Sleep habits in toddlers 18 to 36 months old. *Journal of the American Academy for Child and Adolescent Psychiatry, 26,* 510–515.

Curzi-Dascalova, Lilia (1977). Waking and sleeping EEG in normal babies before 6 months of age. *Revue EEG Neurophysiologie clinique, 7,* 316–326.

Curzi-Dascalova, Lilia, & Majid Mirmiran (1996). Manual of methods of recording and analyzing sleep wakefulness in preterm and full-term infants. INSERM, Paris Editor.

Curzi-Dascalova, Lilia, Patricio Peirano & Françoise Morel-Kahn (1988). Development of sleep states in normal premature and full-term newborns. *Developmental Psychobiology, 21,* 431–444.

Curzi-Dascalova, Lilia, Patricio Peirano, I. Silvestri & G. Korn (1985). Sleep organization in normal premature newborn infants. Polygraphic study. *Revue EEG Neurophysiologie clinique 15,* 237–242.

Curzi-Dascalova, Lilia (1992). Physiological correlates of sleep development in premature and full-term neonates. *Neurophysiologie Clinique, 22,* 151–166.

Curzi-Dascalova, Lilia, J.M. Figueroa, M.Eiselt, E. Christova, A. Virassamy, A.M. Dallest, H. Guimaraes, Christine Gaultier & M. Dehan (1993). Sleep state organization in premature infants of less than 35 weeks' gestational age. *Pediatric Research, 34*(5), 624–628.

Curzi-Dascalova, Lilia (1995). Development of the sleep and autonomic nervous system control in premature and full-term newborn infants. *Archives of Pediatrics, 2,* 255–262.

Dahl, R.E., Mark S. Scher, D.E. Williamson, N. Robles & N. Day (1995). A longitudinal study of prenatal marijuana use. Effects on sleep and arousal at age 3 years. *Archives of Pediatric and Adolescent Medicine, 149,* 145–150.

Dement, William C., & Nathaniel Kleitman (1957). Cyclic variations in EEG during sleep and their relation to eye-movements, body motility and dreaming. *Electroencephalography and clinical Neurophysiology, 9,* 673–690.

Dwyer, T., A.L. Ponsonby, L. Blizzard, N.M. Newman & J.A. Cochrane (1995). The contribution of changes in the prevalence of prone sleeping position to the decline in sudden infant death syndrome in Tasmania. *Journal of the American Medical Association, 273,* 783–789.

Eiselt, M., M. Schendel, H. Witte, J. Dorschel, Lilia Curzi-Dascalova, A.M. D'Allest & U. Zwiener (1997). Quantitative analysis of discontinuous EEG in premature and full-term newborns during quiet sleep. *Electroencephalography and clinical Neurophysiology, 103,* 528–534.

Erkinjuntti, Matti, & P. Kero (1990). SCSB method compared to EEG-based polygraphy in sleep state scoring of newborn infants. *Acta Paediatrica Scandinavica, 70,* 274–279.

Erkinjuntti, Matti, K. Vaahtoranta, J. Alihanka & P. Kero (1984). Use of the SCSB method of monitoring of respiration, body movements and ballistocardiogram in infants. *Early Human Development, 9,* 119–126.

Fagioli, Igino, F. Salomon & Piero Salzarulo (1981). Sleep onset in infants under continuous feeding from birth: 24 hour recordings. *Revue EEG Neurophysiologie clinique, 11,* 37–44.

Fagioli, Igino, & Piero Salzarulo (1982). Sleep states development in the first year of life assessed through 24-h recordings. *Early Human Development, 6,* 215–228.

Fagioli, Igino, Frederic Bes & Piero Salzarulo (1988). 24-hour behavioural states distribution in continuously fed infants. *Early Human Development, 18,* 151–156.

Ficca, Gianluca, Igino Fagioli, Fiorenza Giganti & Piero Salzarulo (1999). Spontaneous awakenings from sleep in the first year of life. *Early Human Development, 55,* 219–228.

Fifer W.P., M. Greene, A. Hurtado, M.M. Myers (1999). Cardiorespiratory responses to bidirectional tilts in infants. *Early Human Development, 55,* 265–279.

Fleming, P.J., P.S. Blair, C. Bacon, D. Bensley, I. Smith, E. Taylor, J. Berry, J. Golding & J. Tripp (1996). Envorinment of infants during sleep and risk of the sudden infant death syndrome: Results of 1993–6 case-control study for confidential inquiry into stillbirths and deaths in infancy. *British Medical Journal, 313,* 191–198.

Fleming, P.J., & P.S. Blair (1997). The role of sleeping position in the aetiology of the sudden infant death syndrome. In McIntosh, N. (Ed.), *Current topics in neonatology*. London: Saunders.

Franco, Patricia, Josè Groswasser, M. Sottiaux, E. Broadfield & André Kahn (1996). Decreased cardiac responses to auditory stimulation during prone sleep. *Pediatrics, 97,* 174–178.

Franco, Patricia, A. Pardou, S. Hassid, P. Lurguin, Josè Groswasser & André Kahn (1997). Auditory arousal thresholds are higher when infants sleep in the prone position. *Journal of Pediatrics, 132,* 240–243.

Gabriel M., B. Grote & M. Jonas (1981). Sleep-wake pattern in preterm infants under two different care schedules during four-day polygraphic recording. *Neuropediatrics, 12,* 366–373, 1981.

Galland, B.C., G. Reeves, B.J. Taylor, & D.P.G. Boltron (1998). Sleep position, autonomic function, and arousal. *Arch. Dis. Child Fetal Neonatal Ed., 78,* 189–194.

Giganti, Fiorenza, Giovanni Cioni, Enrico Biagioni, Maria Teresa Puliti, Antonio Boldrini & Piero Salzarulo (2001). Activity patterns assessed throughout 24-hour recordings in preterm and near term infants. *Developmental Psychobiology, 38,* 133–142.

Gottlieb, G. (1996). A systems view of psychobiological development. In Magnusson, D. (Ed.), *The lifespan development of individuals: Behavioral neurobiological and psychosocial perspectives. A synthesis* (76–104). Cambridge: Cambridge University Press.

Greenough, W.T., & J.E. Black (1992). Induction of brain structure by experience: Substrates for cognitive development. In Gunnar, M. & C.A. Nelson (Eds.), *Behavioral developmental neuroscience, vol. 24. Minnesota symposia on child development.* Hillsdale, NJ: Erlbaum.

Guilleminault, Christiane, Rosalba Peraita, M. Soquet & William C. Dement (1978). Apneas during sleep in infants: Possible relationship with sudden infant death syndrome. *Science Washington DC, 190,* 677–679.

Haddad, G.G., M.A.F. Epstein, Rachel A. Epstein, N.M. Mazza, R.B. Mellins & E. Krongrad (1979). The QT interval in aborted sudden infant death syndrome infants. *Pediatric Research, 13,* 136–138.

Harper, R.M., B. Leake, Toke Hoppenbrouwers, M.B. Sterman, D.J. McGinty & J. Hodgman (1978). Polygraphic studies of normal infants and infants at risk for the sudden infant death syndrome: Heart rate and variability as a function of state. *Pediatric Research, 12,* 778–785.

Hayes, Marie J., Lonnie S. Plante, B.A. Fielding, Savitri P. Kumar, & Maria Delivoria-Papadopoulos M. (1994). Functional analysis of spontaneous movements in preterm infants. *Developmental Psychobiology, 27,* 271–287.

Hayes, Marie J., & Shawn M. Roberts (1996). Early childhood co-sleeping: Parent-child and parent-infant nighttime interactions. Infant Mental Health Journal, *17,* 348–357.

Hayes, Marie J., & D. Mitchell (1998). Spontaneous movements during sleep in children: temporal organization and changes with age. *Developmental Psychobiology 32,* 13–21.

Hayes, Marie J., Akilesh, M., Davare, A., & Parker, K.G. (1999). Comparison of theophylline and caffeine pharmacotherapy on behavioral state and spontaneous movements in infants between 30–35 weeks PCA. *World Federation of Sleep Research Society*, Dresden, Germany.

Hayes, Marie J., K.G. Parker, A.A. Davare & B. Sallinen (2001). Bedsharing, temperament and sleep disturbance in early childhood. *Sleep, 24,* 657–662.

Henslee, J.A., V.L. Schechtman, M.Y. Lee, M.Y., & Harper, R.M. (1997). Developmental patterns of heart rate and variability in prematurely-born infants with apnea of prematurity. *Early Human Development, 47,* 35–50.

Hoffman, H.J., K. Damus, L. Hillman & E. Kongrad (1988). Risk factors for SIDS: Results of the National Institute of Child Health and Human Development SIDS Cooperative Epidemiological Study. *Annals of NY Academy of Science, 533,* 13–20.

Holditch-Davis, Diane, & Evelyn B. Thoman (1987). Behavioral states of premature infants: Implications for neural and behavioral development. *Developmental Psychobiology, 20,* 25–38.

Holditch-Davis, Diane (1990). The development of sleeping and waking states in high-risk preterm infants. *Infant Behavior and Development, 13,* 513–531.

Hoppenbrouwers, Toke, J.E. Hodgman & L. Cabal (1993). Obstructive apnea, associated patterns of movement, heart rate, and oxygenation in infants at low and increased risk for SIDS. *Pediatric Pulmonology, 15,* 1–12.

Hunt, C.E. (1981). Abnormal hypercarbic and hypoxic sleep arousal responses in near-miss SIDS infants. *Pediatric Research, 15,* 1462–1464.

Hunt, C.E., & R.T. Brouillette (1987). Sudden infant death syndrome, 1987 perspective. *Journal of Pediatrics, 110,* 669–678.

Kahn, Andrè, D. Hasaerts & D. Blum (1985). Phenothiazine-induced sleep apneas in normal infants. *Pediatrics, 75,* 844–847.

Kahn, André, A. Sangeleer, & D. Blum (1985). Effects of sleep position upon transcutaneous gas tension in infants. *Archives Française de Pediatrie, 42,* 419–421.

Kahn, André, E. Picard & D. Blum (1986). Auditory thresholds of normal and near-miss SIDS infants. *Developmental Medicine and Child Neurology, 28,* 299–302.

Kahn, André, C. Van de Merckt, M. Dramaix, P. Bagrez, D. Blum, E. Rebuffat & L. Montauk (1987). Transepidermal water loss during sleep in infants at risk for sudden death. *Pediatrics, 80,* 245–250.

Kahn, André, E. Rebuffat, M. Sottiaux, et al. (1991). Arousals induced by proximal esophageal reflux in infants. *Sleep, 14,* 39–42.

Kahn, A., E. Rebuffat, M. Sottiaux, M.F. Muller, A. Bochner & Josè Grosswasser (1990). Brief airway obstruction in infants with breath-holding spells. *Journal of Pediatrics, 117,* 188–193.

Kahn, A., Josè Groswasser, E. Rebuffat et al. (1992). Sleep and cardiorespiratory characteristics of infant victims of sudden death: A prospective case-control study. *Sleep, 15,* 287–292.

Kahn, A., Josè Groswasser, M. Sottiaux et al. (1993). Prone or supine body position and sleep characteristics in infants. *Pediatrics, 91,* 1112–1115.

Kahn, A., P. Franco, S. Scaillet, Josè Groswasser & B. Dan (1997). Development of cardiopulmonary integration and the role of arousability from sleep. *Current Opinion in Pulmonary Medicine, 3,* 440–444.

Keener, M.A., C.H. Zeanah & T.F. Anders (1988). Infant temperament, sleep organization, and nighttime parental interventions. *Pediatrics, 81,* 762–771.

Kinney, H.C., T.J. O'Donnal, P. Kriger & W.S. White (1993). Early development changes in (3H) nicotine binding in human brainstem. *Neuroscience, 55,* 1127–1130.

Kirjavainen, T., D.Cooper, O. Polo & C.E. Sullivan (1996). Respiratory and body movements as indicators of sleep stage and wakefulness in infants and young children. *Journal of Sleep Research, 5,* 186–194.

Kohyama, J., & Y. Iwakawa (1990). Developmental changes in phasic sleep parameters as reflections of the brain-stem maturation: Polysomnographic examinations of infants, including premature neonates. *Electroencephalography and clinical Neurophysiology, 76,* 325–330.

Lijowska, Anna, N.W. Reed, B.A. Chiodini & Bradley T. Thach (1997). Sequential arousal and airway-defensive behavior of infants in asphyxial sleep environments. *Journal of Applied Physiology, 83,* 219–228.

Louis, J., C. Cannard, Helene Bastuji & Marie J. Challamel (1997). Sleep ontogenesis revisited: A longitudinal 24-hour home polygraphic study on 15 normal infants during the first two years of life. *Sleep, 20,* 323–333.

Lozoff, B., A.W. Wolf & N.S. Davis (1985). Co-sleeping in urban families with young children in the United States. *Pediatrics, 74,* 171–192.

Masterson, J., C. Zucker & K.F. Schulze (1987). Prone and supine positioning effects on energy expenditure and behavior of low birth weight neonates. *Pediatrics, 80,* 689–692.

McKenna, J.J., S. Mosko, C. Dungy & J. McAninch (1990). Sleep and arousal patterns of co-sleeping human mother/infant pairs: A preliminary physiological study with implications for the study of sudden infant death syndrome (SIDS). *American Journal of Physical Anthropology, 83,* 331–347.

McKenna, J.J., Evelyn B. Thoman, Thomas F. Anders, Avi Sadeh, V.L. Schechtman & S.F. Glotzbach (1993). Infant-parent co-sleeping in an evolutionary perspective: Implications for understanding infant sleep development and the sudden infant death syndrome. *Sleep, 16,* 263–282.

McKenna, J.J. (1996). Sudden infant death syndrome in cross-cultural perspective: Is infant–parent cosleeping protective? *Annal Review of Anthropology, 25,* 201–216.

McNamara, F., F.G. Issa & C.E. Sullivan (1996). Arousal pattern following central and obstructive breathing abnormalities in infants and children. *Journal of Applied Physiology, 81,* 2651–2657.

McNamara, F., H. Wulbrand & Bradley T. Thach (1999). Habituation of the infant arousal response. *Sleep, 22,* 320–326.

Mograss, M.A., F.M. Ducharme & R.T. Brouillette (1994). Movement/arousals: Description, classification, and relationship to sleep apnea in children. *American Journal of Critical Care Medicine, 150,* 1690–1696.

Mosko, S., C. Richard & J. McKenna (1997). Infant arousals during mother-infant bed sharing: Implications for infant sleep and sudden infant death syndrome research. *Pediatrics, 100,* 841–849.

Myers, M.M., W.P. Fifer, L. Schaeffer, R. Sahni, O. Ohira-Kist, R.I. Stark & K.F. Schulze (1998). Effects of sleeping position and time after feeding on the organization of sleep-wake states in prematurely born infants. *Sleep, 21,* 343–349.

Nayayanan, C.H., M.W. Fox & V. Hamburger (1971). Prenatal development of spontaneous and evoked activity in the rat. *Behaviour, 40,* 100–134.

Parmelee, Arthur H., Jr., W.H. Wenner, T. Akiyama, M. Schultz & Evelyn Stern (1967). Sleep states in premature infants. *Developmental Medicine and Child Neurology, 9,* 70–77.

Phillipson, E.A., & C.E. Sullivan (1978). Arousal: The forgotten response to respiratory stimuli. *American Review of Respiratory Disorders, 118,* 807–809.

Phillipson, E.A., C.E. Sullivan, D.J. Read, E. Murphy & L.F. Kozar (1978). Ventilatory and waking responses to hypoxia in sleeping dogs. *Journal of Applied Physiology, 44,* 512–520.

Prechtl, Heinz F.R. (1974). The behavioral states of the newborn infant (a review). *Brain Research, 76,* 185–212.

Prechtl Heinz F.R., J.G. Nijhuis, C.B. Martin Jr., R.S. Bots (1982). Are there behavioural states in the human fetus?. *Early Human Development, 6,* 177–195.

Prechtl, Heinz F.R. (1997). State of the art of a new functional assessment of the young nervous system. An early predictor of cerebral palsy. *Early Human Development, 50,* 1–11.

Remmers, J.E., W.J. De Grott, E.K. Sauerland & A.M. Anch (1978). Pathogenesis of upper airway occlusion during sleep. *Journal of Applied Physiology, 44,* 931–938.

Richman, N., & P.J. Graham (1971). A behavioral screening questionnaire for use with 3-year-old children. Preliminary findings. *Journal of Child Psychology & Psychiatry, 12,* 5–33.

Robertson, S.S. (1982). Instrinsic temporal patterning in the spontaneous movement of awake neonates. *Child Development, 53,* 1016–1021.

Robertson, S.S. (1987). Human cyclic motility: Fetal-newborn continuities and newborn state differences. *Developmental Psychobiology, 20,* 425–462.

Sadeh, Avi, Peretz Lavie, Anat Scher, Emanuel Tirosh & R. Epstein (1991). Actigraphic home monitoring of sleep disturbed and control infants and young children: A new method for pediatric assessment of sleep-wake patterns. *Pediatrics, 87,* 494–499.

Sadeh, Avi, & Thomas F. Anders (1993). Infant sleep problems: Origins, assessment, interventions. *Infant Mental Health Journal, 14,* 17–34.

Sadeh, A., K.M. Sharkey & Mary A. Carskadon (1994). Activity-based sleep-wake identification: An empirical test of methodological issues. *Sleep, 17,* 201–207.

Sadeh, Avi, Peter J. Hauri, Daniel F. Kripke & Peretz Lavie (1995). The role of actigraphy in the evaluation of sleep disorders. *Sleep, 18,* 288–302.

Sadeh, Avi, C. Acebo, R. Seifer, S. Aytur & Mary A. Carskadon (1995). Activity based assessment of sleep wake pattern during the 1st year of life. *Infant Behavior and Development, 18,* 329–337.

Salzarulo, Piero, Igino Fagioli, F. Salomon, J. F. Duhamel & C. Ricour (1979). Continuous feeding and the wake-sleeping rhythm in children. *Archives Française de Pediatrie, 36,* 26–32.

Salzarulo, Piero, & Igino Fagioli (1992). Post-natal development of sleep organization in man: Speculations on the emergence of the 'S process'. *Neurophysiologie Clinique, 22,* 107–115.

Salzarulo, Piero, & Igino Fagioli (1995). Sleep for development or development for waking?– some speculations from a human perspective. *Behavioural Brain Research, 69,* 23–27.

Salzarulo, Piero, Fiorenza Giganti, Igino Fagioli & Gianluca Ficca (2001). Development of states regulation. In Kalverboer A. & Gramsbergen A. (Eds), *Handbook of brain and behavior in human development* (pp. 725–742). Dordrecht: Kluwer.

Schechtman, V.L., R.M. Harper, K.A. Kluge, A.J. Wilson, H.J. Hoffman & D.P. Southall (1988). Cardiac and respiratory patterns in normal infants and victims of the sudden death syndrome. *Sleep, 11,* 413–424.

Schechtman, V.L., J.A. Henslee & R.M. Harper (1988). Developmental patterns of heart rate and variability in infants with persistent apnea of infancy. *Early Human Development, 50,* 251–262.

Schechtman, V.L., R.M. Harper, A.J. Wilson & D.P. Southall (1991). Sleep apnea in infants who succumb to the sudden infant death syndrome. *Pediatrics, 87,* 841–846.

Schechtman, V.L., R.M. Harper, A.J. Wilson & D.P. Southall (1992). Sleep state organization in normal infants and victims of the sudden infant death syndrome. *Pediatrics, 89,* 865–870.

Schechtman, V.L., S.L. Raetz, R.K. Harper, A. Garfinkel, A.J. Wilson, D.P. Southall, D.P. & R.M. Harper (1992). Dynamic analysis of cardiac R-R intervals in normal infants and in infants who subsequently succumbed to the sudden infant syndrome. *Pediatric Research, 31,* 606–612.

Scher, Anat (1991). A longitudinal study of nightwaking in the first year. *Child: Care, Health Development, 17,* 295–302.

Scher, M.S., G.A. Richardson, P.A. Coble, N.L. Day & D.S. Stoffer (1988). The effects of prenatal alcohol and marijuana exposure: Disturbances in neonatal sleep cycling and arousal. *Pediatric Research, 24,* 101–105.

Scher, M.S., D.A. Steppe, D.L. Banks, R.D. Guthrie & R.J. Sclabassi (1995). Maturational trends of EEG-sleep measures in the healthy preterm neonate. *Pediatric Neurology, 12,* 314–322.

Scher, M.S. (1996). Normal electrographic-polysomnographic patterns in preterm and fullterm infants. *Semeiotics and Pediatric Neurology, 3,* 2–12.

Schulz, Hartmut, Roberto Massetani, Igino Fagioli & Piero Salzarulo (1985). Spontaneous awakening from sleep in infants. *Electroencephalography and clinical Neurophysiology, 61,* 267–271.

Schwartz, P.J., M. Stramba-Badiale, A. Segantini, P. Austoni, G. Bosi, R. Giorgetti, F. Grancini, E.D. Marni, F. Perticone, D. Rosti & P. Salice (1998). Prolongation of the QT interval and the sudden infant death syndrome. *New England Journal of Medicine, 338,* 1709–1714.

Stefanski, Mark, K. Schulze, D. Bateman, R. Kairam, T.A. Pedley, J. Masterson & L.S. James (1984). A scoring system for states of sleep and wakefulness in term and preterm infants. *Pediatric Research, 18,* 58–62.

Siegel, J.M. (1994). The evolution of REM sleep. In R. Lydic & H.A. Baghdoyan (Eds), *Handbook of behavioral state control: Cellular and molecular mechanisms* (87–100).

Steriade, Mircea (1996). Arousal: Revisiting the reticular activating system. *Science, 272,* 225–226.

Sterman, M.B., & Toke Hoppenbrouwers (1971). The development of sleep-waking and rest-activity patterns from fetus to adult in man. In M.B. Sterman, D.J. McGinty & A.N. Adinolfi (Eds). *Brain development and behaviour* (203–229). New York: Academic Press.

Sullivan, C.E., & F.G. Issa (1985). Obstructive sleep apnea. *Clinical Chest Medicine, 6,* 633–650.

Thoman, Evelyn B., & Tynan, W.D. (1979). Sleep states and wakefulness in human infants: Profiles from motility monitoring. *Physiology and Behavior, 23,* 519–525.

Thoman, Evelyn B., & R.C. Glazier (1987). Computer scoring of motility patterns for states of sleep and wakefulness: Human infants. *Sleep, 10,* 122–129.

Thoman, Evelyn B. (1990). Sleeping and waking states in inants: A functional perspective. *Neuroscience and Biobehavioral Review, 14,* 93–107.

Thoppil, C.K., M.A. Belan, C.P. Cowen & O.P. Matthew (1991). Behavioral arousal in newborn infants and its association with termination of apnea. *Journal of Applied Physiology, 70,* 2479–2484.

Visser, G.H.A., G. Poelmann-Weesjes, T.M.N. Cohen & D.J. Bekedam (1987). Fetal behavior at 30 to 32 weeks of gestation. *Pediatric Research, 22,* 655–658.

White, M., M. Beckett, M. O'Regan & T. Matthews (1993). Autonomic function and SIDS. *Acta Paediatrica, 389,* 105–106.

Wolff, Peter H. (1959). Observations on newborn infants. *Psychosomatic Medicine, 21,* 110–118.

Wolke, D., R. Meyer, B. Ohrt & K. Riegel (1995). The incidence of sleeping problems in preterm and fullterm infants discharged from neonatal special care units: an epidemiological longitudinal study. *Journal of Child Psychology, Psychiatry and Allied Disciplines, 36,* 203–223.

Wulbrand, H., G. von Zezschwitz & H.P. Bentele (1995). Submental and diaphragmatic muscle activity during and at resolution of mixed and obstructive apneas and cardiorespiratory arrythmias. *Pediatric Research, 38,* 298–305.

Awakenings from infants' sleep

Some remarks on definitions, methodology and research issues

Gianluca Ficca
Department of Psychology, II University of Naples

Physiological events, like all the other natural processes, need to be operationalized. In other terms, for a given phenomenon, any kind of scientific speculation and construct depends on the possibility of defining it through strict criteria, usable and reproducible in the experimental context and allowing to distinguish it from similar and/or overlapping events.

When talking of awakening, which might seem to be an immediate and easily definable notion, there are actually some entangled conceptual and methodological issues making the picture less clear.

The unsolved questions on awakening definition, yet remaining for the adult, as reminded by Salzarulo (1999), are even more complicate in the research on development, due to the extremely rapid changes, occurring at early ages, in behavioural and psychological processes, as well as in the CNS structures that regulate them.

Therefore, some preliminary remarks on these issues are crucial in the research on awakening and its features (specifically, with regard to its "measurement"). In particular, I will try here to highlight that awakening has to be defined a discrete event, but at the same time that its mechanisms cannot be fully understood without taking into account the dynamic process preceding it. Few attempts have been done so far in this direction, and it might not be pointless to say from the beginning that I will often refer to articles dating back to the sixties and seventies: many important and still crucial intuitions may be found between the lines of the important contributions of that particular period, when the debate on behavioural states was extraordinarily intense and productive.

Awakenings vs. arousal

A first issue that needs to be addressed is the conceptual difference between "arousal" and "awakening". This aspect deserves attention because these are two terms that are very often used as equivalent in scientific literature, especially in the clinical field. Some examples of this frequent use are in Horner (1996) and Thoppil et al. (1991).

The term "arousal" has not been introduced specifically for development, and even in the adult there is a variety of meanings that have been attributed to it. Although some Authors have referred to arousal as a synonymous of "vigilance level", which may be related to attention (Berlucchi, 1996), most of the times the word indicates a transient cortical activation, whatever the previous background level.

The American Sleep Disorders Association (ASDA) definition of arousal, for instance, refers to electroencephalographic changes whose duration may be very short, even not longer than three seconds (ASDA, 1992). In research on infants, a similar definition was given by Scher et al. (1992), referring to a transient desynchronization of the EEG background activity "with more than a 50% reduction in amplitude and more than 90 % reduction of slow EEG frequency activity".

In most of the cases, arousals are associated to impressive changes of autonomic activity, including increases in heart rate, blood pressure and ventilation (Horner, 1996). Recently, it has been underlined that many changes of these parameters, towards activation, are not necessarily concomitant to EEG modifications: this has led some Authors to focus on subcortical events like changes in muscle tone, sighs and heart rate abrupt changes (see for example Ariagno, Mirmiran & Darnall, in a chapter of this book) and other Authors to even trace a pathway that would represent the "arousal sequence" (Thach & Lijowska, 1996).

It goes without saying that the identification of an arousal during infants' sleep is easier when it comes out from Quiet Sleep, that is on a slow background EEG and in the frame of a steady and regular neurovegetative activity, than when it emerges from Active Sleep, characterized by a great amount of phasic events like apnoeas, cardiac arrhythmias and different kinds of sudden movements, e.g. jerky startles (Anders et al., 1971): it is highly debatable whether these state-dependent phenomena may or not be considered arousing events themselves.

However, what matters here is that any change in the arousal level may happen well **within** sleep, often with a more or less quick return to the baseline condition.

Instead, by definition, awakening cannot exist without **the ending of all sleep phenomena** and the wake onset. Strictly speaking (that is, independent from the mechanisms regulating its occurrence), awakening would then be a discrete, single-moment event, and a corollary of this assumption is that there could not be varying degrees of awakening, like implied by those classifications including both "partial" and "full" awakenings (Stepanski et al., 1984), which should be intended as an all-or-none phenomenon. Actually, we will see later that the notion of "partial" awakening could make sense if we take into account the dynamics of the following wakefulness.

Once clarified this apparently obvious but often neglected concept, we can possibly speculate on two consequential theoretical issues.

First, since awakening is the transition between sleep and wakefulness, how can we distinguish between the two? Or, better to say, what are the peculiarities of wakefulness which allow its recognition? If answering to this question is often easier with respect to adult individuals, this is far more difficult for the newborn and even more for the fetus.

Second, does the awakening always emerge from a series of prior arousing events? If this is the case, then the occurrence of this chains of events could be important for the characteristics and the quality of wakefulness following awakening.

Defining and identifying wakefulness in infants

As said before, the identification of an awakening implies that one can establish the criteria to distinguish wakefulness from the other behavioural states and thus to identify its beginning and termination.

A detailed review on the concept of behavioural state goes beyond the objectives of this chapter and may be found elsewhere (Prechtl et al., 1968; Prechtl & O'Brien, 1982; Wolff, 1987). For our purposes, it might be worthwhile reminding that already in 1968, behavioural states were referred to as "*constellations of physiological variables which have to be relatively stable* and ***to reoccur together***" (Prechtl et al., 1968): we can reformulate this by saying that any given variable is meaningless for the identification of a behavioural state unless it is steadily associated to at least another variable and they are simultaneous in time and change together. Thus, although early development is constantly characterized by the progressive appearance of different functions and behaviours, these may be used as state criteria only when: a) they can be recorded and/or observed; b) they are coordinated in recognizable patterns.

Furthermore, associations may happen by chance, due to the random overlapping of independently regulated variables, rather than reflecting a coordinated pattern: Njhuis et al. (1982) underline that "*the lack of a central coordination of these* (variables) *oscillations will lead to a non-synchronized onset and end of such epochs*". This is the reason why a "real" association of physiological variables (in particular, we are interested here to the "real" wakefulness) must meet the additional requirement of a minimum duration.

There are a series of basic questions raised by these assumptions: a) "**How many** variables have to be chosen in order to analyse their pattern of association?" b) "**Which** variables are the most adequate to be looked at for the identification of wakefulness?" and finally c) "**For how long** must this association of variables last to be defined a waking state?"

How many variables?

As far as the first question is concerned, the concept of states as complex ensembles of physiological, behavioural and psychological parameters would tempt to answer that "the more, the better". Nevertheless, the maturation turmoil of the first weeks of life (and thus the rarity of synchronism between different parameters) would hamper any attempt of state designation if one is too conservative about the number of criteria adopted (Curzi-Dascalova & Mirmiran, 1996). Prechtl and O'Brien (1982) suggest that attention is paid not to include too many state criteria in infants' classification of behavioural states. The consequences of this mistake were elegantly described by Anders (1974). When trying to identify only active sleep and quiet sleep on the basis of the concordance of five different criteria, most of the sleep episode was unscorable and finished in the wide category of "indeterminate" states.

This observation introduces to a swampy territory. Actually, a common report from studies on infants at different ages, from the intrauterine life to all across the first year, is that they spend much time in the so-called "ambiguous" sleep (Salzarulo et al., 1980; Fagioli & Salzarulo, 1982). However, as also underlined by Salzarulo & Fagioli (1999), there are two distinct possibilities: one is that there are few specific, reoccurring ensembles of variables, and that a long time is spent in "mixed" states, displaying features which are "in between" two recognizable states (especially Active and Quiet sleep). Another possibility is that an ensemble of variables appears but just for a short period of time, with "transitional" characteristics not fulfilling the preset duration criteria (Dittrichovà, 1969). In my opinion, these two alternative cases should be conceptually and operationally kept apart, since they might have different functional meanings and index different degrees of CNS development. In the former case, in fact, the very immature brain structures create an undifferentiated activity, both at the cortical and the subcortical level. In the latter, instead, there is already an ability to coordinate different physiological variables, even if only for a brief period: we are in the field of the "functional uncertainty" of the CNS, which will also be a distinctive trait of the elderly individual and of some neurological and psychiatric syndromes in the adult (Salzarulo et al., 1997).

Although Anders proposes that three parameters would be sufficient to score sleep states in the first months of life, very few normative studies have tried to precisely address this topic for the experimental studies on infants at different ages, as well as the issue of which variable to select. The choice is extremely important because, in practical terms, it is often very complicate to arrange full polygraphic recordings on infants, and it may sometimes be very convenient to use just one measure as a more or less reliable index of behavioural states (with the added advantage of the simpler methods allowing longer recordings). Ideally, a scale of priority for the selection of variables should be made available, taking into account that each physiological variable is more or less differentiated and recordable at different steps of development.

Which variables?

About this scale of priority, we should start with reminding that physiological signals are not the most reliable and easiest to record at very early ages, because of technical difficulties and, above all, because of their ambiguousness. Both Anders et al. (1971) and Becker & Thoman (1982), for example, claim that waking states are not identifiable by electrophysiological recordings, and point out the necessity of adopting direct observation, which allows the study of behavioural parameters. Despite the improvement of polysomnographic techniques, Kirjavainen et al. recently noticed that the interpretation of polysomnography in infants is controversial, with special respect to the transition periods between sleep and wakefulness (Kirjavainen et al., 1996).

Body motility has been considered a golden standard to discriminate in infants not only between sleep states, but also between sleep and wakefulness. Many Authors emphasize the relevance of body motility in following the developmental trends of sleep and wakefulness (Hayes, 1993; Curzi-Dascalova et al., 1988a). As previously remarked (Giganti et al., symposium " Relationship between sleep-wake states in neonates and adults: importance for identifying regulatory mechanisms and sleep function(s)", 15th Congress of the European Sleep Research Society, Istanbul, September 2000), the most obvious support to this notion is that the distinction for adulthood between REM sleep and NREM sleep, based on eye movements, is replaced in infants by the one between Active Sleep (AS) and Quiet Sleep (QS), with a clear focus on the motor aspects.

The usefulness of body movements as a behavioural index in the earliest epochs of development is suggested by accurate studies, performed through sophisticated techniques like ultrasonography, which have identified quite distinct movements already in the fetus that undergo some changes in their characteristics across age (deVries et al., 1982 and 1985).

At 8 weeks of conceptional age, only generalized movements and startles are detectable, whereas at 19 weeks c.a. there are many other movement patterns. However, these movements result to be diluted in the generalized and intense background motor activity, without any specific time-course or periodicity. In other terms, although its differentiation begins strikingly early, body motility cannot concur to define a proper state of wakefulness until it is not interrupted by quiescent periods. Dreyfus-Brisac claims that it is extremely hazardous to speak about sleep and wakefulness before the 28th week of gestational age and speaks of an "indefinite" state (Dreyfus-Brisac, 1974), similarly to what has been described in the animals at comparable ages: in particular, studies on rats (Jouvet-Mounier et al., 1970) and kittens (Adrien, 1976) have proposed the existence of a particular kind of sleep, concomitant with a frantic generalized motor activity, that was defined by Danielle Jouvet-Mounier "seismic sleep". Therefore, sleep would precede wakefulness across the development, although, for what said before with respect to behavioural states, also the term "sleep" is questionable at such early ages.

The finding of a rhythmic organization of body motility in pre-term infants (Hayes et al., 1993) and of a specific distribution of motility patterns in the diurnal and nocturnal periods (Giganti et al., 2001) also suggests that intense activity patterns, though not being states themselves, can be interpreted as signals of the gradual emergence of a sleep-wake rhythm.

Although wakefulness has been sometimes inferred on the basis of actigraphically detected hand or body movements alone (Sadeh et al., 1991; Sadeh, 1994), it often happens that Active sleep and wakefulness cannot be differentiated without the observation of at least one more behavioural parameter.

In their studies on premature and newborns, Parmelee & Stern (1972) decided to use two measures of state. The first was the combination of eyes opening and amount of body movements, and was based, according to the Authors, on the fact that these criteria may be observed and used over a wide age range. As second measure of state, Parmelee & Stern chose respiratory pattern, but stated that, in fetus and premature of low gestational age, they are "*probably only useful in defining states **during sleep***".

Although in association with respiratory pattern (Thoman & Tynan, 1979; Curzi-Dascalova et al., 1981) and/or heart rate variability (Haddad et al., 1987), body movements were the main state measure in most of the studies on the development of states.

On a sample of ten infants aged 34–40 weeks conceptional age, our group in Florence (Ficca, Giganti & Salzarulo, unpublished data) carried out a preliminary study on the associations between three parameters (eyes opening, body movements and EEG patterns), trying to determine which one, taken separately, was most predictive of concomitant signs of wakefulness displayed by the others. Following Stefanski et al. (1984), the "motility" measure was a combined assessment of both body movements and vocalizations/crying. EEG patterns were conventionally assigned to a state according to the proposals of Nolte & Haas (1978). One main finding was that the opening of the eyes is not always fully discriminating between sleep and wakefulness: in fact, in 6 out of ten infants there were recurring associations of very intense motility with crying, EEG pattern of wakefulness and still closed eyes: likewise, 5 out of ten infants showed epochs with eyes opening but no crying and/or vocalizations. Interestingly, motility pattern before the 38th week of age was predictive of the electrophysiological data more often than the opposite: in fact, the scoring of wakefulness done on the basis of body motility alone was actually consistent with the kind of EEG pattern recorded in about 75% of the epochs, whereas the scoring done on the basis of EEG only led, in almost half of cases, to classify "wakefulness" epochs with weak motility and eyes closed.

The abovementioned scoring system by Stefanski et al. was designed and proposed for determining sleep and wakefulness in both the preterm and the full-term newborn (Stefanski et al., 1984). In this system, EEG patterns are analysed, but a top priority is given to a global assessment of behavioural characteristics, including eye movements and body movements. As for the state we are dealing with, wakefulness may be reflected, according to Stefanski et al., by **nonreflex** movements of the limbs, by opening of the eyes and even by facial activity (frowns, smiles, grunts and so on), and these phenomena do not necessarily have to be all associated. Furthermore, vocalization and crying are considered sufficient to score "wakeful behaviour". There are two main points of this coding system that we repute highly remarkable. One is the introduction in a categorical system of a qualitative assessment of the behavioural indexes. Not only is behaviour a central element of this system, but its components are mainly determined through observation and combined in global patterns. Interestingly, this is not very different, as will be made evident by Giganti & Toselli in a later chapter of this book, from the mother (who obviously cannot rely on polysomnography) **arguing** that a baby is awake from his crying or his opening of the eyes.

The other basic concept evoked by a scoring system such as Stefanski's is that wakefulness differs from sleep because it provides the individual, even immediately after birth, with new properties and with an increasing ability of CNS to interface the inner "milieu" with the outer world. This concept is taken for granted in the adult, for whom it is feasible to identify wakefulness as a state characterized by complex interactions with the environment, by a level of consciousness allowing these interactions and also by the performance of all cognitive processes; in infants, instead, there are less and more confused indexes of this interaction, although it has been a main issue in the research of the past. About forty years ago, Kleitman distinguished a "wakefulness of necessity", a subcortical function, from a "wakefulness of choice", based on cortical activity and characterized by the addition of "a certain level of consciousness" (Kleitman, 1963). Dittrichovà and Lapackovà (1966) tried to trace a profile of the waking state in the first half year of life by choosing as indicators the hand movements with toys suspended over the infant's crib and the vocalization, two indexes considered precursor of play and talking, respectively, and clearly dependent upon the interaction with the outer environment.

It is quite obvious, therefore, that attentional processes and the ability to react to various external stimuli (characterizing what Wolff calls "alert activity") are the most certain signals that an awakening has occurred. In infants, attention may be inferred, by means of direct observation, from peculiar behavioural patterns which can either consolidate across time or be progressively replaced by other features. The basic attention behaviour is the eye scanning, indexed by the number of saccadic movements produced by the subject during the exploration of the environment. Beyond eye movements, other phenomena have been proposed as expressions of information perception and processing, such as non nutritive sucking (Wolff, 1987; for a review, see also Salzarulo et al., 2001).

Index of attentional processes, instead, are not of help in scoring awakenings when infants lie in other kinds of wakefulness such as "*alert inactivity*", with eyes open, but no scanning of the environment, very few body movements, relaxed face and regular respiration (Wolff, 1987).

For how long?

The final issue mentioned at the beginning of this chapter concerns with the minimum duration of the wakeful behaviour which entitles us to speak of waking **state**.

The ability to coordinate and sustain states is progressively increasing across early development (Parmelee & Stern, 1972; Curzi-Dascalova et al., 1988b): therefore, in general lines, it makes sense to adjust this duration as a function of the age of the subjects investigated. For instance, recent studies of our group on pre-term and near-term infants (Giganti et al., 2001) adopted a one-minute criterion, arbitrarily chosen in light of the evidence that there are already reoccurring association of variables, but that they often happen in short bouts.

In most of the studies of the group at the University of Florence on newborn infants, instead, we have used a two-minutes duration criterion to score wakefulness (Salzarulo et al., 1980; Fagioli & Salzarulo, 1982; Salzarulo & Fagioli, 1992; Ficca et al., 1999; Ficca et al., 2000). In other studies, the minimum duration of wakefulness required to score an awakening was even longer (i.e., 5 minutes in Navelet et al., 1982).

This methodological aspect must be acknowledged, because it can partly explain some discrepancies in the data on awakenings found in the literature; however, most likely, the selection of a given criterion does not significantly affect the results, in terms of developmental trends (see also Fagioli, Ficca & Salzarulo chapter later on in this volume).

More difficult is a proper evaluation of some behavioural parameters, with particular respect to ages when the attentional processes are already present and active, occurring within different time windows relative to those usually selected for the definition of states.

Prechtl and O' Brien (1982) already highlighted how, in order to respect the definition of state, sudden and momentary phenomena, e.g. the opening of the eyes, possibly scanning the environment, should be discarded: as an example, they quote the possibility that, having "eyes closed" as a state variable for sleep, rapid eye movements may be accompanied by shortlasting opening of the eyelids. In such a situation, one would share the view of Prechtl & O'Brien, that it would be unproper to consider Active Sleep interrupted by wakefulness only on the basis of this opening. On the other hand, this example makes clear that a rigid scoring rule, strictly based on the duration criteria adopted, runs the risk of overlooking such phenomena, which would be treated only as "noise".

It is in right in these cases that the concept of partial awakening might be introduced: it would be the appearance of clear signals of wakefulness, although a waking state can not be scored because the requirement of stability is not satisfied. A reliable record of all these ensembles of behavioural and physiological events would help in the long term to get normative data on the average degree of stability of these ensembles at different ages.

I would like to close the section by reporting a very good example of a methodologically thorough approach, coming from a study carried out on the human fetus by Nijhuis and collaborators (Nijhuis et al., 1982). The Authors were aware of the difficulty having reliable variables in utero, where EEG cannot be recorded and respiration is not continuously present: therefore, they decided to use only three state criteria and selected the available ones, that is fetal body and eye movements and fetal heart rate pattern. In addition, they arbitrarily set the minimum duration criterion to three minutes. They concluded that before 36 weeks of gestation, although there are cyclic patterns for each variable, sometimes overlapping, there is no sufficiently stable constellation of parameters to identify well organised behavioural states; instead, at 38 and 40 weeks, they managed to distinguish four distinct patterns (states 1F through 4F), showing evidence even for episodes of wakefulness. Interestingly, their results are fully consistent with what observed in low-risk pre-term babies at the same gestational age by Prechtl et al. (1979).

Awakening as an endpoint?

Once that we have defined and identified the awakening, referring to it as to a "single-moment" event, the focus of research can be shifted on the sleep period immediately preceding. On one hand, studying where the awakening emerges from and which circumstances can favour or even predict it, is essential in the experimental field for the understanding of state regulation; on the other, it is also particularly relevant for clinical purposes, because it may help clarify both the reasons of excessive awakenings and of difficulty waking up in threatening situations (e.g., hypoxia).

Of course, a similar consideration might be done for the wake-sleep transition, i.e. the sleep onset, for which nowadays, at least in the adult, there is far more knowledge than on the awakening process. Sleep onset is well announced by the disappearance of alpha waves, by the slowing of EEG rhythms, by slow eye movements, by behavioural signs like the closing of the eyes. As for the awakening process, instead, ending with the scoring of the state "wake", it is largely unknown whether the transition between sleep and wakefulness is "prepared" or announced by any psychophysiological processes, either isolated or in specific and repetitive sequences.

Recently, it has been shown that one main factor related to the emergence of a spontaneous awakening is the sleep state. Results are consistent in indicating REM sleep as the state in which adults' awakenings are more likely to occur (Schulz & Zulley, 1980; Barbato et al., 1994): this predominance is even more marked in early development, especially in the first six months of life (Schulz et al., 1985; Ficca et al., 1999). In another chapter of this volume (Fagioli, Ficca & Salzarulo: "Awakening in infants and the sleep-wake cycle"), the relationships between infants' awakenings and sleep states are discussed in more details: here we want to emphasize the "gating" role towards wakefulness of REM sleep, which in early development coincides with a similar role of "gates to sleep", since the majority of infants' sleep onsets lead to REM sleep (Salzarulo et al., 2000).

However, differences in the propension to awakening as a function of the sleep state would be better understood if we had more knowledge on the sequences of physiological and behavioural events immediately preceding awakening.

The very sparse notions on the issue may partly depend on the methodological difficulty determining which of these events are really related to the awakening process. As a matter of fact, there are basically two hypotheses that can be formulated.

The first, very common in the literature, puts arousals and awakenings at different points of a continuum process. Chugh et al. (1996) speak of a "hierarchy of arousal phenomena", varying from brief electromyograph increases to sleep stage shifts and full awakenings. This is well described also in a paper by Stepanski et al., who differentiated four levels of arousal, ranging from shorter but more frequent events (level 1) to progressively longer but less numerous arousals (level 2 and 3), up to what they call partial and full awakenings.

If one shares this perspective, awakening ends up as a particular "subcategory" of arousal. Although Stepanski et al. classification can turn out to be useful for clinical purposes, there is not yet enough evidence to claim either that awakening is a "longer" arousal, or that it is the natural conclusion of a gradual process starting with an arousal. On the contrary, Stepanski et al. study found that patients with untreated OSAS, who showed significantly more arousals, did not have a higher frequency of awakenings compared to normal subjects (Stepanski et al., 1984).

Studies investigating the profile of gross body movements in the first six months of life have failed in finding a higher prevalence of awakenings within 60 seconds after the movements (Vecchierini-Blineau et al., 1984). This leads to the second hypothesis, proposed amongst others by Scher et al. (1992): the awakening (note that they use the term "behavioural arousal to awakening") abruptly ends all sleep activity, and may involve different alerting mechanisms from transient electrographic microarousals. This would have an immediate clinical fallout, because the debate on "arousability" would not necessarily coincide with the problem of "ability waking up".

Conclusions

Awakening is an event that one can look at from two different perspectives.

The first is the mere identification of the "gate" between sleep and wakefulness. In the experimental approach to the development of states, it is indispensable to detect these gates, to locate them in time, to analyse the changes in their frequency and features as a function of age. If we adopt these perspective, there is a need for very precise criteria to clearly distinguish these moments from other events with probably different meanings: this implies also that in every research dealing with awakening one should preliminarily select and unambiguously define the variables of interest, the procedures for their recordings and the time windows of the analysis.

From another perspective, however, the interest on the awakening process should naturally push further research on the various sequences of events before awakening and on the characteristics of wakefulness afterwards. As a matter of fact, both issues could be tightly related to the still poorly known functioning of sleep-wake regulatory systems across the development.

Acknowledgements

I wish to thank my colleagues Igino Fagioli and Fiorenza Giganti for long and fruitful discussions.

References

Adrien, Joelle (1976). Le sommeil du nouveau-né. *La Recherche, 63*, 74–76.

Anders, Thomas F., R. Emde & Arthur H. Jr. Parmelee (1971). *A manual for standardized terminology, techniques and criteria for the scoring of states of sleep and wakefulness in newborn infants.*:Los Angeles: Brain Information Service, School of Health Sciences, UCLA.

Anders, Thomas F. (1974). The infant sleep profile. *Neuropädiatrics, 5*, 425–442.

A.S.D.A. (1992). EEG arousals: scoring rules and examples. A preliminary report from the sleep disorders atlas task force of the American Sleep Disorders Association. *Sleep, 15*, 174–184.

Barbato, Giuseppe, Charles Barker, Charles Bender, Holly A. Giesen & Thomas Wehr (1994). Extended sleep in humans in 14 hour nights (LD 10:14): relationship between REM density and spontaneous awakening. *Electroencephalography and Clinical Neurophysiology, 90*, 291–297.

Becker, Patricia T. & Evelyn B. Thoman (1982). Waking activity: the neglected state of infancy. *Developmental Brain Research, 4*, 395–400.

Berlucchi, G. (1996). One or many arousal systems? Reflection on some of Giuseppe Moruzzi's foresights and insights about the intrinsic regulation of brain activity. *Archives Italiennes de Biologie, 135*, 5–11.

Chugh, Deepak K., Terri E. Weaver & David F. Dinges (1996). Neurobehavioral consequences of arousal. *Sleep, 19*, S198–S201.

Curzi-Dascalova, Lilia, C. Gaudebout & Colette Dreyfus-Brisac (1981). Respiratory frequencies of sleeping infants during the first months of life: correlations between values in different sleep states. *Early Human Development, 5*, 39–54.

Curzi-Dascalova, Lilia, Patricio Peirano & Françoise Morel-Kahn (1988a). Body motility and sleep states development in newborns. In Koella, W.P., F.Obal, H. Schulz, P. Visser (Eds), *Sleep '86* (229–231), Stuttgart/New York: Gustav Fischer Verlag.

Curzi-Dascalova, Lilia, Patricio Peirano & Françoise Morel-Kahn (1988b). Development of sleep states in normal premature and full-term newborns. *Developmental Psychobiology, 21*, 431–444.

Curzi-Dascalova, Lilia, & Majid Mirmiran (1996). *Manual of methods of recording and analyzing sleep-wakefulness states in preterm and full-term infants.* Paris: INSERM.

De Vries, Johanna I.P., G.H.A. Visser & Heinz F.R. Prechtl (1982). The emergence of fetal behaviour. I: qualitative aspects. *Early Human Development, 7*, 301–322.

De Vries, Johanna I.P., G.H.A. Visser & Heinz F.R. Prechtl (1985). The emergence of fetal behaviour. II: quantitative aspects. *Early Human Development, 12*, 99–120.

Dittrichovà, Jaroslava (1969). Development of sleep in infancy. In Robinson, R.J. (Ed.), *Brain and early behavior* (193–200). London: Academic Press.

Dittrichovà, Jaroslava, & V. Lapackovà (1964). Development of the waking state in young infants. *Child Development, 35*, 365–370.

Dreyfus-Brisac, Colette (1968). Sleep ontogenesis in early human prematurity from 24 to 27 weeks of conceptional age. *Developmental Psychobiology, 1*, 162–169.

Fagioli, Igino, & Piero Salzarulo (1982). Sleep states development in the first year of life assessed through 24-hour recordings. *Early Human Development, 6*, 215–228.

Ficca, Gianluca, Igino Fagioli, Fiorenza Giganti & Piero Salzarulo (1999). Spontaneous awakenings from sleep in the first year of life. *Early Human Development*, *55*, 219–228.

Ficca, Gianluca, Igino Fagioli & Piero Salzarulo (2000). Sleep organization in the first year of life: developmental trends in the quiet sleep-paradoxical sleep cycle. *Journal of Sleep Research*, *9*, 1–4.

Giganti, Fiorenza, Giovanni Cioni, Enrico Biagioni, Maria Teresa Puliti, Antonio Boldrini & Piero Salzarulo (2001). Activity patterns assessed throughout 24-hour recordings in preterm and near term infants. *Developmental Psychobiology*, *38*, 133–142.

Haddad, G.G., H.J. Jeng & T.L. Lai (1987). Heart rate variability during respiratory pauses in puppies and dogs. *Pediatric Research*, *22*, 306–311.

Hayes, Marie J., Lonnie Plante, Savitri P. Kumar & Maria Delivoria-Papadopoulos (1993). Spontaneous motility in premature infants: features of behavioral activity and rhythmic organization. *Developmental Psychobiology*, *26*, 279–291.

Horner, Richard L. (1996). Autonomic consequences of arousal from sleep: mechanisms and implication. *Sleep*, *19*, S193–S195.

Jouvet-Mounier, Danielle, L. Astic & D. Lacote (1970). Ontogenesis of the states of sleep in rat, cat, and guinea pig during the first postnatal month. *Developmental Psychobiology*, *2*, 216–239.

Kirjavainen, Turkka, David Cooper, Olli Polo & Colin E. Sullivan (1996). Respiratory and body movements as indicators of sleep stage and wakefulness in infants and young children. *Journal of Sleep Research*, *5*, 186–194.

Kleitman, Nathaniel (1963). *Sleep and wakefulness*. Chicago: University Press.

Navelet, Yvonne, Odile Benoit & G. Bouard (1982). Nocturnal sleep organization during the first months of life. *Electroencephalography and Clinical Neurophysiology*, *54*, 71–78.

Nijhuis, J.G., Heinz F.R. Prechtl, C.B. Martin Jr., & R.S.G.M. Bots (1982). Are there behavioural states in the human fetus? *Early Human Development*, *6*, 177–195.

Nolte, Renate, & Gerard Haas (1978). A polygraphic study of bioelectrical brain maturation in preterm infants. *Developmental Medicine and Child Neurology*, *20*, 167–182.

Parmelee, Arthur H. Jr., & Evelyn Stern (1972). Development of states in infants. In Clemente, C.D., D.P. Purpura, F.E. Meyer (Eds), *Sleep and Maturing Nervous System* (199–228). New York: Academic Press.

Prechtl, Heinz F.R. (1974). The behavioural states of the newborn infant (a review). *Brain Research*, *76*, 185–212.

Prechtl, Heinz F.R., Yoshio Akiyama, P. Zinkin & D.K. Grant (1968). Polygraphic studies of the full term newborn. I: Technical aspects and quantitative analysis. In Bax M.C., Mac Keith R.C. (Eds), *Studies in infancy* (1–21) London: Heinemann.

Prechtl, Heinz F.R., J.W. Fargel, H.M. Weinmann & H.H. Bakker (1979). Postures, motility and respiration of low risk preterm infants. *Developmental Medicine and Child Neurology*, *21*, 23–27.

Prechtl, Heinz F.R., & Michael John O'Brien (1982). Behavioural states of the full-term newborn: the emergence of a concept. In Stratton, P. (Ed.), *Psychobiology of the human newborn*, New York: John Wiley and Sons.

Rechtschaffen, Allen, & A. Kales (Eds) (1968). *A manual of standardized terminology, techniques and scoring system for sleep stages of human subjects*. Washington: Public Health Service, US Government Printing Office.

Sadeh, Avi (1994). Assesment of intervention for infant night waking: parental reports and activity-based home monitoring. *Journal of Consulting Clinical Psychology*, *62*, 63–68.

Sadeh, Avi, Peretz Lavie, Anat Scher, Emanuel Tirosh & Rachel Epstein (1991). Actigraphic home-monitoring of sleep-disturbed and control infants and young children: a new method for pediatric assesment of sleep-wake patterns. *Pediatrics* 87, 494–499.

Salzarulo, Piero (1999). *La fine del sonno*. Torino: Bollati Boringhieri.

Salzarulo, Piero, & Igino Fagioli (1992). Sleep-wake rhythms and sleep structure in the first year of life. In Stampi, C. (Ed.), *Why we nap*. Boston: Birkhäuser, pp. 50–57.

Salzarulo, Piero, Igino Fagioli, F. Salomon, Claude Ricour, G. Raimbault, S. Ambrosi, O. Cicchi, J.F. Duhamel & M.T. Rigoard (1980). Sleep patterns in infants under continuous feeding from birth. *Electroencephalography and Clinical Neurophysiology*, *49*, 330–336.

Salzarulo, Piero, Giuliana Formicola, Pasquale Lombardo, Sara Gori, Luigi Rossi, Luigi Murri & Carlo Cipolli (1997). Functional uncertainty, aging and the memory processes during sleep. *Acta Neurologica Belgica*, *97*, 118–122.

Salzarulo, Piero, & Igino Fagioli (1999). Changes of sleep states and physiological activities across the first year of life. In Kalverboer, A., M.L. Genta, B.Hopkins (Eds), *Current issues in developmental psychology: a biopsychological perspective* (53–74). Dordrecht: Kluwer.

Salzarulo Piero, Fiorenza Giganti, Gianluca Ficca, Igino Fagioli, Monica Toselli (2000). Gates to awakening in early development. *Clinical Neurophysiology*, 53: S352–S354.

Salzarulo, Piero, Fiorenza Giganti, Igino Fagioli & Gianluca Ficca (2001). Development of state regulation. In Gramsbergen, A., A. Kalverboer (Eds), *Handbook of brain and behaviour in human development* (pp. 725–742). Dordrecht: Kluwer.

Scher, Mark, Doris A. Steppe, Ronald E. Dahl, Shoba Asthana & Robert D. Guthrie (1992). Comparison of EEG sleep measures in healthy full-term and preterm infants at matched conceptional ages. *Sleep*, *15*, 442–448.

Schulz, Hartmut, & Jürgen Zulley (1980). The position of final awakening within the ultradian REM/NREM sleep cycle. *Sleep Research*, *9*, 124.

Schulz, Hartmut, Roberto Massetani, Igino Fagioli & Piero Salzarulo (1985). Spontaneous awakening from sleep in infants. *Electroencephalography and Clinical Neurophysiology*, *61*, 267–271.

Stefanski, Mark., Karl F. Schulze, D. Bateman, R Kairam, T.A. Pedley, J. Masterson & S.L. James (1984). A scoring system for states of sleep and wakefulness in term and preterm infants. *Pediatric Research, 18*, 58–62.

Stepanski, E., J. Lamphere, P. Badia, E. Zorich & T. Roth (1984). Sleep fragmentation and daytime alertness. *Sleep*, *7*, 18–26.

Thach, Bradley, & Anna Lijowska (1996). Arousal in infants. *Sleep*, *19*, S271–S273.

Thoman, Evelyn B., & W.D. Tynan (1979). Sleep states and wakefulness in human infants: profiles from motility monitoring. *Physiology and Behavior*, *23*, 519–525.

Thoppil, C.K., M.A. Belan, C.P. Cowen & O.P. Mathew (1991). Behavioural arousal in newborn infants and its association with termination of apnea. *Journal of Applied Physiology*, *70*, 2479–2484.

Vecchierini-Blineau, Marie Françoise, Beatrice Nogues, S. Louvet & O. Desfontaines (1994). Maturation de la motilité généralisée, spontanée au cours du sommeil, de la naissance à terme à l'âge de 6 mois. *Neurophysiologie Clinique, 24*, 141–154.

Wolff, Peter H. (1987). *The development of behavioral states and the expression of emotions in early infancy*. Chicago: University of Chicago Press.

Arousals in infants during the first year of life

Argument for new definitions and criteria

Ariagno R.L., Mirmiran M., and Darnall R.A.
Stanford University, Department of Pediatrics /
Department of Pediatrics and Physiology, Dartmouth Medical School

Introduction

The purpose of this chapter is to review what is known about arousal in preterm and term infants (see also Curzi et al. chapter "Spontaneous Arousal and Awakening in Preterm and Full-Term Infants) and to defend the need for new definitions and criteria which can be used in future investigations.

Arousals, brief awakenings and subtle central nervous system adjustments are normal phenomena during sleep. However, EEG events have been given the most emphasis for scoring arousals in adult subjects. The International Pediatric Wake-Up Club following a series of collaborative discussions and meetings over the last several years is preparing a "A Consensus on the Scoring of Arousals in Healthy Preterm and Term Infants During the First Year". The Curzi-Dascalova et. al chapter in this volume reports on the use of these criteria for the first time in a group of healthy preterm and term infants. The Consensus stated that the arousal definitions from the Sleep Disorders Task Force of the ASDA (1992) are not adequate for the assessment of arousal in infants because they do not include all of the sub-cortical components usually seen in the response during the first year of life.

The phenomena of arousal and awakening, particularly in infants during the first year of life, has become more important as a research area since there is general agreement that understanding these mechanisms is essential to understand the adaptive physiology of infants during development and illness

(Schulz et al., 1985; McNamara et al. 1998; Ficca et al. 1999; Davidson-Ward & Keens, 2000). Furthermore, the failure of these mechanisms i.e., failure to arouse or awaken may help explain the mechanism of sudden infant death syndrome (SIDS). We hypothesise that the sub cortical central nervous system adjustments for physiologic functioning and homeostasis may be more predominant early in life and may also represent the basic protective responses to life-threatening stimuli during sleep. Since most SIDS deaths may begin with a failure to arouse from sleep and associated insufficient cardiorespiratory changes, it is necessary to understand the brain mechanisms that modify arousal during a critical period of development (i.e., during the first year of life).

Why are specific infant criteria for arousal necessary?

The first departure from the ASDA EEG arousal criteria is that both cortical and sub-cortical/brainstem responses may be essential components which are overlooked and thus not analysed. Furthermore, the sub-cortical responses i.e., the "non cortical components" may be more typical and of greater importance for appreciating the brain mechanisms operating in the immature or developing infant during the first year of life. At some later age or time in development the EEG/cortical response may become the most effective way to achieve an adaptive response to physiologic or pathologic challenges. However, for preterm and term infants during the first several months of life, many arousal responses may have no EEG component or a very brief one of 1–3 sec. Moreover an adaptive response to a physiologic or pathologic stimulus/challenge (e.g., increased breathing in response to hypoxia) may occur without an arousal or awakening and be better categorized as a 'reflex response'.

Preterm infants

There are approximately 300,000 low birth weight preterm infants born in the United States per year (7.6% of all live births). Modern advancements in neonatal care have led to survival rates exceeding 90% in infants with birth weights > 1000 grams. Preterm infants are at 3–7 times higher risk of SIDS compared with term infants (Grether et al., 1989). The sleep of infants who are in a Neonatal Intensive Care Unit (NICU) is often disrupted by clinical interventions. We hypothesise that this sleep interruption may be associated with higher arousal thresholds (i.e., decreased responsiveness) for life threatening stimuli. In support of this idea, Scher et al. found fewer and shorter arousals during the 12 hour nighttime sleep recording in preterm (<32 w GA) infants recorded at corrected term age compared with full term infants (Scher et al., 1992, 1994).

Spontaneous vs. provoked arousals

Most of the information about arousal in infants is based on the responses to provoked (exogenous) stimuli e.g., hypoxia and or hypercapnea, tactile, and auditory stimuli. These studies show a higher arousal threshold at 2–4 months of age which further increased when the infant is sleeping prone, compared to younger and older infants (Newman et al., 1986; 1989, Horne et al., 2000). There are few studies of spontaneous arousals and minimal data for the preterm infant. Since the preterm infant is at higher risk for SIDS the development of arousal mechanisms should be studied in this group of infants as well. It is generally accepted that the SIDS event usually occurs during sleep. If arousal and awakening are basic protective mechanisms for survival a failure of these responses could explain in part why SIDS occurs. Infants who are at increased risk for SIDS (e.g., following an "apparent life threatening event" i.e., ALTE) have increased arousal thresholds for respiratory, tactile, thermal and auditory stimuli. Thus spontaneous arousal or awakening from sleep, or the infant's ability to make a transition from one sleep state to another when confronted with a life-threatening challenge, may be deficient (Newman et al., 1989). McNamara, Thach and colleagues have found that the frequency of spontaneous arousals, not associated with apnea, were more frequent once every 3–6 per min. in 2–3 month old infants compared with once every 6 to 10 per min in children 4.6 years old (McNamara et al., 1996). The higher frequency of arousals in young infants supports that these are components of a basic protective mechanism and not simply a response to apneic events. In a later study, this group examined arousal responses to tactile stimuli in infants (McNamara et al., 1998). By recording movement, cardiorespiratory changes and EEG desynchronization they could differentiate 3 types of arousals: 1) Spinal arousal which included only body movement, 2) Brainstem arousal which accompanied body movement and cardiorespiratory changes, and 3) Cortical arousal which was evoked later and required much more powerful stimuli included body movement, cardiorespiratory changes and EEG desynchronization. This classification needs to be systematically applied to spontaneous arousals. This would be important to study since it is not yet clear what the function of these different arousals are or whether specific type of arousal is necessary. We hypothesise that for a hypoxic/hypercapnic stimulus at least a 'brainstem response' is required to increase ventilation but an arousal which includes body movement, heart rate and cortical changes (desynchrony or even an awakening) may be needed to augment an inadequate response to prevent SIDS.

Infant arousal studies have shown "spontaneous" arousals with and without respiratory changes (McNamara et al., 1996; Wulbrand et al., 1998; Davidson-Ward & Keens 2000; Schramm et al., 2000; Vecchierini et al., 2001). Provoked arousals have been studied following auditory, visual, tactile or proprioceptive stimuli (Dittrichova et al., 1977; Kahn et al., 1986; Thach & Lijovska, 1996; Read et al., 1998). Criteria for arousal definition in these studies have been variable (Curzi-Dascalova et al., 2000). Arousability is affected by birth weight, gestational and post-natal age (Horne et al., 2000; Reed et al., 1998), by sleeping position and sleep stages (Franco et al., 1996; Skadberg & Markestad, 1997; Goto et al., 1999; Galland et al., 1998, 2000), by prenatal exposure to drugs (Bard et al., 2000) and by passive smoking (Franco et al., 1999). Time of the day influences sleep and waking pattern particularly in infants older than 1 month of age (Ariagno et al., 1997). Other studies in newborns have been focused on evoked potential (Monod & Garma, 1971; Todorovich et al., 1987), on cardiac response to ocular compression (Philips et al., 1964; Ramet et al., 1988) or on respiratory challenges (Wulbrand et al., 1997; Thoppil et al., 1991; Tirosh et al., 1996; Curzi-Dascalova et al., 2000; Davidson Ward & Keens, 2000).

Computer scoring of EEG arousal

Automatic analysis of EEG component of sleep and arousal parameters in newborns has been difficult (Apkarian et al., 1991; Curzi-Dascalova & Mirmiran 1996). Scher et al. (1997) used computer classification of states in healthy preterm neonates and confirmed automatic analysis with visually defined EEG desynchronization during spontaneous arousals in active sleep (AS). This study concluded that it was difficult to detect automatically EEG defined arousals from normal discontinuous infant EEG patterns particularly during quiet sleep (QS). Recently described methods using spectral Wavelet analysis of the EEG, may provide an improved approach for automatic detection of arousals (see below).

Definition of arousals

Type of stimulus

Arousal events may be categorized according to the stimulus, spontaneous or provoked ("evoked"), sleep state and sleep position. The spontaneous (i.e., intrinsic or endogenous stimulus) may be associated with a physiological (e.g., decreased lung volume during active sleep) or a pathologic (e.g., gastroesophageal reflux or obstructive apnea) change. The provoked (i.e., extrinsic or exogenous stimulus) may be applied intentionally (e.g., touch or sound) or may be incidental in the environment, e.g., increased ambient temperature or random noise.

Level of response

Arousal events may be further categorized according to the level of response. As described above some investigators have observed and defined a hierarchy of responses to calibrated tactile stimulus applied to the plantar surface of the foot. The simplest sub cortical response is *spinal*, i.e. a foot twitch and leg withdrawal. The next two levels are also sub cortical: *respiratory*, i.e. augmented breath or increase in respiratory rate for several breaths then a return to baseline or a *startle* which is characterized by a jerky body movement, extension and abduction of arms, ending with bowing of the arms over the chest when the baby is supine or body jerk and head lift for the infant who is sleeping prone. Finally, the *cortical response* is noted as an abrupt change in EEG pattern with frequencies of alpha (9–13 Hz) or >16 Hz for 1 sec. Curzi-Dascalova et al. (see this volume) did not observe these stereotypical responses with spontaneous arousal in preterm infants at term corrected age or in term newborns in the first 10 days of life. However McNamara et al. report that as many as 92% of spontaneous cortical arousals during REM and 86% of these episodes during QS included changes in breathing, a startle and EEG responses. Another 5%–12% of responses included a startle and cortical components. In our studies in preterm infants before discharge as well as at 1 and 3 month corrected age we observed EEG responses in only a small percentages of spontaneous arousals. In our experience startles occur in a minority of arousals and many startles during QS do not appear to be associated with other arousal components. Startles have usually been considered by pioneers in sleep research as a characteristic of quiet sleep state (Anders et al., 1971). In contrast the gross body movement component seen in arousals is usually a coordinated gradual type of movement with a slow onset.

In another study in 10–12 w old term infants, Wulbrand et al. report suppression of spindles as a characteristic arousal response to both spontaneous and evoked startle and sigh. They used inter-spindle interval as a measure of arousal. Using the 3 s EEG desynchronization criteria of the ASDA, only 60% of sigh and startles events were considered arousals, however 100% of these arousal events could be identified if one used spindle suppression criteria. A significant drawback of this approach is that spindles usually develop around 2 months of age. Spindles are not frequent and not confined to a specific portion of quiet sleep until 6 months of age which makes them a less consistent criteria for arousal at least during the 1st 6 months of life.

Whether the neuronal mechanisms underlying spontaneous and provoked arousals are similar is still unknown. Also it is unclear whether the responses are different according to sleep state or time of day. Sleep position does appear to affect the response as is seen with the startle.

Components of the arousal and/or sub-cortical responses

EEG changes. Cortical arousals include EEG desynchronization shortly preceding, during and/or within 5 s following general body movements and heart rate changes (usually acceleration). These EEG changes include suppression of delta, a reduction in amplitude and an increase in the frequency of EEG. In young infants with trace alternant or a discontinuous EEG, these changes may be more difficult to detect. Suppression of spindles during arousal in QS is another EEG finding which may be observable after 2 months of age. Cortical arousals are usually accompanied with cardiorespiratory changes and general body movements in preterm and term infants.

Cardiac changes. Heart rate acceleration is the most consistent finding observed. The amplitude of this acceleration increases with post conceptional age. Heart rate decelerations during arousal are less frequent and may be due to a vagal rebound following an acceleration. Because of the high between-subject and between-state variability, heart rate changes should be normalized for basal pre-arousal heart rate level. Heart rate variability (HRV) during arousal can be assessed by using both time and frequency domain analysis of ECG. Time domain analysis of R–R intervals include square root of the mean of the sum of the squares of differences between adjacent R–R intervals (RMSSD) and standard deviation of all R–R intervals (SDNN). Frequency analysis of R–R intervals include low frequency (LF) and high frequency (HF) range. Power in the low frequency range (0.04–0.14 Hz) may be predominantly associated with sympathetic control and in the high frequency range parasympathetic control. RMSSD is frequently increased during arousal followed by increased SDNN, LF and HF. (Task Force of the European Society of Cardiology and the North American Society of Pacing and Electrophysiology. 1996). It is important to note that most arousal episodes are too brief for meaningful frequency analysis and they are usually not stationary. Nevertheless, a change in heart rate variability may be part of the infant arousal. HRV changes can also be seen during non arousal periods (e.g., HRV is significantly higher during REM compared to QS). Differentiating HRV changes which are part of an arousal vs. variability within a state will be necessary. Studies in piglet have shown that increased blood pressure is another early sign of arousal (BuSha B. et al., 2001).

Respiratory changes. Changes in breathing rate are usually characterized by a deceleration, which may include a sigh. Respiratory variability during the arousal may also be obvious by visual scoring. However, respiratory changes may be less clear during active or indeterminant sleep which is characterized by irregular respiration. Additionally, detection of respiratory efforts is complicated by the artifact associated with body movements.

Sub-cortical or brainstem events are characterized by cardiorespiratory changes described above and usually includes general body movements in young infants. An arousal without body movements is very rare in infants before 3 or 6 months of age in contrast to adult subjects. On the other hand, general body movements or isolated startles which are not accompanied by other changes such as heart rate, breathing frequency, EEG or phasic increase in chin EMG (unless associated with sucking on a pacifier) would not be sufficient for identification of sub-cortical event or arousal. The spinal responses reported by the McNamara group in response to tactile stimuli always occurred without heart rate change by definition. We have rarely seen body movements without changes in heart rate. Since spontaneous startles commonly occur during QS we propose that they are probably a characteristic of the state and should not be considered as an arousal unless they are accompanied by other arousal components.

Behavioural manifestation of arousal in addition to general body movements include brief eye opening, cry and head turning. They do not always accompany brief arousals although they are always present during awakening (60 sec. or longer). Nevertheless, these behavioural changes are very helpful in defining episodes of arousals where general body movement artifacts make cortical EEG and respiratory changes unreliable in a given episode. The ECG signal is usually less affected by movement but one should be aware that a few beats artifacts in ECG in a short episode of arousal may influence the results of HRV analysis.

Duration of the response

We believe that arousals can be as short as 1–3 s with a maximum 59 s. following a period of at least 10 seconds of baseline sleep. Any arousal event lasting 1 minute or longer should be considered an awakening.

Definition of arousal and sub-cortical event using non-automated method

An **arousal** would be defined by an EEG change lasting at least 1-3 sec (desynchronization and/or suppression of spindles) after an uninterrupted sleep period of at least 10 sec. accompanied by at least two of the following 4 criteria.

A **sub-cortical event** would be scored if there are no changes in the EEG but at least two of the following changes are observed for at least 3 sec.

- ECG: heart rate acceleration; increased heart rate variability
- Respiratory deceleration including sigh and increased respiratory variability
- General body movement including but not limited to startle
- A phasic increase in chin EMG amplitude (unless associated with sucking on a pacifier).

Defining arousals using automated arousal Analysis

In the Piglet

Using spectral analysis of 5-second epochs of EEG data periods of QS can easily be identified by initial elevations in delta power (0.5–4Hz) followed by delta suppression. Piglets cycle through QS → AS → Wakeful/Drowsy → QS approximately every 20 minutes. QS periods last on average 6–9 minutes and are interrupted by arousals characterized by a startle or turning of the head, brief eye-opening, decreases in delta power and in most cases stereotypical changes in heart rate and blood pressure. The frequency of these events is 2–4 events per minute. We have used both spectral analysis and discrete wavelet transforms of the EEG to identify cortical arousals. Figure 1 shows changes in EEG delta power, heart rate (HR), and mean arterial blood pressure (MAP), de-

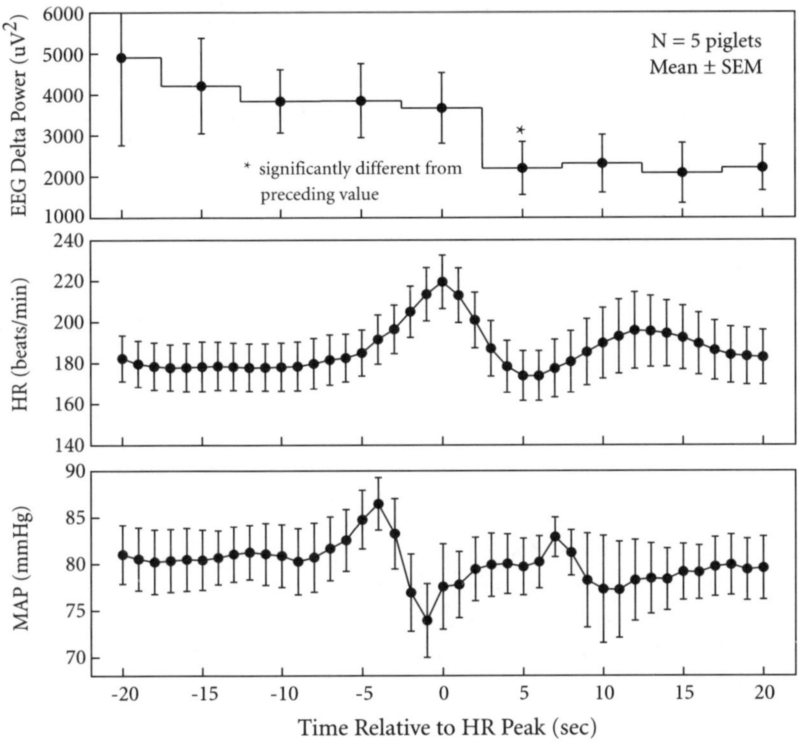

Figure 1. Plot (mean ± SEM) of EEG Delta Power (uV^2), heart rate (HR) in beats/min, mean arterial pressure (MAP) in mmHg at time (in seconds) relative to HR Peak derived from 75 isolated or first in series arousals during NREM sleep in 5 piglets using spectral analysis.

rived from 75 isolated first series (see definition below) arousals aligned by the peak in heart rate in 5 piglets using spectral analysis with 5-second epochs. Using this method, the resolution of the EEG frequency changes is limited to the epoch length. The advantage of wavelet analysis is that it can identify changes in low frequency EEG activity (LFA) with a resolution of 1 second. The wavelet method can be automated by constructing "arousal" thresholds for LFA. Defining the amount of time a signal must be below threshold can then identify arousals. When using the wavelet method the definition for arousal included measurement of a preceding baseline period of QS for at least 10 seconds and a decrease in delta activity (i.e., equivalent of delta power) below threshold for at least 4 seconds. Similar thresholds can be defined for mean arterial pressure (MAP) to allow independent identification of hemodynamic and EEG changes.

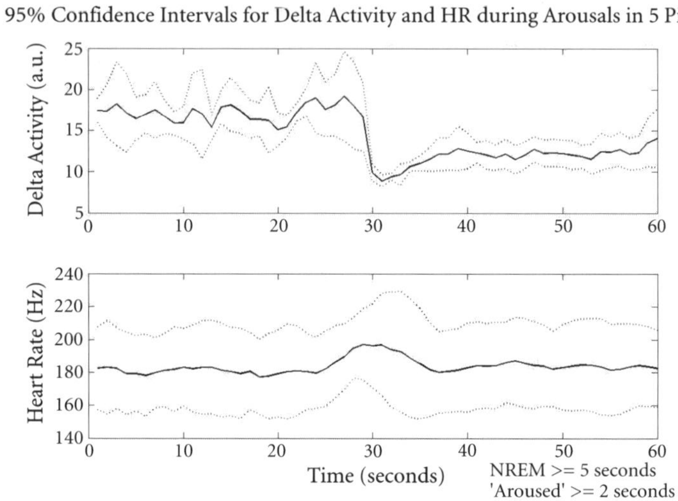

Figure 2. Plot of mean and 95% confidence Intervals for low frequency EEG activity (equivalent to delta power) in arbitrary units (a.u.) and Heart rate in Hz during over time (seconds) for 73 arousals ($\geq$ 4 sec) during NREM sleep ($\geq$ 10 seconds preceding arousal) in 5 piglets. In this analysis data were aligned with the point at which low frequency EEG activity decreased below threshold. Note the similarity with plot of human infant in Figure 3.

Figure 2 shows the mean changes in low frequency EEG activity (LFA) and heart rate derived from 75 arousals in 5 piglets using wavelet analysis. In this figure, each arousal was aligned with the point at which EEG LFA dropped below threshold value.

When EEG and MAP changes were independently identified using wavelets there were more MAP events identified than EEG events. Sixty-two percent of EEG arousals were associated with MAP and HR changes. When EEG and hemodynamic events occurred together, hemodynamic events always preceded EEG changes (see Figure 1 and 2). In addition, three temporal patterns of arousals were identified: 1) isolated or first in a series of events, 2) multiple events (events preceded by an event separated by an interval of < 20 seconds) and 3) events associated with the termination of apnea. Apnea was associated with approximately 25% of the events and the average apnea duration was 14.8 $\pm$0.9 seconds. Isolated or first in series events were always associated with an abrupt decrease in low frequency EEG activity, whereas in multiple events, low frequency activity was already decreased from a previous event. The time courses of the hemodynamic and EEG events were different with the recov-

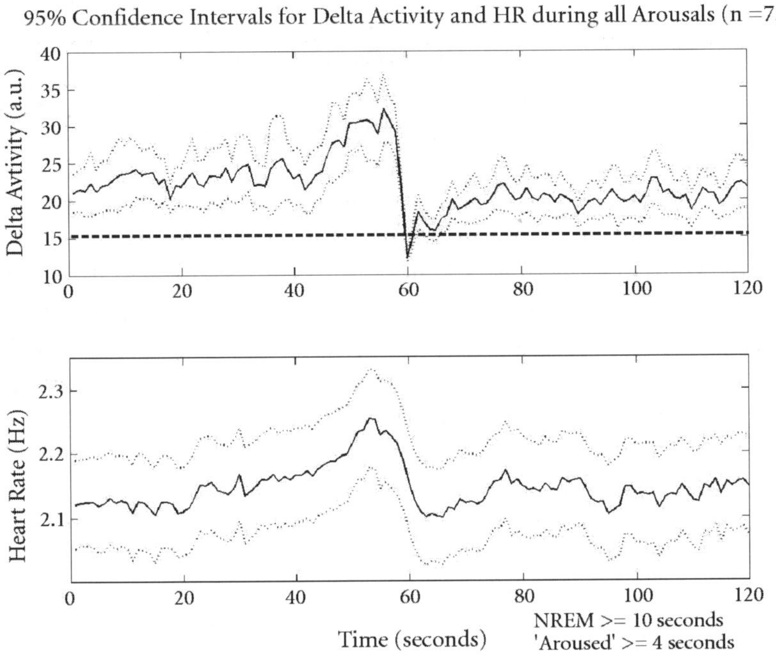

Figure 3. Plot of mean and 95% confidence Intervals for low frequency EEG activity (equivalent of delta power) in arbitrary units (a.u.) and Heart rate in Hz over time (seconds) for 73 arousals ($\geq$ 4 sec) during NREM sleep ($\geq$ 10 seconds preceding arousal) in a preterm human infant (GA 36 wks) at 3 months corrected age. In this analysis data were aligned with the point at which low frequency EEG activity decreased below the 'wakefulness' threshold (shown as a dotted line). Note the similarity with plot of Piglet arousal in Figure 2.

ery of the decrease in EEG low frequency activity lagging behind that of the changes in blood pressure or heart rate (BuSha, et al., 2001).

In the human infant

In a preliminary study, we applied our piglet wavelet analysis to data obtained from a preterm infant at 3-month old corrected age. Figure 3 shows the mean and 95% confidence limits for EEG delta activity and HR derived from 73 spontaneous EEG events automatically defined by threshold criteria. Note the similarities between the human arousal and the piglet arousals shown in Figure 2. The HR changes occur antecedent to the decrease in Delta activity in both species.

Thus in piglets and in human infants, EEG and hemodynamic events are usually coupled. The finding that hemodynamic events precede EEG events when they occur together supports the idea that the initiation of arousal from sleep may begin in the brainstem or midbrain, irrespective of whether the arousal is spontaneous or the result of a provoked stimulus. On the other hand, it is also clear that cortical EEG events and brainstem responses are not always coupled. We therefore favor the term **'cortical arousal'** for isolated EEG events, **'autonomic arousal'** for isolated HR and MAP events, and **'integrated arousal'** when they all occur together. These definitions are consistent with the findings of others and do not imply any particular mechanisms. They incorporate EEG events coupled to and possibly triggered by brainstem events, but recognize the possibility that arousing stimuli may originate by multiple mechanisms, some without accompanying markers of brainstem activation. In defining arousal events, the wavelet-based method has much to offer. It is observer independent, and visually identifying brief changes in EEG frequency in isolation is difficult. Reasonable observers can easily disagree about what constitutes an EEG event. In our wavelet analysis, the definition of an EEG event was arbitrary, and the threshold we selected may not have been the best threshold to use. Only with a larger study population, a statistically defensible threshold could be defined and we very much favor continued work to develop a consensus for quantitative EEG analysis in neonates.

Summary and conclusions

Why are specific/unique criteria for arousal identification in infants needed?
As discussed above the ASDA criteria emphasize EEG changes which define the cortical response. In infants using EEG criteria alone to define arousals overlooks the respiratory, heart rate, blood pressure and EMG components (sub-cortical events). In the developing infant sub-cortical events which do not progress to cortical arousal may be more common and may represent an important basic mechanism for maintaining physiological function and homeostasis. Ideally, brain stem 'reflexes' such as ventilatory and cardiovascular responses to hypoxia or hypercapnia, without an arousal component, should not in themselves be identified as or considered as an arousal or sub-cortical event. This differentiation may be difficult and requires further study.

How will the new criteria be used?
A consensus for the identification of cortical arousals and sub-cortical events or autonomic arousals in infants during the first year of life would allow better comparison of data between investigators. The number and quality of the arousal and sub-cortical events are important. The developmental differences in spontaneous and provoked arousal responses may also help our understanding of brain development and homeostasis and pathophysiology of SIDS.

Future research needed
Research will be needed to apply a new arousal classification to determine the correlation with normal development and abnormality with illness. Comparison of the new definitions for arousal and sub-cortical events using non-automated and automated methods with traditional arousal scoring should be done to determine what addition information and understanding of the developing infant brain is achieved. Ideally, the use of an automated arousal analysis could make the evaluation of arousal i.e., cortical and sub-cortical events ('autonomic and integrated arousals') more objective. However, more research would be needed to differentiate variability within state from arousal and sub-cortical events as seen with non automatic analysis methods. Finally, more research, discussion and consensus are needed to decide when the ASDA criteria for arousal are applicable and appropriate for the pediatric subject.

Acknowledgement

We give our thanks to B. BuSha for the wavelet analysis for the piglet and the human infant sleep.

References

Apkarian, P., M. Mirmiran, & R. Tijssen (1991). Effects of behavioural state on visual processing in neonates. *Neuropediatrics, 22*, 85–917.

Anders, T., R. Emde & A. Parmelee (1971). *A Manual of Standardized Terminology, Technique and Criteria for Scoring States of Sleep and Wakefulness in Newborn Infants* UCLA Brain Information Service BRI Publications Office, NINDS Neurological Information Network, Los Angles.

Ariagno, R.L., E.B. Thoman, M.A. Boeddiker, B. Kugener, J.C. Constantinou, M. Mirmiran & R.B. Baldwin (1997). The effect of individualized developmental care on sleep and development of very low birth weight premature infants. *Pediatrics, 100*, e9, 1–7.

Bard, K.A., C.D. Coles, K.A. Platzman & M.E. Lynch (2000). The effect of prenatal drug exposure, term status, and care giving on arousal modulation in 8-week-old infants. *Developmental Psychobiology, 36*, 194–211.

BuSha, B., J.C. Leiter, A.K. Curran, A. Li, E.E. Nattie & R.A. Darnall (2001). Spontaneous arousals during quiet sleep in piglets: A visual and wavelet-based analysis. *Sleep, 24*, 499–513.

Clairambault, J., L. Curzi-Dascalova, F. Kauffmann, C. Médigue, & C. Leffler (1992). Heart rate variability in normal, sleeping full-term and preterm neonates. *Early Human Development, 28*, 169–183.

Curzi-Dascalova, L., & M. Mirmiran (1996). Manual of methods of recording and analyzing sleep-wakefulness states in preterm and full-term infants. Paris: INSERM.

Curzi-Dascalova, L., F. Kauffmann, C. Gaultier, A. Regina & C. de Amorim (1999). Heart rate modifications related to spontaneous body movements in sleeping premature and full-term newborns. *Pediatric Research, 45*, 515–518.

Curzi-Dascalova, L., J. Bloch, M. Vecchierini, A. Bedu & P. Vignolo (2000). Physiological parameters evaluation following apnea in healthy premature infants. *Biology of the Neonate, 77*, 203–211.

Davidson-Ward, S.L., & T.G. Keens (2000). *Maturation of the arousal response. Sleep and Breathing in Children; A developmental approach.* Loughlin GM, Carroll JL and Marcus CL (Eds). (79–97) New York: Marcel Dekker Inc.

Dittrichova, J., K. Paul & E. Pavlikova (1977). Responsiveness to stimulation during paradoxical sep in infants. *Early Human Development, 1*, 213–225.

Ficca, G., I. Fagioli, F. Giganti, & P. Salzarulo (1999). Spontaneous awakenings from sleep in the first year of life. *Early Human Development, 55*, 219–228.

Franco, P., J. Groswasser, M. Sottiaux, E. Broadfield & A. Kahn (1996). Decreased cardiac responses to auditory stimulation during prone sleep. *Pediatrics, 97*, 174–178.

Franco, P., J. Groswasser, S. Hassid, J.P. Lanquart, S. Scarlett & A. Kahn (1999). Prenatal exposure to cigarette smoking is associated with a decrease in arousal in infants. *Journal of Pediatrics, 135*, 34–38.

Galland, B.C., D.P. Bolton, B.J. Taylor, R.M. Sayers & S.M. Williams (2000). Ventilatory sensitivity to mild asphyxia. *Archives of Disease in Childhood, 83*, 423–428.

Galland, B.C., R.M. Hayman, B.J. Taylor, D.P.G. Bolton, R.M. Sayers & S.M. Williams (2000). Factors affecting heart rate variability and heart rate responses to tilting in infants aged 1 and 3 months. *Pediatric Research, 48*, 360–368.

Galland, B.C., G. Reeves, B.J. Taylor & D.P.G. Bolton (1998). Sleep position, autonomic function, and arousal. *Archives of Disease in Childhood, Fetal and Neonatal Ed, 78*, F189–F194.

Goto, K., M. Mirmiran, M.M. Adams, R.V. Longford, R.B. Baldwin, M.A. Boeddiker & R.L. Ariagno (1999). More awakenings and heart rate variability during supine sleep in preterm infants. *Pediatrics, 103*, 603–609.

Grether, J.K., & J. Schulman (1989) Sudden infant death syndrome and birth weight. *Journal of Pediatrics, 114*, 561–567.

Horne, R., S.C., David J. Sly, S.M. Granage, B. Chau & T. Michael Adamson. (2000). Effect of prematurity on arousal from sleep in the newborn infant. *Pediatric Research, 47*, 468–474.

Kahn, André, E. Picard & D. Blum (1986). Auditory arousal thresholds of normal and near-miss SIDS infants. *Developmental Medicine and Child Neurology, 28*, 299–302.

Lewis, K.W., & E.M. Bosque (1995). Deficient hypoxia awakening response in infants of smoking mothers: possible relationship to sudden infant death syndrome. *Journal of Pediatrics, 127*, 691–699.

McNamara, F., H. Wulbrand & B.T. Thach (1998). Characteristics of the infant arousal response. *Journal of Applied Physiology, 85*, 2314–2321.

McNamara, F, F.G. Issa, & C.E. Sullivan (1996). Arousal pattern following central and obstructive breathing abnormalities in infants and children. *Journal of Applied Physiology, 81*, 2651–2657.

Monod, N., & L. Garma (1977). Auditory responsivity in the human premature. *Biology of the Neonate, 17*, 292–316.

Newman, N.M., J.A. Trinder, K.A. Phillips, K. Jordan & J. Cruickshank (1989). Arousal deficit: mechanism of the sudden infant death syndrome? *Australian Pediatric Journal, 25*, 196–201.

Newman, N.M., J.K. Frost, L. Bury, K. Jordan & K. Phillips (1986). Responses to partial nasal obstruction in sleeping infants. *Australian Pediatric Journal, 22*, 111–116.

Phillips, S.J., J. Frederic, J. Agate Jr., W.A. Silverman & P. Steiner (1964). Autonomic Cardiac reactivity in premature infants. *Biology of the Neonate, 6*, 225–249.

Ramet, J., J.-P. Praud, A. M. d'Allest, A. Carofilis, M. Dehan, C. Guilleminault & C. Gaultier (1988). Effect of maturation on heart rate response to ocular compression test during rapid eye movement sleep in human infants. *Pediatric Research, 24*, 477–488.

Read, Paul A., R.S. C. Horne, S.M. Cranage, A.M. Walker, D.W Walker & T.M. Adamson (1998). Dynamic changes in arousal threshold during sleep in the human infant. *Pediatric Research, 43*, 679–703.

Scher, M.S., G. Dokianakis, D.A. Steppe, D.L. Banks & R. J. Sclabassi (1997). Computer classification of state in healthy preterm neonates. *Sleep, 20*, 132–141.

Scher, M., M. Sun, D. Steppe, D. Banks, R. Guthrie & R. Sclabassi (1994). Comparison of EEG sleep state-specific spectral values between healthy full-term and preterm infants at comparable postconceptional ages. *Sleep, 17*, 47–51.

Scher, M., D. Steppe, R. Dahl, S. Asthana & R. Guthrie (1992). Comparison of EEG sleep measures in healthy full-term and preterm infants at matched conceptional ages. *Sleep, 15*, 442–448.

Schramm, D., B. Scheidt, A. Hübler, J. Frenzel, K. Holthausen & O. Breidbach (2000). Spectral analysis of electroencephalogram during sleep-related apneas in pre-term and term born infants in the first weeks of life. *Clinical Neurophysiology, 111*, 1788–1791.

Schulz, H., R. Massetani, I. Fagioli & P. Salzarulo (1985). Spontaneous awakening from sleep in infants. *Electroencephalography and clinical Neurophysiology, 61*, 267–271.

Skadberg, B.T., & T. Markestad (1997). Behaviour and physiological responses during prone and supine in early infancy. *Archive of Disease in Childhood, 76*, 320–324.

Sleep Disorders Atlas Task Force of the American Sleep Disorders Association (1992). EEG arousals: scoring rules and examples. *Sleep ,15*, 173–184.

Task Force of the European Society of Cardiology and the North American Society of Pacing and Electrophysiology (1996). Heart rate variability. *Circulation, 93*, 1043–1063.

Thach, B.T., & A. Lijowska (1996). Arousal in infants. *Sleep, 19*, S271–S273.

Thoppil, C.K., M.A. Belan, C.P. Cowen, & O.P. Mathew (1991). Behavioural arousal in newborn infants and its association with termination of apnea. *Journal of Applied Physiology, 70*, 2479–2484.

Tirosh, E., D. Liban & D. Bader (1996). The effect of maternal smoking during pregnancy on sleep respiratory and arousal pattern in neonates. *Journal of Perinatology, 16*, 435–438.

Todorovich, R.D., D.H. Crowell & L.E. Kapuiniai (1987). Auditory responsivity and intrauterine growth retardation in small for gestational age human newborns. *Electroencephalography and Clinical Neurophysiology, 67*, 204–212.

Vecchierini, M.F., L. Curzi-Dascalova, H. Trang-Pham, J. Bloch & C. Gaultier (2001). Patterns of EEG frequency, movement, heart rate, and oxygenation following isolated short apneas in infants. *Pediatric Research, 49*, 220–226.

Wulbrand, H., F. McNamara & B. T. Thach (1998). Suppression of σ spindle electroencephalographic activity as a measure of transient arousal after spontaneous and occlusion-evoked sighs and startles. *Pediatric Research, 44*, 767–773.

Wulbrand, H., F. McNamara & B.T. Thach (1997). Indicators of arousal activity in the infant's ascending reticular activating system: sigh, startles, EEG spindle suppression and heart rate changes. *Pediatric Pulmonology, 24*, 453–457.

Wulbrand, H., F, McNamara & B.T. Thach (1997). Occurrence of arousal related reflexes, sigh and startle during airway occlusion in infants. *American Journal of Respiration and Critical Care Medicine, 155*, A775.

Spontaneous arousal and awakening in preterm and full-term infants

Lilia Curzi-Dascalova, Heinz Zotter, Ronald L. Ariagno, and Majid Mirmiran

INSERM, Hôpital Robert Debré, Paris / Department of Pediatrics, University of Graz / Dept. Pediatrics, Stanford University, USA / Netherlands Institute for Brain Research, Amsterdam

Introduction

The purpose of this chapter is to present preliminary results from a collaborative study which combined polysomnography recordings from preterm and term neonates from several investigators in Europe and the USA to improve the uniformity of scoring for arousal and awakening events.

Arousal and brief awakenings related to subtle central nervous system changes are normal phenomena during sleep. These events may be *spontaneous* i.e., without any obvious cause or a response to endogenous stimuli e.g., a sigh, apnea or gastroesophageal reflux. These events may also be *provoked* by an exogenous stimulus such as a noise or touch. It is generally accepted that the arousal definitions from the ASDA Report (1992) are not adequate for the assessment of infants. To answer the question of when these criteria are appropriate for the pediatric subject will require research and consensus. The phenomena of arousal and awakening, particularly in infants during the first year of life, has become more important as a research area since there is general agreement that understanding these mechanisms is essential to understand the adaptive physiology of infants during development and illness.

Most of the previous data which has been reported concern babies who have been recorded during the first months of age. Data from the literature describe "spontaneous" arousals occurring after breathing abnormalities or without any detectable events (Schulz et al., 1985; McNamara et al., 1996; Wulbrand et al., 1998; Ficca et al., 1999; Schramm et al., 2000; Vecchierini et al., 2001) as well as provoked arousals following auditory, light, tactile or proprioceptive stimuli (Dittrichova et al., 1977; Kahn et al., 1986; Thach and Lijovska, 1996; Read et al., 1998). The criteria used for arousal definition are highly variable (ref. in the Arousal and Awakening in human Development Symposium documents, WFSRS meeting, Dresden, 1999, Curzi-Dascalova et al, 2000). It has been demonstrated that arousability is affected by birth weight, gestational and post-natal age (Horne et al., 2000), by sleeping position (i.e., prone versus supine, Franco et al., 1996; Goto et al., 1999; Galland et al., 2000), by prenatal exposure to drugs (Bard et al, 2000) and smoking (Lewis et al., 1995; Franco et al., 1999; Kahn et al., 2000).

As far as we know, the recent study of Giganti et al. (1999) is the only one investigating awakenings of newborns across a 24 hour period. These preliminary data did not show significant modifications in number or duration of awakening between 34 and 40 weeks post-conceptional age (PCA). There are limited data on arousability in newborns: evoked potential study (Monod and Garma, 1971; Todorovich et al., 1987); cardiac response to ocular compression (Philips et al., 1964; Ramet et al., 1988); respiratory variability (Thoppil et al., 1991; Tirosh et al., 1996; Curzi-Dascalova et al., 2000). Automatic analysis of EEG arousal in newborns has been used by some investigators. Recently Schramm et al. (2000) reported decreased EEG amplitude associated with apnoeas during active sleep (AS). These authors investigated premature and full-term infants but it is not clear at which age they were studied (range from 25 to 100 weeks PCA; no between-age comparisons were given). Scher et al. (1997) used a computer classification of states in healthy preterm neonates which was confirmed visually. EEG desynchronization was associated with arousal during AS. This careful study concluded that it was difficult to distinguish arousals from normal discontinuous EEG patterns during quiet sleep (QS) using an automatic method of analysis.

The aim of our preliminary collaborative investigation was to examine changes in various physiological variables as part of the definition of arousal. We have tried to evaluate the use of the arousal related parameters recently proposed for older infants (Consensus of the Pediatric European Wake-Up Club, in preparation; also see Arousal and Awakening in Human Development Symposium summary, WFSRS meeting, Dresden, 1999; Kahn et al., 2000). In addition, data from the Stanford study are presented to show the influence of prone and supine sleeping position on spontaneous arousals in preterm infants. The European collaborative investigation used recordings of infants who were supine. The methods for scoring arousals are from the evolving Consensus of the Pediatric Euopean Wake-Up Club. By convention arousals lasting for at least one minute were scored as awakenings, although there is still debate on this issue. The advantage of using a unique approach for scoring arousals in infants is that a better understanding of the developing infant will be possible. The data presented in this chapter are preliminary and further research to compare the traditional method for scoring arousals (Stanford data) and a new definition for arousals will be needed. Also it will be necessary to define the conditions of the study such as sleep position, which will affect the results.

Arousal characteristics in preterm and full-term infants: European Data Bank

The recordings used in this study are part of the European Data Bank on Arousal in Newborn Infants. We arbitrarily selected arousals which were initiated by spontaneous bilateral or generalized body movements for analysis.

Subjects

Healthy asymptomatic infants (born at 30–40 weeks gestational age) were studied in supine position at neutral ambient temperature. Sixty-four arousals (arbitrarily a minimum of 2 were selected for AS and QS in each baby) were analysed in 10 preterm and 5 term infants who were recorded during the 1st 10 days of life (48 hours to less than 10 days of age, Paris data). Ten arousals were analysed in 9 additional preterm infants at 37–41 weeks PCA (Graz data); Table 1.

Table 1. Number of infants and arousal episodes according to sleep states

Postconceptional Age in weeks	N infants	Number of arousals analysed		
		Total	In Active Sleep	In Quiet Sleep
NB 31–33w	6	24	12	12
NB 34–36w	4	16	8	8
NB 37–41w	5	24	12	12
Prem. → 37–41w	9	10	8	2
TOTAL	24	74	40	34

Note: newborn, i.e. less than 10 days of age by the time of recording (Paris data) Prem.→ 37–41w: prematurely born infants recorded when reaching 37–41w postconceptional age (Graz data).

Polysomnographic recordings were performed during daytime sleep, between two feedings. The method of polysomnography and sleep states scoring have been previously described (Curzi-Dascalova & Mirmiran, 1996). Body movements were detected using actimeters and or movement related artefacts on polysomnography. All arousal periods included body movement. None of these arousals were followed by sleep state change or awakening.

Methods of analysis

By definition, body movements were present in all cases studied. The other parameters analysed are as follows:

EEG amplitude and frequency have been evaluated by visual inspection (in the Paris data), comparing EEG pattern during or immediately after the arousal with the EEG pattern observed during the 20 sec. preceding any given arousal. Changes lasting ≥ 1 sec were scored. A 20 sec baseline period allowed analysis of normal fluctuations of EEG patterns, especially during quiet sleep (Curzi-Dascalova and Mirmiran, 1996). The EEG amplitude and frequency variations were scored as increased, decreased, or unchanged. Studies comparing visual with computer analysis of EEG showed excellent agreement with visually classified EEG frequency (variability between these methods ranged from 0.7 to 1.2 Hz; Curzi-Dascalova et al., 2000; Vecchierini et al., 2001). Episodes in which body movements were associated with EEG artefacts were excluded.

Respiratory rate and heart rate changes during the arousal were analysed separately for two time periods, 5 sec. and 20 sec. pre and post arousal (Fig. 1). This allowed evaluation of the best period in which to describe the arousal (see results). Changes were normalised for the baseline as: change = ((value before the arousal – value during or after the arousal)/value before the arousal)x100. In presenting the data with this normalization, acceleration is expressed as negative values and deceleration in positive values.

Statistical analysis were performed using: a) Chi-square test for qualitative EEG changes; b) ANOVA; c) Linear regression model and d) Wilcoxon rank-sum test. A p value of ≤ 0.05 was considered statistically significant. Median and range of changes are indicated in the results. Means are used for graphic illustrations presented in Fig. 3 and 5.

Results

Seventy four arousals have been analysed: 64 in 15 preterm/term infants recorded the 1st 10 days of life (at 31 to 41w PCA) and 10 in 9 preterm in-

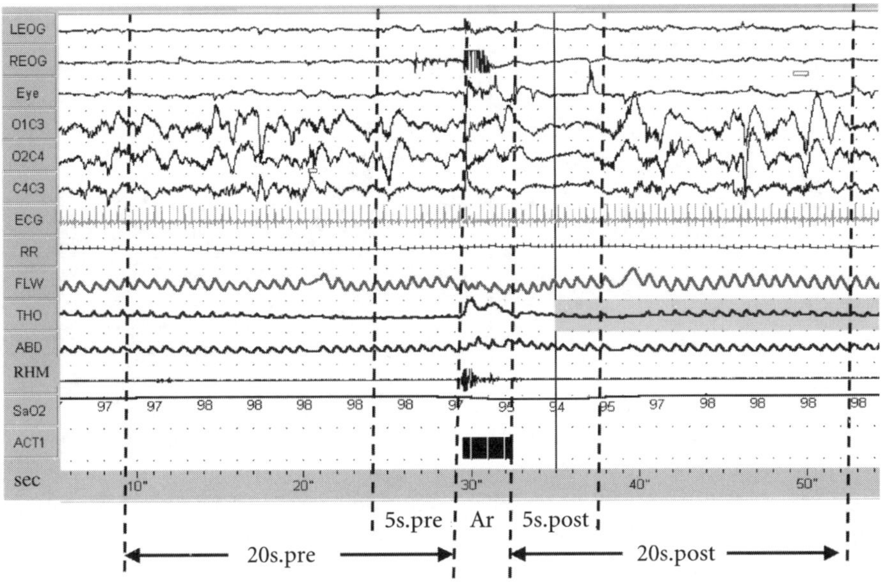

Figure 1. Example of active sleep digitised recordings in a 3 days old, 34w postconceptional age (PCA), healthy premature baby with schema for 5 and 20 sec analysed periods.
LEOG, REOG: left and right electro-oculogram; eye: eye movements recorded using a piezo transducer (Sleep Watch, Respironics); C301 and C402: EEG recordings; RR: cardiotachography based on instantaneous heart rate measurement; flow: nasobuccal airflow detected by thermistors; tho and abd: thoracic and abdominal respiratory movements detected by strain gauges; RHM and ACTI1: right hand and left leg movements, respectively, detected by a piezo transducer and a commercial (Alice 4) actimeter; sec: time in seconds.
Ar: arousal period; 5, 20s. pre: analysed periods preceding arousal; 5, 20s post: analysed periods following arousal.

fants recorded when reaching term age (Table 1). Analyses were done to assess: a) arousals in preterm/term infants in the first 10 days of life; b) preterm infants at 37–41w PCA.

a. Arousals in preterm/term infants during the 1st 10 days of life

Arousals that were analysed lasted from 2.5 to 59 sec (median = 7sec; Fig. 2) not dependent on PCA (F = 0.6, p = 0.4) or sleep-state (F = 1.2, p = 0.3).

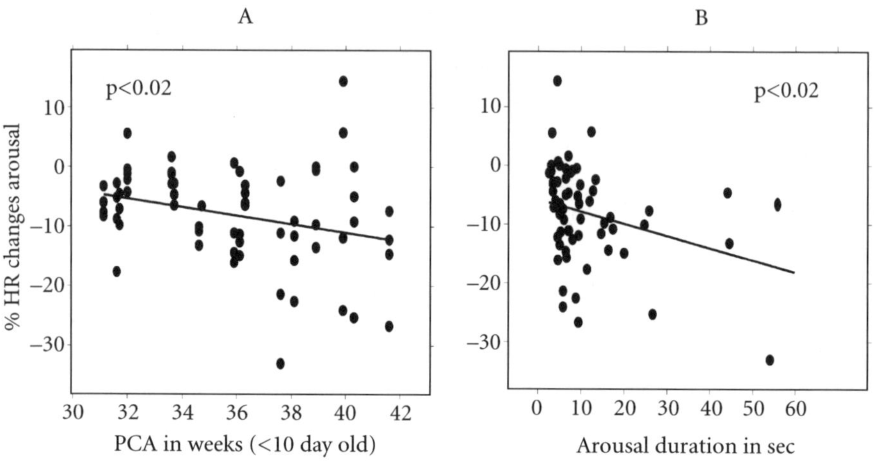

Figure 2. Correlation between hear rate changes during arousal and post conceptional age, PCA (in A) and arousal duration (in B) in infants recorded during the neonatal period (after 48 hours and by 10 days of age). Changes are difference between values recorded during arousal and the 5 sec preceding arousal. Each point correspond to one arousal data.
% HR changes arousal = percentage of changes normalised for pre-arousal base heart rate values as follows: change = ((value before the arousal – value during or after the arousal)/value before the arousal) × 100.

EEG amplitude and frequency could be analysed during 60 of the 64 arousal events. Forty-seven of these arousals were accompanied by EEG changes, mainly consisting of EEG amplitude decrease accompanied by an EEG frequency increase. Increase in EEG amplitude was observed in only 4 cases, and an EEG frequency decrease in only one other case. Thirteen arousals were not accompanied by any EEG changes: 11 in 6 preterm infants 31–33w PCA and 2 in 2 term infants of 39 and 40w PCA Sleep state had no significant effect on the EEG changes observed ($p = 0.5$).

Respiratory frequency changes were variable and could not be counted in many cases because of body movement artefacts.

– Respiratory frequency during arousal (31/64 cases analysed), as compared with the 5 sec. preceding arousals was accelerated in 19 and decelerated in the remainder 12 cases (median = 16.1%; range from –47.7% acceleration to 47.7% deceleration). Respiratory changes were not dependent on PCA

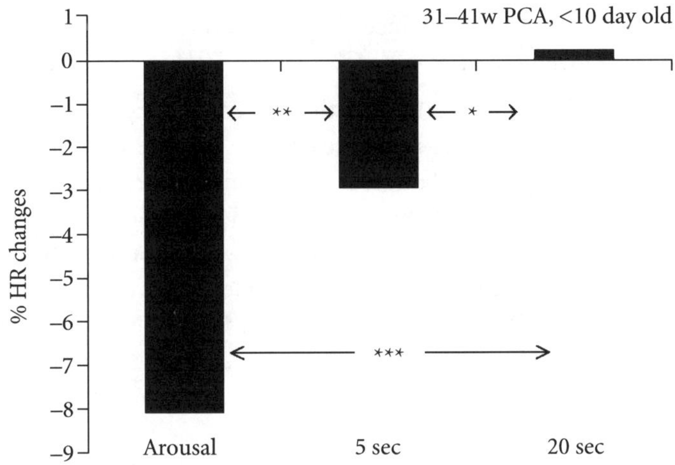

Figure 3. Percent heart rate changes induced by arousal, according to 5 and 20 sec periods taken into account in infants recorded during the neonatal period.
Arousal = difference between arousal period and the 5 sec preceding arousal.
5 sec = difference between the 5 sec. preceding and the 5 sec following arousal.
20 sec = difference between the 20 sec. preceding and the 20 sec following arousal.
See legend Fig. 2 for abbreviations and formula used to normalize the data.
*$p < 0.003$; **$p < 0.001$; ***$p < 0.0001$.

($F = 1.6$, $p = 0.2$), subject ($F = 1.3$, $p = 0.3$), arousal duration ($F = 0.7$, $p = 0.4$) or sleep-state ($F = 2.7$, $p = 0.1$) factors.

- Respiration within the 5 sec following as compared with 5 sec preceding arousals (45/64 cases analysed) was accelerated in 18 cases, not changed in 5 and decelerated in 22 others (median = 0). Data obtained were not dependent on PCA ($F = 0.02$, $p = 0.9$), the subject ($F = 1.1$, $p = 0.4$), or arousal duration ($F = 2$, $p = 0.2$). Respiration was usually decelerated in AS (median = 12.5%) and accelerated in QS (median = –3.2%), between-state difference being statistically significant ($F = 6.8$, $p < 0.02$).
- Respiration within the 20 sec following as compared with the 20 sec preceding arousals (40/64 cases analysed) was accelerated in 17 cases and decelerated in the other 23 cases (median = 4.1%), independently from subject ($F = 1.6$, $p = 0.1$), PCA ($F = 2.6$, $p = 0.1$), arousal duration ($F = 0.5$, $p = 0.5$) or sleep-state ($F = 0.1$, $p = 0.7$). Differences between data based on 5 sec and 20 sec period analysis did not reach statistical significance ($p < 0.09$).

In contrast with respiratory recording, *heart rate* recordings were usually not affected by movement artefacts.

- Arousal periods, as compared with the preceding 5 sec baseline, were usually accompanied by heart rate acceleration (56 of 63/64 cases that were analysed); there were no changes in 2, and in 5 other cases heart rare was decelerated. (median = –7.1%, ranged from –33% acceleration to 14.4% deceleration). Heart rate changes were independent of the subject ($F = 1.5$, $p = 0.3$) and sleep-state ($F = 0.5$, $p = 0.5$). Heart rate changes (mainly frequency increase) significantly depended on PCA ($F = 5.4$, $p < 0.03$) and arousal duration ($F = 6.0$, $p < 0.02$). Figure 2 shows relationship between the amplitude of heart rate changes on one hand and PCA and arousal duration on the other hand.
- Heart rate within the 5 sec following as compared with the 5 sec preceding arousals (61/64 cases) was accelerated in 40 cases, not changed in 5 and decelerated in 16 cases (median = –2.3, ranged from –18.6% of acceleration to 13.2% of deceleration). These were not dependent on PCA ($F = 0.1$, $p = 0.8$), subject ($F = 0.5$, $p = 0.9$), arousal duration ($F = 1.8$, $p = 0.2$) or sleep-state ($F = 0.5$, $p = 0.5$).
- Heart rate within the 20 sec following as compared with the 20 sec preceding arousals (61/64 cases analysed) was accelerated in 24 cases, non modified in 5 cases and usually slightly decelerated in the other 32 cases (median = 0.3%), independent of PCA ($F = 0.3$, $p = 0.6$), of the subject ($F = 0.5$, $p = 0.9$), arousal duration ($F = 2.9$, $p = 0.09$) and sleep-state ($F = 1.7$, $p = 0.2$).
- Heart rate changes found during arousal, 5 sec. and 20 sec after arousal were significantly different. Means and statistical differences between these values are shown in Figure 3.

b. Arousals in prematurely born babies recorded when reaching 37–41w PCA.

Ten arousals were recorded in 9 babies (Table 1) born at 32 to 35 weeks of gestation, when reaching 37–41w PCA (ranges of postnatal age: 12 to 47 days). Arousals analysed lasted from 20 to 59 sec (median = 27 sec).

Respiratory frequency was decelerated during 9 out of ten arousal periods analysed as compared with the 5 sec preceding each arousal (median = 27.1%, range = from –3.7 % of acceleration to 53.8% of deceleration). Respiration was also usually decelerated during the 5 sec following as compared with the 5 sec preceding arousal (median = 25.9%, range from –11% of acceleration to 62.5% of deceleration), and during the 20 sec following as compared with the 20 sec

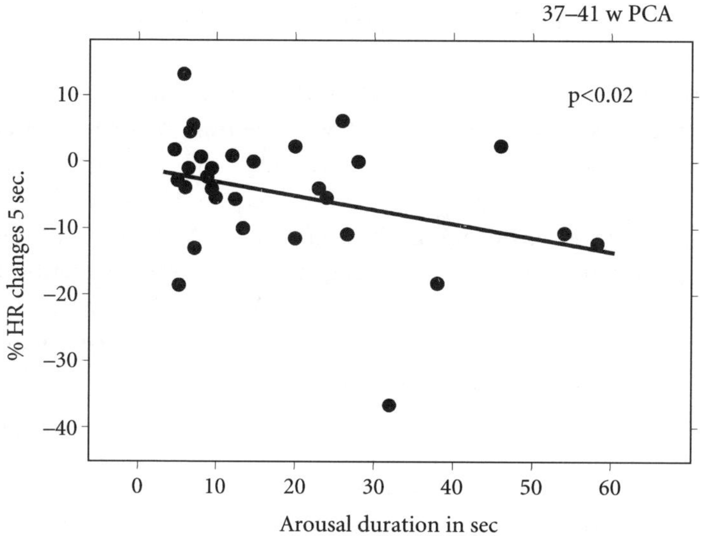

Figure 4. Correlations between HR changes during the 5 seconds following arousal and arousal duration in 37–41w PCA infants (term and preterm infants at term PCA). See legend Figure 2 for formula used to normalize the data.

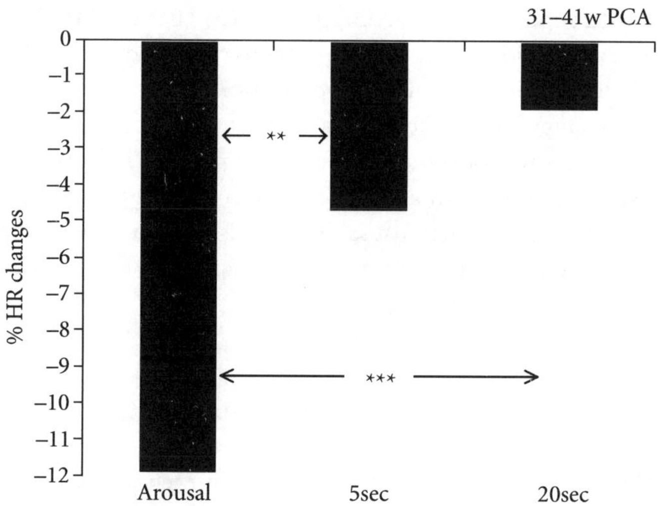

Figure 5. Normalized heart rate changes induced by arousal, according to reference periods taken into account in 37–41w PCA infants (newborn and premature reaching term infants). See Fig. 3 legend for description of 5 and 20 sec. analysis.

preceding arousals (median = 18.1%, range from –18.5% acceleration to 65,3% deceleration).

Heart rate during arousals was always accelerated as compared with the 5 sec. preceding arousals (median = –6.9, range from –35.7 to –5.1 acceleration). It was usually faster within the 5 sec following as compared with the 5 sec preceding arousal (median = –4.7, range from –36.6% acceleration to 6.2% deceleration), as well as during the 20 sec following compared with the 20 sec preceding arousals (median = –2.1, range from –21.9% acceleration to 5.7% deceleration).

Changes of respiratory frequency and heart rate modifications related to arousal in preterm infants reaching term age were similar to those observed in premature and full-term newborn infants during the first 10 days of life (see above).

A relationship between arousal duration and HR acceleration (example on Figure 4) was observed. These data confirmed the higher magnitude of HR changes concomitant with arousal and less changes when analysing the 20 sec following arousal (Figure 5).

c. *Comparison between term infants and preterm infants at corrected term age.*

Each of the 10 arousals recorded in preterm infants reaching 37–41w PCA (Graz data) was paired with 2 arousals recorded in the same sleep state in a term infant with similar (<1 week difference) PCA (Paris data). Doctor Zotter who scored Graz data identified EEG changes as clear or questionable. Because of larger subjectivity in visual EEG appreciation, only respiratory frequency and heart rate changes were taken into account for the comparison.

Duration of recorded arousals was longer in preterm infants reaching term compared with the term neonates. There was a greater respiratory deceleration within the 5 sec following arousal in preterm compared with term infants ($p < 0.04$). However, all other comparisons of respiratory and HR changes were not significant.

Arousals and awakenings in supine versus prone position: Stanford data

At Stanford site we have analyzed the duration of each arousal episode based on continuous observation of movement time (via time-lapse video) and/or simultaneous presence of artifacts on at least one polygraph recording channel in 16 asymptomatic preterm infants (27–36w PCA). Arousal was defined as the occurrence of one of the following criteria: 1) body movement lasting 10 s or more; 2) cry; 3) eye opening lasting at least 5 s. A minimum of 30 sec. of continuous intervening sleep was necessary before scoring the subsequent arousal episode. An arousal period lasting for 60 s or more was defined as an awakening. Each infant served as his/her own control and was recorded in both supine and prone positions. The mean number of arousals or awakenings in 16 preterm infants at term age during all AS or QS episodes in supine and prone are reported.

Effect of prone supine position on arousal and awakening in preterm infants at term age. For the group there were no significant differences between the mean number of arousal in supine vs. prone during all AS episodes (23 vs. 19 respectively) or during QS (10 vs. 8). However, the differences between the number of arousals between the two sleep states were significantly higher during AS compared with QS both in supine as well as in prone (paired t test, $p = 0.01$). Overall, the number of awakenings were greater in supine compared to the prone sleep position. Number of awakening in AS was 11 in supine vs. 7 in prone ($p = 0.02$). Number of awakening in QS was 6 in supine vs. 1 in prone ($p = 0.01$). The effect of sleep position on awakening remained significant when both sleep states were combined ($p = 0.04$).

Comments and conclusions

The preliminary data from the European Data Bank on Arousal in Newborn Infants demonstrated changing physiological variables, usually taken as indicators of arousal, to spontaneous body movements in preterm infants (from 31 wks) during AS and QS. The response and the amplitude of change seems to increase with PCA (based on EEG and HR analysis). The responses of preterm babies at term corrected age was similar to term infants at similar PCA (based on respiratory and heart rate analysis).

These preliminary observations have the methodological limitation of examining the response to body movement (spontaneous) which arguably may initiate the arousal, the view for this study or alternatively could be part of the arousal. It is difficult to determine what is due to the movement per se or the response to an endogenous stimulus. In our investigation we analysed what occurred in relation to body movement and it was assumed that this was a spontaneous event. We could evaluate modifications of other physiological parameters concomitant or closely following movements. Another limitation was the visual detection of EEG changes. Visual assessment of changes is more obvious when familiar with the neonatal EEG but still influenced by subjectivity. Some recent studies suggest that computer identified EEG changes could be used to detect arousal in newborn babies during AS, but there are no data available on QS (Scher et al., 1997; Schramm et al., 2000; Wulbrand et al., 1998).

Many of the discussions at the Paediatric Wake-up Club working group meetings were focussed on choice of the best parameters and epoch duration which would be most useful for arousal definition and detection. The above data give some insight on these questions.

- From 31w PCA, changes in EEG amplitude and frequency could be observed during arousals. In both AS and QS EEG modifications were usually seen after 34w PCA with some rare exceptions in full-term newborn babies. EEG modifications mainly consisted in amplitude decrease and frequency increase. Slowing and increase in EEG amplitude were rarely seen.
- Movement frequently distorted the respiratory signal and thus the appreciation of changes in respiratory frequency related to movement arousals were variable.
- Heart rate changes related to arousals were the most constant and easy to detect. Heart rate acceleration was the most frequently observed and the amplitude of this acceleration increased with PCA. Heart rate decelerations were rarely seen. These decelerations may be related to vagal rebound after acceleration. This hypothesis was not tested in the present study. Due to the high between-subject and between-state variability of heart rate, modifications detected should be normalized for basal pre-arousal heart rate level (Clairambault et al., 1992). The results above agree with previous published data (Curzi-Dascalova et al., 1999) in which we found that the heart rate return to basal level was rapid, and that heart rate changes observed during movement arousal were decreasing within the following 5 sec. Extending the period to 20 sec. for the analysis following the arousals obscured the heart rate change noted close to arousal in the 5 sec. analysis. Our results support that significant changes in physiological variables are usually observed during and within 5 sec of the arousal event. Perhaps a time domain analysis would provide a better assessment of these changes.

The increased number of awakenings during supine as compared with prone sleep in addition to increased heart rate variability (present data and Goto et al., 1999) may represent an adaptive protective response for the developing infant. It is well established that supine sleep position is associated with lowering the risk and incidence of sudden infant death syndrome (SIDS) in many countries by almost 50%. We believe that this decreased threshold for arousal during supine sleep may indeed serve as a mechanism by which many cases of SIDS are prevented through arousal from a life threatening provoking event.

In conclusion, our investigation demonstrated that preterm infants from 31 w PCA, in both AS and QS and term neonates do physiologically respond to spontaneous generalized body movements and that preterm infants at 35–38 weeks PCA have more arousals and greater heart rate variability in supine than in prone sleep position. The amplitude of response increases with PCA and was similar for preterm infants at term PCA when compared to term infants. Finally, these preliminary results showed that the physiological response to spontaneous generalized body movement during the neonatal period is a change in EEG, respiration and heart rate seen during or shortly after arousals.

References

ASDA Report (1992). EEG arousals: Scoring rules and examples. *Sleep, 15*, 173–184.

Bard, K.A., C.D. Coles, K.A. Platzman & M.E. Lynch (2000). The effect of prenatal drug exposure, term status, and carevigiving on arousal modulation in 8-week-old infants. *Developmental Psychobiology, 36*, 194–211.

Clairambault, Jean., Lilia Curzi-Dascalova, François Kauffmann, Clair Médigue, & Christoph Leffler (1992). Heart rate variability in normal, sleeping full-term and preterm neonates. *Early Human Development, 28*, 169–183.

Curzi-Dascalova, Lilia & Majid Mirmiran (1996). Manual of methods of recording and analyzing sleep-wakefulness states in preterm and full-term infants. Paris: INSERM.

Curzi-Dascalova, Lilia, François Kauffmann, Claude Gaultier & Regina A. Caldas de Amorim (1999). Heart rate modifications related to spontaneous body movements in sleeping premature and full-term newborns. *Pediatric Research, 45*, 515–518.

Curzi-Dascalova, Lilia, Juliette Bloch, Marie-Françoise Vecchierini, Antoine Bedu & Patricia Vignolo (2000). Physiological parameters evaluation following apnea in healthy premature infants. *Biology of the Neonate, 77*, 203–211.

Dittrichova, Jaroslava, K. Paul & E. Pavlikova (1977). Responsiveness to stimulation during paradoxical sleep in infants. *Early Human Development, 1*, 213–225.

Ficca, Gianluca, Igino Fagioli, Fiorenza Giganti, & Piero Salzarulo (1999). Spontaneous awakenings from sleep in the first year of life. *Early Human Development, 55*, 219–228.

Franco, Patricia, José Groswasser, Martine Sottiaux, Ema Broadfield & André Kahn (1996). Decreased cardiac responses to auditory stimulation during prone sleep. *Pediatrics, 97*, 174–178.

Franco, Patricia, José Groswasser, S. Hassid, J. P. Lanquart, S. Scarlett, André Kahn (1999). Prenatal exposure to cigarette smoking is associated with a decrease in arousal in infants. *Journal of Pediatrics, 135*, 34–38.

Galland, B.C., D.P. Bolton, B.J. Taylor, R.M. Sayers & S.M. Williams (2000). Ventilatory sensitivity to mild asphyxia. *Archive of Disease in Childhood, 83*, 423–428.

Giganti, Fiorenza, Gianluca Ficca, Enrico Biagioni, Giovanni Cioni, Maria Teresa Puliti, Igino Fagioli & Piero Salzarulo (1999). Awakenings in pre-term and near-term infants. *Sleep Research Online, 2* (suppl 1), 201.

Goto, Kazuya, Majid Mirmiran, Marian M. Adams, Robyn V. Longford, Roger B. Baldwin, Margaret A. Boeddiker & Ronald L. Ariagno (1999). More awakenings and heart rate variability during supine sleep in preterm infants. *Pediatrics, 103*, 603–609.

Horne, Rosemary S.C., David J. Sly, Susan M. Granage, Bonnie Chau, & T. Michael Adamson. (2000). Effect of prematurity on arousal from sleep in the newborn infant. *Pediatric Research, 47*, 468–474.

Kahn, André, E. Picard & D. Blum (1986). Auditory arousal thresholds of normaland near-miss SIDS infants. *Developmental Medicine and Child Neurology, 28*, 299–302.

Kahn, André, José Grosswasser, Patricia Franco, S. Scaillet, T. Sawaguchi, I. Kelmanson, A. de Broca, B. Dan & L. Servais (2000). Factors influencing the determination of arousal thresholds in infants – a review. *Sleep Medicine, 1*, 273–278.

Lewis, K.W. & E.M. Bosque (1995). Deficient hypoxia awakening response in infants of smoking mothers: possible relationship to sudden infant death syndrome. *Journal of Pediatrics, 127*, 691–699.

McNamara, Frances, Faiq G. Issa, & Colin E. Sullivan (1996). Arousal pattern following central and obstructive breathing abnormalities in infants and children. *Journal of Applied Physiology, 81*, 2651–2657.

Monod, Nicole, & Lucile Garma (1977). Auditory responsivity in the human premature. *Biology of the Neonate, 17*, 292–316.

Phillips, Steven J., Frederic J. Agate Jr., Willam A. Silverman & Philip Steiner (1964). Autonomic Cardiac reactivity in premature infants. *Biology of the Neonate, 6*, 225–249.

Ramet, J., J.-P. Praud, A. M. d'Allest, A. Carofilis, M. Dehan, Christian Guilleminault & Claude Gaultier (1988). Effect of maturation on heart rate response to ocular compression test during rapid eye movement sep in human infants. *Pediatric Research, 24*, 477–488.

Read, Paul A., Rosemary S. C. Horne, Susan M. Cranage, Adrian M. Walker, David W. Walker & T. Michael Adamson (1998). Dynamic changes in arousal threshold during sleep in the human infant. *Pediatric Research, 43*, 679–703.

Scher, Marc S., George Dokianakis, Doris A. Steppe, David L. Banks & Robert J. Sclabassi (1997). Computer classification of state in healthy preterm neonates. *Sleep, 20*, 132–141.

Schramm, D., B. Scheidt, A. Hübler, J. Frenzel, K. Holthausen & O. Breidbach (2000). Spectral analysis of electroencephalogram during sleep-related apneas in pre-term and term born infants in the first weeks of life. *Clinical Neurophysiology, 111*, 1788–1791.

Schulz, Hartmut, Roberto Massetani, Igino Fagioli & Piero Salzarulo (1985). Spontaneous awakening from sleep in infants. *Electroencephalography and Clinical Neurophysiology, 61*, 267–271.

Thach, Bradley T., & Anna Lijowska (1996). Arousal in infants. *Sleep, 19*, S271–S273.

Thoppil, C.K., M.A. Belan, C.P. Cowen, & O.P. Mathew (1991). Behavioral arousal in newborn infants and its association with termination of apnea. *Journal of Applied Physiology, 70*, 2479–2484.

Tirosh, Emanuel, Dan Liban & David Bader (1996). The effect of maternal smoking during pregnancy on sleep respiratory and arousal pattern in neonates. *Journal of Perinatology, 16*, 435–438.

Todorovich, Rod D., David H. Crowell & Linda E. Kapuiniai (1987). Auditory responsivity and intrauterinr grouth retardation in small for gestational age human newborns. *Electroencephalography and Clinical Neurophysiology, 67*, 204–212.

Vecchierini, Marie-Françoise, Lilia Curzi-Dascalova, Ha Trang-Pham, Juliette Bloch & Claude Gaultier (2001). Patterns of EEG frequency, movement, heart rate, and oxygenation following isolated short apneas in infants. *Pediatric Research, 49*, 220–226.

Wulbrand, Henning, Frances McNamara & Bradley T. Thach (1998). Suppression of ś spindle electroencephalographic activity as a measure of transient arousal after spontaneous and occlusion-evoked sighs and startles. *Pediatric Research, 44*, 767–773.

Awakening and sleep–wake cycle in infants

Igino Fagioli, Gianluca Ficca, and Piero Salzarulo
Department of Psychology, University of Florence /
Department of Psychology, II University of Naples

Introduction

Pioneering studies showed that the behavioural states of sleep and wakefulness appear early during ontogeny in humans (Dreyfus-Brisac, 1970; Prechtl, 1974; Prechtl & O'Brien, 1982), and that physiological and behavioural characteristics of each state undergo several age-related changes.

Developmental changes are very fast in the first few months of life, and sleep-wake rhythm organisation approaches the one of adulthood already by the second semester of life (Fagioli & Salzarulo, 1982; Coons & Guilleminault, 1982; Salzarulo & Fagioli, 1992a; Salzarulo & Fagioli, 1999). These studies have pointed out the necessity of investigating not only the characteristics of states, but also the modalities of transition between states.

States transitions can be classified in three categories: 1) the transitions within sleep, i.e. between different sleep states, 2) the transitions from wakefulness to sleep, i.e. the sleep onset, and 3) the transitions between sleep and wakefulness, i.e. the awakenings. Whereas the first two types of transition have been extensively described (for the sleep transitions, see Monod & Curzi, 1973; and for the sleep onset, Salzarulo & Fagioli, 1980; Fagioli et al., 1981b), fewer studies were devoted to the issue of awakenings, and these were clinical more frequently than normative.

Describing the features of awakening in early development, however, is of utmost importance in order to clarify, on one side, the mechanisms determining the changes of infants sleep-wake rhythm and, on the other, the reasons for excessive awakenings in several clinical conditions.

This paper will first provide an overview of the main changes with age in the characteristics of awakenings, such as their number and duration, mainly studied through long-lasting (24-hour or nocturnal period) recordings. The mechanisms underlying most of awakenings' developmental changes are still largely unknown, and only few experimental results can be explained in light of the already existing models of sleep regulation. We will speculate on those factors, such as the gradual development of the central nervous system, that may contribute in shaping the sleep-wake cycle and awakening timing and modalities across the first epochs of life. Additionally we will also try to pinpoint some elements possibly essential to account for the characteristics of sleep-wake alternate occurrence in infants in the framework of a model for state regulation.

Methodological aspects

Preliminarily, we should remark that the data presented below come from studies which differ for some methodological aspects.

A first issue concerns the number of states defined and scored. Indeed, whereas there is a general agreement on the presence of the two main sleep states (NREM, or Quiet, sleep, and REM, or Active, sleep), some Authors (Monod & Curzi, 1973; Fagioli & Salzarulo, 1982, Coons & Guilleminault, 1982; Hoppenbrouwers et al., 1988, Louis et al., 1997) take separately into account those epochs sharing the characteristics of two different states, classifying them as *ambiguous* or *indeterminate* or *transitional* sleep.

Furthermore, the minimum duration required to score a state can differ a lot, ranging from 1 or 2 minutes (Ficca et al., 1999; Louis et al., 1997) to 5 (Navelet et al., 1984).

Finally, the frame of reference for the awakening time should be mentioned: in fact, each awakening can be either referred to the "external" timing (i.e., the clock time) or more simply considered within the frame of sleep and wakefulness alternate occurrence, that is in the way it interrupts sleep at different hierarchical organisational levels: the sleep episode, the NREM-REM cycle, the single sleep state (Salzarulo et al., 1999).

Main developmental changes

Number of awakenings

Two polygraphic studies assessed the number of awakenings across the 24-hour. Salzarulo & Fagioli (1992a) estimated the mean number of awakenings to be about 9 at one month and 4.5 at one year. Louis et al. (1997) also reported a sharp decrease in the number of awakenings from three months to one year of life (mean values respectively being 12 and 8), although they did not find any further decrease in the second year of life.

These two researches also checked whether the distribution of awakenings was different as a function of the time of day: to this aim, the 24-hour period was split in a "night" and a "day" period, defined according to the clock time (being 8 p.m. and 8 a.m. the limits) in Salzarulo & Fagioli (1992a), and to the light-off and light on given by parents in Louis et al. (1997). Both studies clearly showed that the decrease in the number of the overall 24-hour awakenings throughout the first year of life was mostly accounted for by the their decrease at night-time.

This evidence, paralleling the precocious process of sleep consolidation during night-time, (Kleitman, 1963; Parmelee et al., 1964; Fagioli & Salzarulo, 1982; Coons & Guilleminault, 1984), suggested the hypothesis that the nocturnal period could be characterised by peculiarities acquired very early during development and led several studies to specifically focus on the changes with age of nocturnal wakefulness. The trend to the decrease in the number of night awakenings was a common report of these studies, and could account for the reduction of both the total amount of intra-sleep wakefulness (Anders, 1978; Navelet et al., 1982; Hoppenbrouwers, 1988; Louis et al., 1997; Ficca et al., 1999) and of night-time wakefulness (Fagioli & Salzarulo, 1982; Fagioli et al., 1988; Giganti et al., 2001).

Slight discrepancies in the absolute numbers from literature data are probably due to methodological differences reminded in the previous paragraph. For instance, the Figure 1 displays that the mean number of awakenings per night, as expectable, is inversely related to the minimal duration criterion used by the authors. Nevertheless, what matters here is that, irrespective of the different methods, there is an extremely high consistency, between independent studies, of the trends with age in the occurrence of awakenings.

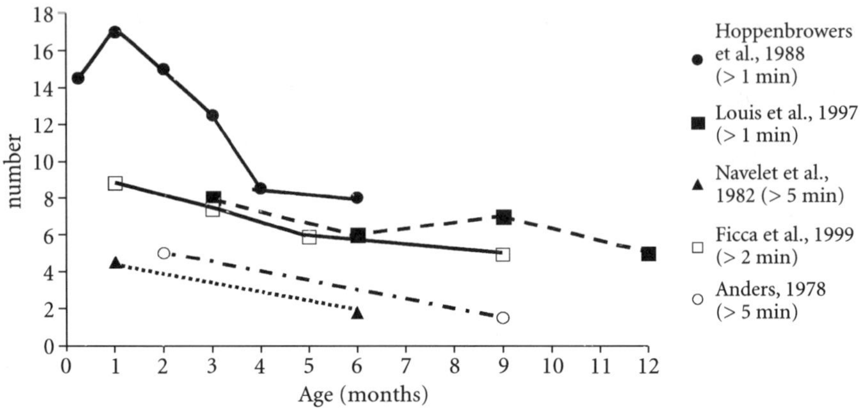

Figure 1. Number of night awakenings (y axis) as a function of age (x axis) reported in five studies.

Duration of awakenings

An important aspect of the sleep-wake cycle is represented by the events following awakening: in particular, the reciprocal interaction between the increasing ability to sustain wakefulness and the propensity to sleep re-onset is responsible for the duration of the awakening. Quite obviously, the mean duration of wakefulness following awakenings reported in the different studies partly depends on the criterion of the minimal duration for states' scoring (Figure 2). For instance, the mean duration of nocturnal awakenings observed by Ficca et al. (1999), based on a 2-min criterion, was higher than those by Hoppenbrouwers et al. (1988) and by Louis et al. (1997), both based on a 1-min criterion.

As for its developmental trend (Figure 2), the mean duration of awakenings slightly increases with age according to Hoppenbrouwers et al. (1988), whereas Louis et al. (1997) and Ficca et al. (1999) did not find any significant change: only the study by Navelet et al. (1982) reported a clear age-related decrease, which is difficult to account for. Again, the different criteria for the minimum duration of the waking state (5 minutes) could contribute to explain the result.

A reanalysis of the data by Fagioli & Salzarulo (1982), using a criterion for the minimal duration for sleep and wakefulness of 15 minutes (Salzarulo & Fagioli, 1992a), showed that the mean duration of the waking episodes during daytime increased from about 90 min in the young subgroup (aged between 1 and 3 months: mean age 2 months) to 170 min in the older subgroup (4 months to one year old: mean 7 months), whereas during night-time, mean duration of waking episodes slightly lengthened from 70 to 80 min. Moreover,

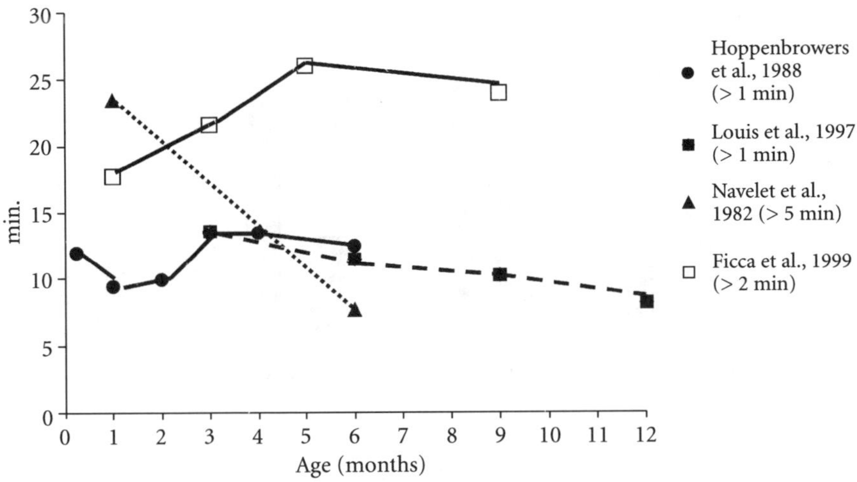

Figure 2. Mean duration of night awakenings (y axis) as a function of age (x axis) reported in four studies.

the "fragmented sleep-wake pattern", characterised by the alternate occurrence of two or more periods of sleep and wakefulness longer than 2 min and shorter than 15 min, significantly decreased with age, but did not show a different distribution between daytime and night-time. A re-analysis of Louis et al. (1997) data showed that the mean duration of the diurnal waking episodes increased from 95 to 123 min between 3 and 9 months, whereas the duration of nocturnal awakenings slightly decreased from 13.6 to 10.3 min. The comparison of the data of these two researches suggests that during daytime there is a generalised increase in the duration of the waking episodes, irrespective of the criterion for the minimum duration. At night-time, instead, an opposite trend is shown by longer and shorter waking episodes: the former tend to further increase their mean duration, similarly to what happens at daytime, whereas the latter show a trend to become even shorter.

A reanalysis of the data from Ficca et al. (1999) on nocturnal awakenings was aimed at assessing the respective contribution provided by the awakenings of different duration to the overall waking time at different ages (Figure 3). The largest part of the waking time was determined by waking bouts lasting between 32 and 64 min in infants younger than 2 months and by awakenings longer than 64 min in infants 2 to 5 months old. Interestingly, the time spent in waking bouts lasting more than 64 min strongly decreases after six months of life, when they occur in less than half of the infants.

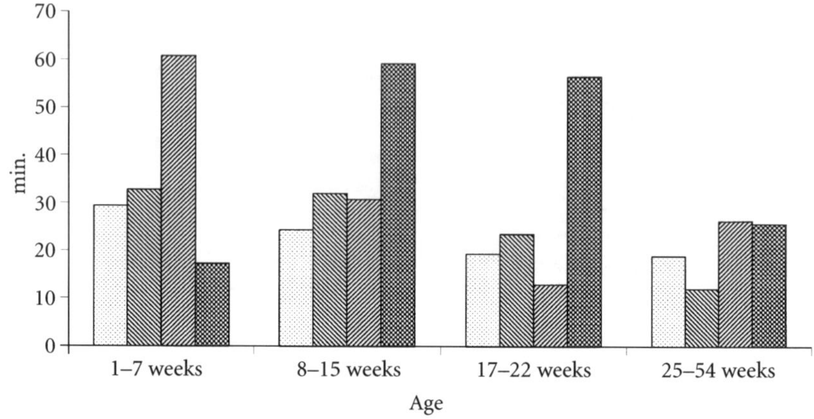

Figure 3. Time spent in wakefulness per night (y axis) as a function of age (x axis) and of the duration of the awakening (⬚ 2–16 min.; ▧: 16–32 min.; ▨: 32–64 min.; ▩: > 64 min.).

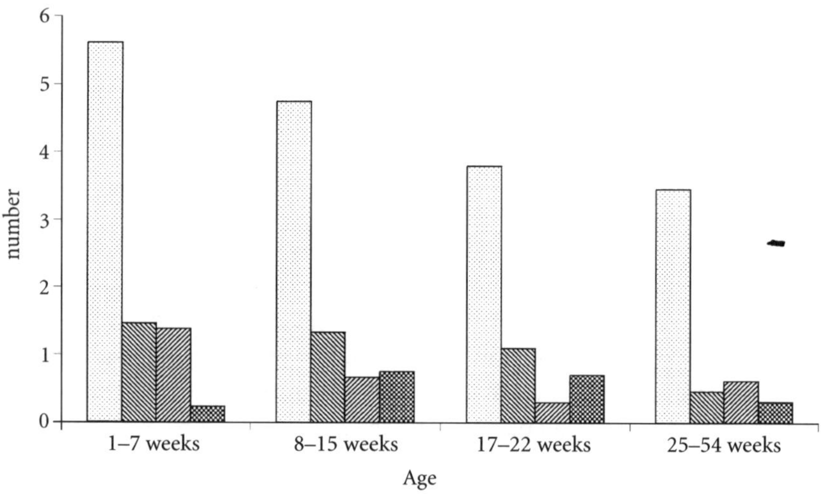

Figure 4. Number of awakenings per night (y axis) as a function of age (x axis) and of the duration of the awakening (⬚ 2–16 min.; ▧: 16–32 min.; ▨: 32–64 min.; ▩: > 64 min.).

The distribution of the number of nocturnal awakenings according to both their duration and age has been evaluated again through a re-analysis of the data from Ficca et al. (1999). During the night-time short waking episodes largely predominate at all ages and the number of long awakenings increases after 2 months (Figure 4). The data concerning diurnal awakenings reported by Wolff (1984: 146, 148) show on the contrary a strong decrease of short awakenings and an increase of longest ones between 1 and 2 months of age. Although the comparison between nocturnal and diurnal data should be interpreted cautiously, since they come out from two different researches, it could be suggested that the changes in the distribution of the duration of diurnal waking bouts precedes that of nocturnal ones.

Periodicity of awakenings

Ficca et al. (1999: 223–225) highlighted that also the overnight distribution of the awakenings show age-related modifications. Infants younger than four months showed one main peak at the 5th hour and two minor peaks at the 2nd and at the 7th hour. Older infants displayed a polymodal distribution, more evident after 6 months of age, with several alternating peaks and troughs. The different distribution of awakenings through the night, compared to previous ages, shown by the qualitative analysis in infants older than 6 months, adds another argument in favour of the hypothesis that this age represents a "turning point" of many parameters.

Parallel to the change in awakening distribution over time, also the periodicity of awakenings appears to undergo age-related changes. Mean recurrence time of all awakenings shows significant changes with age, going from one awakening every 56 min to one every 89 min. However, if the awakening out of NREM sleep are taken separately from those out of REM sleep, a different course over age is shown. A substantially stable pattern is found for the recurrence time of awakenings from REM, with values ranging between 77 and 100 min. On the contrary, the recurrence time of the awakenings from NREM sleep shows a non-linear trend, decreasing until the 5th month of life and going up again after the 6th month (Figure 5). The 1:2 ratio in infants older than 6 months between the mean recurrence time of awakenings from REM and of those from NREM, resembles (albeit with a twofold increase: 100:200 minutes vs. 50:100 minutes) the similar coupling exhibited by the ratio between REM recurrence time and Slow Wave Sleep recurrence time in infants (Bes et al., 1991). This intriguing early feature has been emphasised (Ficca et al., 1999): the ultradian rhythms of some neurophysiological activities are multiple of each other at early ages, and become synchronised later on during the development.

Studies on the 24 hour distribution of wakefulness showed that the evening hours are those most frequently characterised by the behavioural waking state

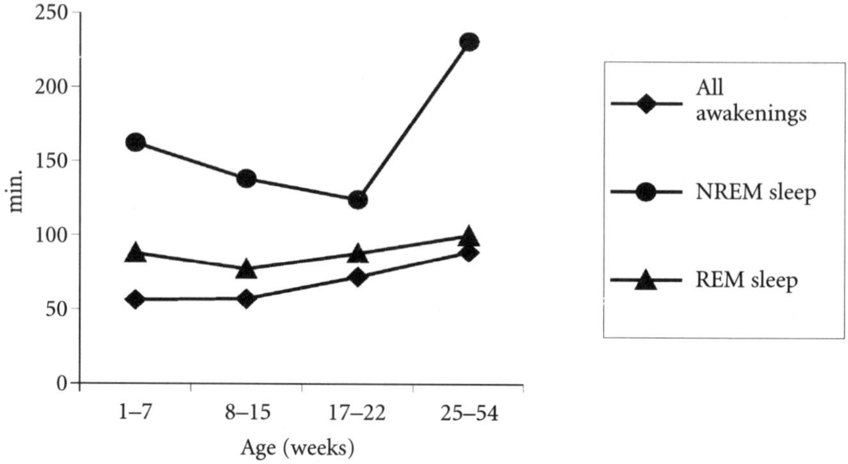

Figure 5. Mean recurrence time of night awakenings as a function of age (x axis) and of the sleep state from which the infants woke up (redrawn from Ficca et al., 1999).

early in development (Giganti et al., 2001) and that its time placement corresponds to the forbidden zone for sleep observed in the adult (Lavie et al., 1986). Those results prompt further research on the relationship between waking and physiological mechanisms, possibly related to circadian factors, inducing spontaneous awakening during development.

Physiological processes preceding awakening

What said before about the duration of waking bouts is a first evidence that each spontaneous awakening may have its own peculiar features. Most likely, also the physiological events preceding the transition towards wakefulness may show remarkable differences.

It is important to look at the state from which the awakening emerges. This implies carrying out two distinct kind of analysis: one assesses the absolute number of awakenings out of each state, another one takes into account that the number of awakenings from a given sleep state is a function of the time spent in that state. A ratio between the two expresses the probability of waking up from that state. Indeed, some data on the number of awakenings may be interpreted in light of differences in the proportion of sleep states.

The decrease in the number of night-time awakenings in older infants is due to a decrease of the awakenings from REM sleep and Ambiguous sleep, but not from NREM sleep (Figure 6). In fact, the number of awakenings out

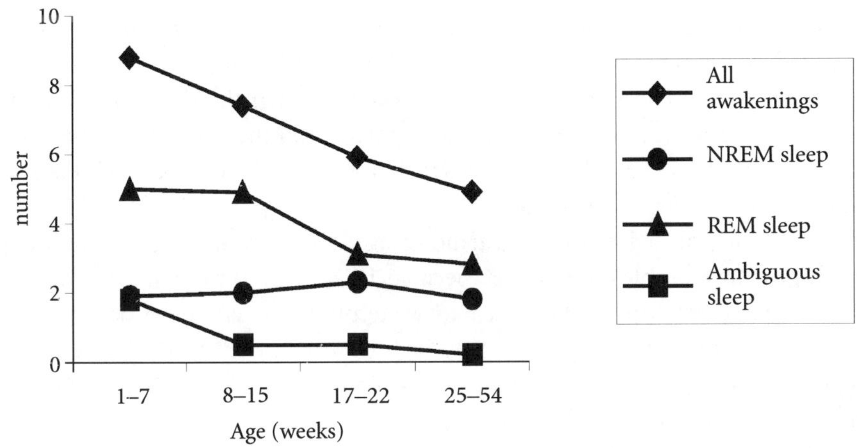

Figure 6. Number of night awakenings as a function of age (x axis) and of the sleep state from which the infants woke up (redrawn from Ficca et al., 1999).

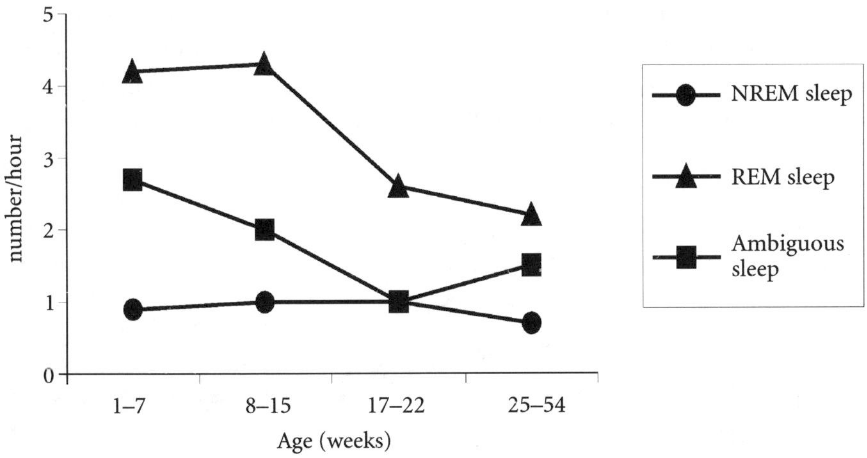

Figure 7. Frequency (number/ total time of each sleep state) of awakenings as a function of age (x axis) and of the type of sleep from which infants wake up (redrawn from Ficca et al., 1999).

of NREM remains stable across the first year of life, whereas awakenings out of REM sleep reduce at about the fourth month of life and from that age on do not exceed those from NREM, as it was before, and awakenings from Ambiguous sleep are to values close to zero already after 2 months of age. The probability to wake up turned out to be higher from REM sleep than from NREM sleep across the whole first year of life (Figure 7). The difference become less pronounced in infants older than 6 months, with a trend failing to reach statistical significance. The comparisons between ratios confirm the decrease with age in the awakenings out of REM sleep, and partially in those out of Ambiguous sleep; those out of NREM sleep shows very stable (both absolute and relative) values across the first year of life.

As it was pointed out by Salzarulo et al. (2000), awakening during early development resembles sleep onset, because REM sleep is the state where most of the transitions from either sleep to wakefulness or viceversa occur. REM sleep would then play a "gating" role in both directions. With age, a major change affects the prevalent state for sleep onset, becoming NREM in the adult, with no similar change in the modality of awakening.

The duration of wakefulness following awakening, in infants younger than 6 months, is longer when the awakening comes from NREM sleep. At later ages, awakenings from NREM significantly shorten, so that their duration become similar to the one of awakenings from REM sleep (Figure 8).

Another aspect of awakenings, their time of occurrence during the sleep bout, was analysed: the duration of each state was assessed in infants 2 weeks to 13 months old according to the occurrence of either an awakening or another sleep state (Schulz et al., 1985). REM sleep followed by awakening re-

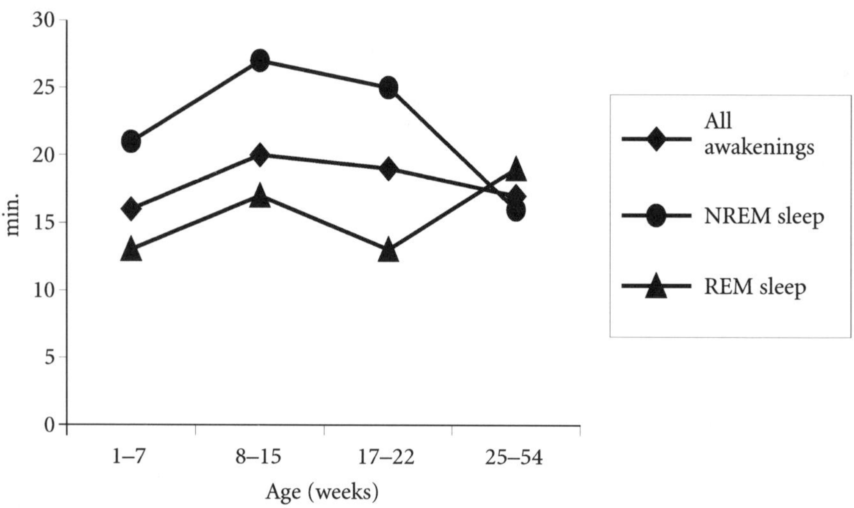

Figure 8. Mean duration of night awakenings as a function of age (x axis) and of the sleep state from which the infants woke up (redrawn from Ficca et al., 1999).

sulted shorter (median 5 min), than REM sleep periods followed by another sleep state (median = 12), whereas NREM sleep periods duration was independent on the following state, either waking or sleep (in both cases the median duration was about 30 min).

The interest for the sleep state from which the awakenings emerge is also in their link with the NREM-REM cycle. In the adult the completion of the NREM-REM cycle was considered the gate for awakening. Across the first year of life there is an increase in the proportion of awakenings out of NREM sleep. Therefore, according to our definition of sleep cycle (Fagioli et al., 1981a) its disruption should follow. What is observed is no change in the number of cycles with increase of their duration and an improvement of sleep organisation, as expressed by the increasing ratio of sleep time spent in cycle/ total sleep time (Salzarulo & Fagioli, 1999; Ficca et al., 2000a). This might have important functional consequences, since a role of NREM-REM cycle has been hypothesised for physiological anabolic processes (Fagioli et al., 1981a; Salzarulo & Fagioli, 1995) and psychological functions, such as memory (Mazzoni et al., 1999; Salzarulo et al., 1997; Ficca et al., 2000b).

Factors involved in awakening regulation

What said so far suggests that the phenomenon of awakening in infants shows clear links with the time of day, the time course of sleep states and their alternate occurrence in NREM-REM cycles, and that the impressive changes in the awakening features reflect a continuous reshaping during development of the complex psychophysiological regulatory mechanisms. A still open question is whether the main mechanisms regulating the sleep-wake rhythm in the adult are already active in infancy and to what extent they can predict awakening modalities.

The alternate occurrence of sleep and wakefulness in the adult is commonly explained in the frame of the two-process model (Borbély, 1982; Daan et al., 1984; Achermann & Borbély, 1990; Achermann et al., 1993). This model assumes that the timings of spontaneous sleep onset and spontaneous awakening result from the interaction between a homeostatic (Feinberg, 1974) *Process S* and a circadian *Process C*. The process S (S = sleep) is built up following an exponential kinetics during the waking period, and decays during sleep at a faster rate, but always following an exponential kinetics. Slow wave activity (SWA) of NREM sleep indexes process S during sleep. Process C (C = circadian) fluctuates with a maximum in the afternoon and a minimum in the early morning and determines the parallel time course of the thresholds H and L. Threshold H represents the minimum level of process S necessary to fall asleep spontaneously: it is high in the late afternoon, when falling asleep is very difficult, and low in the early morning, when the "propensity" to fall asleep is very high. Threshold L represents the level of process S which has to be attained during sleep for the occurrence of a spontaneous awakening.

It is very difficult to assess whether processes similar to C and S are to be found in the infant and, if so, in which way they interact. Very sparse data are available on circadian rhythms, reflecting process C, during the first year of life. In pre-term infants, Mirmiran and Kok (1991) found circadian rhythms of body temperature and heart rate, but not of rest-activity cycles: the Authors claim that the continuous light could impair the emergence of circadian rhythms. According to Hellbrugge (1960) circadian rhythms are evident no earlier than the sixth month of life. The emergence after the 4th month of a circadian profile of heart rate (Fagioli & Salzarulo, 1985), could be related to the feeding schedules (Salzarulo et al., 1985).

Several characteristics of sleep organisation in infants, e.g. the differences in physiological activities between the first NREM-REM sleep cycle and the following, have been considered a "sketch" of the adult's Process S (Salzarulo & Fagioli, 1992b; Bes et al., 1994). These features led to further explore the psychophysiological regulation of sleep–wake rhythm in early development, and, in particular, those mechanisms which could underlie the presence of nocturnal awakenings.

The frequent occurrence of awakenings, interrupting night sleep (as well as the naps interrupting wakefulness during the daytime) could be explained by three hypothetical mechanisms (Fagioli et al., 1995), non necessarily mutually exclusive, in the framework of the two-process model (Borbély, 1982; Daan et al., 1994):

1. the "instantaneous build-up rate" or "rise rate" of the process S during wakefulness and the "instantaneous breakdown rate" or "decay rate" during sleep (respectively in Daan et al., 1984, and Achermann & Borbély, 1990) would be faster in infants and slow down with age, as can be argued also from Bes et al. (1994);
2. the maximum amount of process S sustainable during wakefulness, without falling asleep (i.e., the *threshold H* level: Daan et al., 1984), would increase with age;

3. additionally, the process C fluctuations might be less ample in infants than in adults, as a consequence of the lower amplitude of the circadian rhythms.

The first two hypotheses imply that, in infants, both the faster increase of process S during wakefulness and the lower level of the threshold H (responsible for the sleep fragmentation in condition of continuous bed rest according to Daan et al., 1984) would entail an earlier sleep onset, i.e. shorter waking episodes relative to adults; likewise, the faster decay of process S during sleep would entail shorter sleep episodes. This would result in the occurrence of several sleep and waking episodes in the 24-hour period and thus in the typical polyphasic sleep-wake organisation observed in infants.

The occurrence of two sleep episodes in the night is frequent in infants (it was found in about 40% of the recordings in a group of 35 infants: unpublished data) and is observed also in adults put in particular environmental conditions (Zulley & Carr, 1993; Wehr et al., 1994). The analysis of the EEG background activity of two sleep episodes separated by a spontaneous nocturnal waking episode (lasting up to nearly 4 hours in infants) 2 to 11 months old allowed to test the hypotheses described before.

The study was carried out through the measurement of a parameter, computed by automatic analysis (Haustein et al., 1986; Bes et al., 1988), which reflects the degree of synchronisation of EEG background activity. For each NREM period, three indicators of the time course of the EEG parameter were defined, according to Achermann & Borbély (1987) method: the *range* (difference between the values of EEG parameter at the beginning of the NREM sleep period and at the trough), the *trough latency* (after NREM sleep onset), and the *rate of synchronisation* (range/trough latency). The rate of synchronisation has been assumed as a good indicator of the level of process S, according to the recent elaboration (Achermann & Borbély, 1990; Achermann et al., 1993) of the two-process model, where the authors state that "*the rate of the build up of SWA and the plateau level are determined by the process S*" (Achermann et al., 1993: 98).

The rate of EEG synchronisation of the first and second NREM period of the first sleep episode was higher than that of the corresponding NREM periods of the second sleep episode, and the value of the first NREM period of the second sleep episode was higher than that of the second NREM period of the first sleep episode (Fagioli & Salzarulo, 1997: 623, Figure 1, lower panel). Since those values of the rate of synchronisation are an estimate of the level of the process S, and they follow the S process time course in a simulation of the biphasic night sleep obtained only by a lowering of the threshold H (Daan et al., 1984: R165, Figure 3, lower central figure), this result is compatible with the hypothesis of a lower level of the threshold H in infants. To test the hypothesis that the amplitude of circadian rhythms might be reduced, we should compare the rate of synchronisation between infants and adults both displaying a spontaneous biphasic sleep organisation; the model would predict a lower difference between the first and the second sleep episode (Daan et al., 1984: R165, Figure 3, lower left figure). Unfortunately, such data are not up to now available.

Nevertheless, a model could be proposed which takes into account the hypotheses suggesting increased rise rate and breakdown rate of the process S and a lowered threshold H, in infants. The time course of the process S and of the H and L thresholds and the resulting sleep and wakefulness occurrence in the adults, according to Daan et al. (1984), are shown in the upper panel of Figure 9. Changes in the mathematical coefficients in the equations of the model according to the previously reported hypotheses (i.e., by enhancing the coefficient of the S process build-up during wakefulness and the coefficient of its dissipation during sleep, and by lowering the mean value of the threshold H), allow to simulate both sleep-wake organisation (Fagioli & Salzarulo, 1982; Salzarulo & Fagioli, 1999), and the results concerning EEG dynamics (Fagioli et al., 1995; Fagioli & Salzarulo, 1997), as shown in the lower panel of the Figure 9.

With the coefficients modified this way, the model predicts in fact one short nap in the afternoon and two nocturnal sleep episodes of similar duration, separated by a long period of wakefulness; moreover it accounts for the results on the rate of synchronisation (Fagioli & Salzarulo, 1997: 625, Figure 1, lower panel).

Whereas the modification in the mathematical constants of the equations of the model allows to simulate the sleep-waking organisation observed at early ages, the frequent occurrence of brief awakenings during the night-time is more difficult to account for. A possible explanation for the latter might be related to time course of the curve of the process S, which for long time during sleep runs closer to the L threshold in infants than in adults (see Figure 9); this hypothesis should be confirmed through empirical evidence.

Pollak (1994) suggested some points to explain the distribution and the duration of the awakenings at early ages. In his work he analysed the distribution of sleep and waking states, assessed through behavioural observation of one infant during the first 6 months of life through an original statistical approach, the fractional analysis. He found that the two measures provided by this method, the percentage of sleep time and the sleep and wakefulness con-

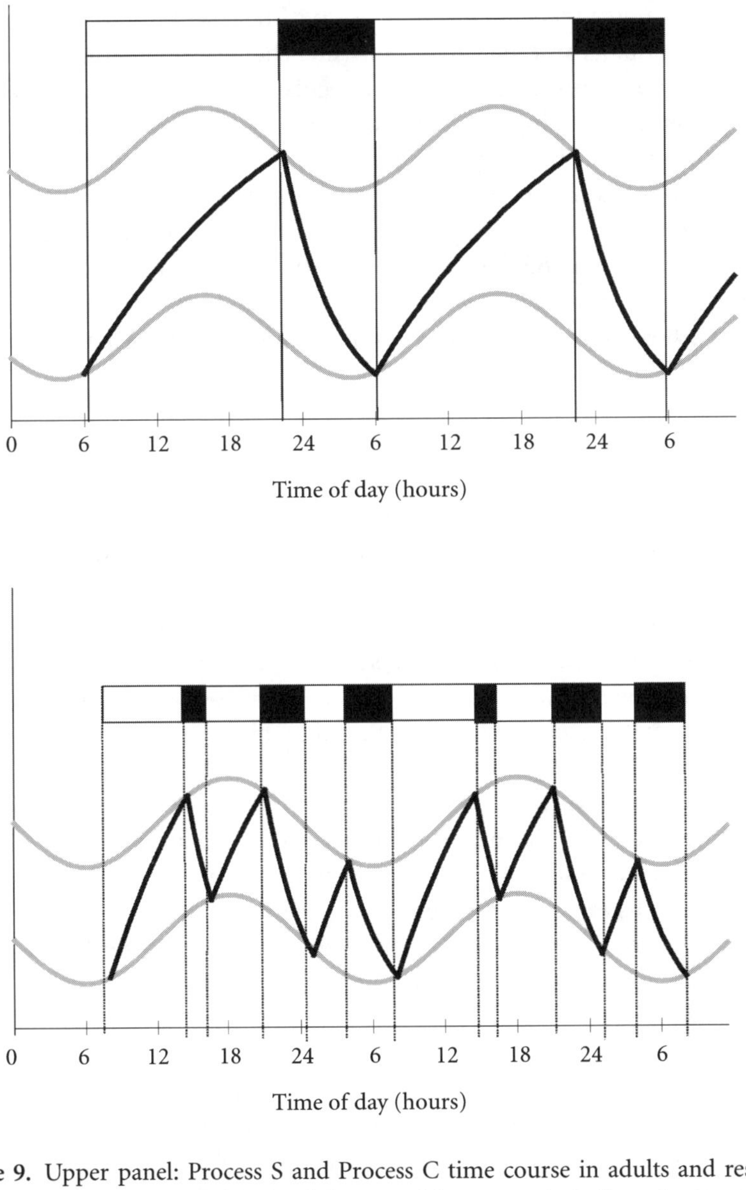

Figure 9. Upper panel: Process S and Process C time course in adults and resulting sleep-wake organisation: waking and sleep resulting respectively from the intersection of declining S process (black) curve and the threshold L (grey, lower sinusoidal curve) and from the intersection of the increasing S process curve and the threshold H (grey, upper sinusoidal curve) are represented by white and black rectangles in the upper part of the Figure (redrawn from Daan et al., 1984). Lower panel: Processes S and C and sleep-wake organisation in infants according to the hypotheses (see text).

solidation, change independently with ageing. To account for sleep wake characteristics in infants and their developmental changes, the maturation of separate underlying neuronal mechanisms, regulating respectively circadian timing and sleep and waking alternate occurrence was invoked. In particular it was assumed that: *i)* the circadian pacemaker is reset by daytime and night-time stimuli only after maturation; *ii)* the percentage of sleep is related to the metabolic rate which decreases with growth. This preliminary study, though based on data coming out from one observation on a single infant, although very long, suggests to perform further research aiming at the construction of a model which could integrate evidences from different approaches.

Conclusion

Several characteristics of the awakenings in infants show clear developmental trends: the number of awakenings decreases, the duration of wakefulness increases and their distribution becomes more and more differentiated between day and night-time. Young infants wake up more often during REM sleep than NREM sleep, but the difference is less ample later on, when the number of awakenings out of REM sleep reduces. Furthermore, the awakenings from NREM sleep get shorter, reaching by the end of the first year a duration similar to those from REM.

Globally, there has been an improvement in the understanding of factors regulating awakenings: for instance, the study of EEG dynamics during NREM sleep provides a clue to explain some aspects which are rather stable between 2 and 12 months of age: *i)* the frequent occurrence, from two months of age onward, of a biphasic nocturnal sleep, with a long lasting awakening in the middle of the night, and *ii)* EEG characteristics of the following sleep (Fagioli & Salzarulo, 1997 and 1998).

Other aspects of awakenings have been shown to change throughout the first year of life, such as the frequency of brief awakenings, which is high in very young infants and decreases with age, or the relationships between the awakening and the NREM-REM sleep cycle. These features own peculiar developmental trends, not yet described by any theoretical and/or mathematical model of sleep-wake rhythms in infants. Further research should focus on the interaction between CNS maturation, on one hand, and the environmental influences, on the other, in order to clarify their role on physiological and behavioural characteristics of the awakening process in early development.

Acknowledgements

Partially supported by a grant of University of Florence ("Progetti Strategici") to Piero Salzarulo.

References

Achermann, Peter, & Alexander A. Borbély (1987). Dynamics of EEG slow wave activity during physiological sleep and after administration of benzodiazepines hypnotics. *Human Neurobiology 6,* 203–210.

Achermann, Peter, & Alexander A. Borbély (1990). Simulation of human sleep: Ultradian dynamics of electroencephalographic slow-wave activity. *Journal of Biological Rhythms, 5,* 141–157.

Achermann, Peter, Derk-Jan Dijk, Daniel P. Brunner & Alexander A. Borbély (1993). A model of human sleep homeostasis based on EEG slow-wave activity: quantitative comparison of data and simulations, *Brain Research Bullettin, 31,* 97–113.

Anders, Thomas (1978). Home-recorded sleep in 2- and 9-months old infants. *American Academy of Child Psychiatry, 17,* 421–432.

Bes, Frederick, Paolo Baroncini, Christine Dugovic, Igino Fagioli, Hartmut Schulz, Bernard Franc & Piero Salzarulo (1988). Time course of EEG activity during night sleep in the first year of life based on automatic analysis. *Electroencephalography and clinical Neurophysiology, 69,* 501–507.

Bes, Frederick, Igino Fagioli, Patricio Peirano, Hartmut Schulz & Piero Salzarulo (1994). Trends in EEG synchronization across nonREM sleep in infants. *Sleep, 17,* 323–329.

Bes, Frederick, Hartmut Schulz, Yvonne Navelet & Piero Salzarulo (1991). The distribution of slow wave sleep across the night: a comparison for infants, children and adults. *Sleep, 14,* 5–12.

Borbély, Alexander A. (1982). A two process model of sleep regulation. *Human Neurobiology, 1,* 195–204.

Coons, Susan, & Christian Guilleminault (1982). Development of Sleep-Wake Patterns and Non-rapid Eye Movement Sleep Stage during the First Six Months of life in normal infants, *Pediatrics, 79,* 793–798.

Coons, Susan, & Christian Guilleminault (1984). Development of consolidated sleep and wakeful periods in relation to day/night cycle in infancy. *Developmental Medicine of Child Neurology, 26,* 169–176.

Daan, Serge, Domien G.M. Beersma & Alexander A. Borbély (1984). Timing of human sleep: recovery process gated by a circadian pacemaker. *American Journal of Physiology, 246*: R161–R178.

Dreyfus-Brisac, Colette (1970). Ontogenesis of sleep in human prematures after 32 weeks of conceptional age. *Developmental Psychobiology, 3,* 91–121.

Fagioli, Igino, Frederik Bes & Piero Salzarulo (1988). 24-hour behavioural states distribution in continuously fed infants. *Early Human Development, 18,* 151–156.

Fagioli, Igino, Frederik Bes, Patricio Peirano & Piero Salzarulo (1995). Dynamics of EEG background activity level within quiet sleep in successive cycles in infants, *Electroencephalography and clinical Neurophysiology, 94,* 6–11.

Fagioli, Igino, Claude Ricour, Françoise Salomon & Piero Salzarulo (1981a). Weight changes and sleep organization in infants. *Early Human Development, 5,* 395–399.

Fagioli, Igino, Françoise Salomon & Piero Salzarulo (1981b). L'endormissement chez l'enfant en nutrition continue depuis la naissance: enregistrements de vingt-quatre heures, *Revue E.E.G. Neurophysiologie, 11,* 37–44.

Fagioli, Igino, & Piero Salzarulo (1982). Sleep States Development in the first year of life assessed through 24-hour recordings. *Early Human Development, 6*: 215–228.

Fagioli, Igino, & Piero Salzarulo (1985). Behavioural states and development of the circadian periodicity of heart rate, in P. Koella, E. Rüther & H. Schulz (Eds), *Sleep 1984* (287–289). Stuttgart–New York: Gustav Fischer Verlag.

Fagioli, Igino, & Piero Salzarulo (1997). Dynamics of EEG background activity level during quiet sleep in multiple nocturnal sleep episodes in infants. *Electroencephalography and clinical Neurophysiology, 103,* 6–11.

Feinberg, Irwin (1974). Changes in sleep cycle pattern with age, *Journal of Psychiatry Research, 10,* 283–306.

Ficca, Gianluca, Igino Fagioli, Fiorenza Giganti & Piero Salzarulo (1999). Spontaneous awakenings from sleep in across the first year of age. *Early Human Development, 55,* 219–228.

Ficca, Gianluca, Igino Fagioli & Piero Salzarulo (2000a). Sleep organisation in the first year of life: Developmental trend in quiet sleep–paradoxical sleep cycle. *Journal of Sleep Research, 9,* 1–4.

Ficca, Gianluca, Pasquale Lombardo, Luigi Rossi & Piero Salzarulo (2000b). Morning recall of verbal material depends on prior sleep organization. *Behavioral Brain Research, 112,* 159–163.

Giganti, Fiorenza, Igino Fagioli, Gianluca Ficca & Piero Salzarulo (2001). Polygraphic investigation of 24-hour waking distribution in infants. *Physiology and Behaviour, 73*: 621–624.

Haustein, Werner, June Pilcher, Joakim Klink & Hartmut Schulz (1986). Automatic analysis overcomes limitations of sleep stage scoring. *Electroencephalography and clinical Neurophysiology, 64,* 364–374.

Hellbrugge, Theodore (1960). The development of circadian rhythms in infants. *Cold Spring Harbor Symposium of Quantitative Biology, 25,* 311–323.

Hoppenbrouwers, Toke, Joan Hodgman, Kazuko Arakawa, Sue Ann Geidel & M.B. Sterman (1988). Sleep and waking states in infancy: normative studies. *Sleep, 11,* 387–401.

Kleitman, Nathaniel (1963). *Sleep and wakefulness.* 2nd ed. Chicago: The University Press.

Lavie, Peretz (1986). Ultrashort sleep-waking schedule. III "Gates" and "Forbidden zones" for sleep. *Electroencephalography and clinical Neurophysiology, 63,* 414–425.

Louis, Jacqueline, Christine Cannard, Hélène Bastuji & Marie-Josèphe Challamel (1997). Sleep ontogenesis revisited: a longitudinal 24-hour home polygraphic study on 15 normal infants during the first two years of life. *Sleep, 20*: 323–333.

Mazzoni, Giuliana, Sara Gori, Giuliana Formicola, Carlo Gneri, Roberto Massetani, Luigi Murri & Piero Salzarulo (1999). Word recall correlates with sleep cycles in elderly subjects. *Journal of Sleep Research, 8*,185–188.

Mirmiran, Majid, & J.H. Kok (1991). Circadian rhythms in early human development. *Early Human Development*, 26, 121–128.

Monod, Nicole, & Lilia Curzi-Dascalova (1973). Les états transitionnels de sommeil chez le nouveau-né à terme. *Revue EEG Neurophysiologique, 3*, 87–96.

Navelet, Yvonne, Odile Benoit & Ginette Bouard (1982). Nocturnal sleep organization during the first months of life, *Electroencephalography and clinical Neurophysiology, 54*, 71–78.

Parmelee, Arthur H., Waldemar H. Wenner & Helen R. Schulz (1964). Infant sleep patterns from birth to 16 weeks of age. *Journal of Pediatrics, 65*, 576–582.

Pollak, Charles P. (1994). Regulation of sleep rate and circadian consolidation of sleep and wakefulness in an infant, *Sleep, 17*, 567–575.

Prechtl, Heinz F.R. (1974). The behavioural states of the newborn infant (a Review), *Brain Research, 76*, 185–212.

Prechtl, Heinz F.R., & Michael J. O'Brien (1982). Behavioural states of the full-term newborn. The emergence of a concept. In P. Stratton (Ed.), *Psychobiology of the Human Newborn* (53–73). New York: John Wiley and Sons, Ltd.

Salzarulo, Piero, & Igino Fagioli (1980). Waking-sleeping transition during human ontogenesis. In L. Popoviciu, B. Asgian, G. Badiu (Eds), *Sleep 1978* (29–35). Basel: Karger.

Salzarulo, Piero, & Igino Fagioli (1992a). Sleep-wake rhythms and sleep structure in the first year of life. In C. Stampi (Ed.), *Why we nap* (50–57). Boston: Birkhauser.

Salzarulo, Piero, & Igino Fagioli (1992b). Post-natal development of sleep organization in man: speculations on the emergence of the "S". *Neurophysiologie Clinique, 22*, 107–115.

Salzarulo, Piero, & Igino Fagioli (1995). Sleep for development or development for waking? – Some speculations from a human perspective. *Behavioral Brain Research, 69*, 23–27.

Salzarulo, Piero, & Igino Fagioli (1999). Changes of sleep states and physiological activities across the first year of life. In A.F. Kalverboer, M. L. Genta, J.B. Hopkins, (Eds), *Current issues in developmental biopsychology* (53–73). Dordrecht: Kluwer.

Salzarulo, Piero, Igino Fagioli & Fiorenza Giganti (1999). Organizzazione e disorganizzazione del sonno nel corso dello sviluppo. In A. Tartara, R. Manni, M.G. Terzano (Eds), *Il sonno in Italia 1998* (20–23). Milano: Poletto Edizioni.

Salzarulo, Piero, Igino Fagioli & Claude Ricour (1985). Long term continuously fed infants do not develop heart rate circadian rhythm, *Early Human Development, 12*, 285–289.

Salzarulo, Piero, Fiorenza Giganti, Gianluca Ficca, Igino Fagioli & Monica Toselli (2000). Gates to awakening in early development. *Clinical Neurophysiology, 53 Suppl.* Z. Ambler, S. Nevsimalova, Z. Kadanka, P.M. Rossini (Eds), 352–354.

Salzarulo, Piero, Giuliana Formicola, Pasquale Lombardo, Sara Gori, Luigi Rossi, Luigi Murri, & Carlo Cipolli (1997). Functional uncertainty, aging and memory processes during sleep. *Acta Neurologica Belgica, 97*, 118–122.

Schulz, Hartmut, Roberto Massetani, Igino Fagioli & Piero Salzarulo (1985). Spontaneous awakening from sleep in infants. *Electroencephalography and clinical Neurophysiology, 61*, 267–271.

Wehr, Thomas A. (1993). In short photoperiod, human sleep is biphasic, *Journal of Sleep Research, 1*, 103–107.

Wolff, Peter. H. (1984). Discontinuous changes in human wakefulness around the end of the second month of life; a developmental perspective. In H.F.R. Prechtl (Ed.), *Continuity of neural functions from pre-natal to post-natal life* (144–158). Oxford: Blackwell.

Zulley, Jurgen & David Carr (1993). Forced splitting of human sleep in free-running rhythms. *Journal of Sleep Research, 1*, 108–111.

Awakenings in school-age children

O. Bruni, S. Miano, E. Verrillo, S. Galiffa, and S. Ottaviano
Center for Pediatric Sleep Disorders, University "La Sapienza", Rome

Introduction

During development, sleep architecture shows dramatic modifications in different sleep parameters (sleep duration, distribution of sleep states, sleep states amount, stage-related sleep onset, etc.). Although several researches evaluated the polysomnographic aspects of sleep in infants and children, analysing the sleep architecture and researching for normative data (Schulz et al., 1985; Carskadon et al., 1987; Carskadon, 1992; Coble et al., 1987; Louis et al., 1997; Ficca et al., 1999), few studies have been carried out on spontaneous awakenings especially in school-age children. Spontaneous awakenings, lasting at least 2 minutes, during nocturnal sleep is a frequent event in early development, coinciding with a polyphasic sleep-wake rhythm (Ficca et al., 1999). Hoppenbrowers et al. (1988) presented normative data on infants and described more frequent nocturnal awakenings during the first 3 months of life. Giganti et al. (1999), in a preliminary study on pre-term infants, showed few changes in the number and duration of awakenings between 34 weeks and the term.

The developmental trend of awakenings is a decrease with age, continuing at slower rate until it reaches values not far from adulthood; then, the rate of awakenings increase again in elderly people (Ficca et al., 1998).

In infancy, most of the awakenings occur more frequently out of REM sleep like in young adults (Campbell, 1985; Ficca et al., 1999; Schultz et al., 1985) whereas in the elderly awakenings occur during Stage 2 NREM as well as in REM (Salzarulo et al., 1999). It is interesting to note that also the onset of sleep is the same: REM in the first year and Stage 2 NREM in the elderly (Salzarulo et al., 2000).

It has been demonstrated that infants awake preferentially out of REM sleep and less often out of non-REM sleep, even taking the proportion of sleep states into account. It is proposed that the specific desynchronized pattern of brain activity during REM sleep (similar to EEG pattern of wake) facilitates the transition from sleep into the waking state, particularly in the youngest infants (Schulz et al., 1985).

Ficca et al. (1999) studying 48 healthy infants in 4 age groups (from 1 to 54 weeks) confirmed that infants awake more often from REM than from quiet sleep (QS) but showed that this difference tend to reduce in older infants. The absolute number of awakenings per night in the whole sample was 6.8 (2.0 out of quiet sleep, 4.0 out of REM sleep and 0.8 out of ambiguous sleep). In the older age group the mean number of awakenings was 4.9 (1.8 out of quiet sleep, 2.8 out of REM sleep and 0.2 out of ambiguous sleep).

Another interesting result was that awakenings out of QS were followed by longer periods of wakefulness than those out of REM sleep. The duration of the bouts of wakefulness following awakenings remained stable with age all along the first year of life. In the two younger groups, the distribution of the awakenings showed two main peaks and one main peak differently located during the night; a polymodal pattern appears in older infants. Further, since in infants successive sleep bouts have a similar internal architecture, night sleep interruptions may represent "final awakenings" of each sleep bout, that corresponds to a periodicity which is around 100 minutes by the end of the first year of life (Ficca et al., 1999).

It is possible that the process underlying awakenings in infancy and elderly is different. In the first year of life sleep is still unstable and homeostatic factors and circadian drive are not completely consolidated; further, specific pattern of brain activity during REM sleep facilitates the transition from sleep to the waking state (Schulz et al., 1985; Ficca et al., 1999). In the elderly, instead, the increase of awakenings reflects a sleep disorganization with prolonged wakefulness after sleep onset (Salzarulo et al., 1999).

It is very difficult to find data on awakenings in older children and especially in school-aged ones. Since it has been always considered the period of more stable sleep, it has been often ignored by researchers. Recently some Authors underlined the necessity to study sleep in school-age children, because it could be associated with several important factors for children quality of life as low school performances, behavior disorders, socioeconomic difficulties (Rona et al., 1998; Owens et al., 2000; Paavonen et al., 2000). They use either objective or subjective instruments to evaluate sleep in school-age: subjective measures (questionnaires, sleep diaries, interviews) have focused on observable aspects of sleep, but problems as nocturnal awakenings may escape notice, while objective measures, as polysomnography, actigraphy and video, capture more information about them; however studies through objective measure of spontaneous awakenings in school-age children are very rare.

Studies using subjective instruments

In a longitudinal study, frequent nocturnal awakenings were reported in 14% of children at 6 years of age and in 8% at 8 years (Klackenberg, 1971). Salzarulo and Chevalier (1983) found a prevalence of awakenings in a sample of children between 6–10 years of 23.5%, using interview and questionnaire.

A study using the Children's Sleep Behavior Scale found that 14.9% of children under 8.5 years, 11,6% between 8.5 and 11.5 years, and 6.2% over 11.5 year, were reported by parents to wake up six times or more in the previous 6-months period (Fisher et al., 1989).

Kahn reported a prevalence of poor sleep in 14% of elementary school children, considering a poor sleeper a child with awakenings lasting more than 30 minutes in a night, for at least 2 times/week, and associated with a shorter duration of total sleep. This prevalence of insomnia is unexpectedly strong in the preadolescent latency age and it is similar to that of children aged 2–4 (Kahn et al., 1989).

In our previous questionnaire-based study on a sample of 6–14 aged children, we found that nocturnal awakenings (>2 per night for at least 2 time a week) were present in 6.9% of cases (Bruni et al., 1994).

In another research on children aged 5 to 12 years, prevalence of awakenings, for more than 3 nights per week, was 6.5% (Blader et al., 1997).

In an epidemiological Swedish study of 5–8-year-old children, 15.5 % of the children had nocturnal awakenings at least 3 nights per week (Smedje et al., 1999), with a persistence of these disorders in 47.4 % of the children after 14 months (Smejde, 2000) confirming Klackenberg's (1971) findings.

Paavonen et al. (2000) reported a prevalence of nocturnal awakenings in 8–9 aged children of 7%.

Owens et al. (2000) considered the presence of an awakening during the night followed by co-sleeping or waking 1 or more times per night; they found a prevalence of insomnia in 6.7 % of children between 4–11 years and they also noted a higher frequency of nocturnal awakenings reported by older children vs. parents (14.6% vs. 4.6%).

Although different methodologies of collecting data had been employed in the different abovementioned researches, almost all recent studies agreed on a percentage of nocturnal awakenings of about 7%, showing that, even in the age considered as the "gold standard for sleep quality", awakenings are still present.

Studies using objective instruments

Despite the increase of polysomnographic applications on children sleep, the number of normative data published on school children are relatively small. Data on spontaneous awakenings in school age children, based on polygraphic recordings, are rare and dealing with single aspects of wakefulness during sleep.

Coble et al. (1987) collected and analysed polysomnographic reports on a sample of 43 latency-aged children (6–12 yr, 21 males e 22 females). Children were predominantly Caucasian and from middle and upper class families, they were scheduled to sleep for 3 consecutive week nights during school year. The mean duration of awake time was 8.2 minutes in 6–7 years aged children, of 4.3 minutes in 8–9 years aged, of 3.7 minutes in 10–11 years aged; number of arousals was 3.2 at 6–7 yr, 4.7 at 8–9 yr and 3.8 at 10–11 yrs. The time spent asleep showed a steady decline with increasing age from 9 hours and 30 minutes to 9 hours and 8 hours respectively, whereas specific measures of sleep continuity remains constant, with high sleep efficiency of 95% in all children (Coble et al., 1987).

Sleep of 16 preadolescent children were analysed in 3 consecutive nights, polysomnographic data reported a mean duration of wake after sleep onset of 12 minutes for males and 16 for females, with a number of arousals of 5.2 and 3.6 respectively (Carskadon et al., 1987).

In another group of prepubertal to adolescent children it has been found that wake after sleep onset was 28 minutes in the first day, 11 minutes in the second day and 16 minutes in the third day (Carskadon, 1992).

From these normative data we cannot evaluate the frequency of spontaneous awakenings but only the polysomnographic parameters of wake after sleep onset and of number of arousals.

To our knowledge, no systematic studies on the features of awakenings in school age children have been carried out.

A contribution to awakenings in school-aged children (Personal study)

Although the sleep of the school-aged children has been considered as the "gold standard" of sleep quality (Carskadon et al., 1987) because of its length, continuity and restorative features, either objective and subjective studies have demonstrated that awakenings are still present in this period of age. Since no polysomnographic researches have been carried out on awakenings in this age group, we evaluated the characteristics of spontaneous awakenings in this age group through night polysomnography.

Material and method

We retrospectively analysed the polysomnograms of 19 healthy children (11 M; 8 F; mean age 10 years and 7 months; range 6.2–13.6 yrs) used as control group for a previous study. They underwent a polysomnographic study (PSG) in the Sleep Laboratory of our Department after a one night adaptation.

Two or four EEG channels (C4-A1, C3-A2, O1-A2 and O2-A1), left and right electro-oculograms, chin EMG, EKG, respiratory flow, abdominal respiratory effort and oxygen saturation were used for scoring sleep and rule out respiratory disorders. Gold-plated surface electrodes were applied to the scalp using the collodium technique according to the International 10–20 System.

Sleep recordings were started at the habitual patients' bedtime and continued until spontaneous awakening.

Records were visually scored in 30 seconds epochs according to the standard criteria of Rechtschaffen and Kales.

Awakenings were polygraphically identified by a combination of electrophysiological and behavioral signals and considered if followed by four epochs of wakefulness (2 minutes) and the preceding period analysed was 5 minutes of stable sleep.

The decision to set the minimum duration interval for awakening computation at 2 min is derived from Salzarulo et al. (1999) according to Garma et al. (1981) and it is exactly the same as the criterion used by Schulz et al. (1985) with groups of younger subjects.

In order to study the characteristics of the awakenings, the following variables were evaluated:

a. nocturnal distribution of intra-night awakenings
b. duration of intra-night awakenings

c. preceding sleep stages of intra-night awakenings
d. preceding sleep stages of final awakening
e. awakening/stage ratio (number of awakenings/time spent in each single stage)
f. sleep stages following the awakenings
g. mean duration of awakenings per stages
h. duration of sleep stages preceding the awakenings
i. effects of the preceding sleep state on the duration of awakenings
j. awakening recurrence time (the time interval between the occurrence of one awakening and that of the following one). The same procedure was adopted to determine the recurrence time for awakenings out of each sleep state.

Statistical analysis. A frequency analysis was performed in order to evaluate the distribution of awakenings per sleep stages. A chi-square test was used to assess differences in the distribution of awakenings between first second and third part of the night.

To assess the effect of the length of sleep stage preceding awakenings on the duration of the awakening a Spearman correlation analysis was carried out.

A univariate analysis with one-way ANOVA was used to evaluate the role of the sleep state preceding the awakenings, mainly the effects of part of the night and the preceding sleep stage on the duration of the bouts of wakefulness following awakenings and the effects of part of the night on the recurrence time of awakening.

For these purposes we use the criteria used by Schulz et al. (1985): in order to exclude differences in the frequency of awakenings from being a mere by-product of differences in the relative length of sleep states, a ratio of the number of awakenings in a given sleep state to the overall duration of that state throughout the night was calculated and was named awakening index.

All statistical analyses were performed on a personal computer using the commercially available package program Statistica (TM) (Statsoft Inc., Tulsa, OK).

Results

Absolute number of awakenings and relationship with sleep stages

A total of 50 awakenings were recorded, with a mean number of awakenings per subject equal to 2,6 (range 1–5). Each subject presented at least 1 awakening per night; 11 subjects had 1–2 awakenings and 8 subjects had 3–5 awakenings.

The main sleep stage preceding intra-night awakenings was stage 2NREM (31 awakenings = 62%); a lower number of awakenings raised from stage 3–4NREM (10 awakenings = 20%) and less awakenings occurred out of stage REM (6 awakenings = 12%) or 1NREM (3 awakenings = 6%). The main sleep stage following awakenings was stage 1NREM (44 = 88%), stage 2NREM (5 = 10%) and stage REM (1 = 2%).

Final awakenings were preceded by stage 2NREM in 10 cases (52.6%), by stage 1NREM in 5 (26.3%), by stage 3–4NREM in 2 (10.5%) and by stage REM in the remaining 2 subjects (10.5%).

Overnight distribution of awakenings

The overnight distribution of all awakenings showed that there is one main peak of awakenings between midnight and 1 AM and a lower plateau from 3 to 5 am (Fig. 1).

Nocturnal timing of awakenings in relation to preceding sleep stage (Fig. 2) showed a non-specific distribution of awakenings with no significant differences between first, second and third part of the night (chi-square = 9.27; $p = 0.16$). Although there was a trend toward a decrease of number of awakenings during the night, the relative percentage showed that awakenings out of 3–4 NREM are mostly represented in the first and third part of the night and 1 NREM in the second part of the night, while awakenings out of stage 2NREM and stage REM showed a non-specific distribution.

Awakening/stage ratio

The awakening/stage ratio (number of awakenings in a given sleep stage/total duration of the same stage) was 0.0057 for Total Sleep Time, 0.0049 for NREM1; 0.0085 for NREM2, 0.0041 for NREM3–4 and 0.0043 for REM, demonstrating that stage 2NREM predisposed to awakening in this age group.

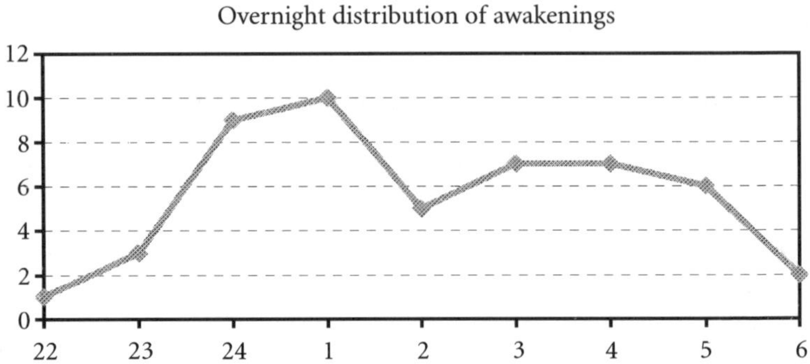

Figure 1. Distribution of awakenings through the night (on x axis time in hours, on y axis absolute number of awakenings for each hour).

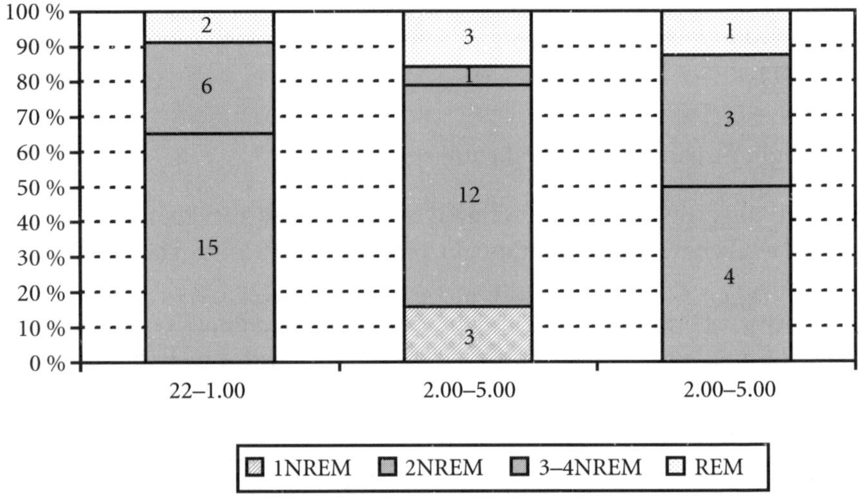

Figure 2. Overnight distribution of awakenings per stage represented as percentage for each third of the night.

Mean duration of awakenings

Mean duration of wakefulness following awakenings was 6.21 minutes; the length remained stable during the night (Table 1) with only a slight decrease in the third part of the night. Statistical analysis did not show significant effect of the part of the night on the duration of awakenings ($F = 0.56$; $p = 0.57$).

The preceding sleep stages affected the duration of the wakefulness following awakenings (Table 2): if 3–4NREM preceded awake, the event lasted more

Table 1. Mean (SD) duration in minutes of awakenings according to part of the night

	N° of awakenings	Duration
First	23	6.78 (3.9)
Second	19	6.1 (5.7)
Third	8	4.81 (2.45)
Whole night	50	6.21 (4.51)

Table 2. Mean (SD) duration in minutes of awakenings according to preceding sleep stage

	N° of awakenings	Duration
Stage NREM 1	3	4.33 (0.58)
Stage NREM 2	31	6.10 (4.0)
Stage NREM 3-4	10	9.20 (6.15)*
Stage REM	6	2.76 (1.17)

* stage 3–4NREM vs. stage REM; $p < 0.005$

than if REM or NREM 1 or 2 preceded it. The duration of wakefulness increased progressively with the depth of NREM sleep with lower length if awakenings followed REM sleep ($F = 3.19$; $p = 0.032$) with a significant effect of stage 3–4NREM vs. REM ($p = 0.005$).

Recurrence time of awakenings

Mean recurrence time of awakenings during the whole night was 118 (SD 113) minutes. Considering the timing of appearance of awakenings from the sleep onset, it was 158 (SD 127) minutes for the first awakening, 221 (SD 121) minutes for the second awakening and 234 (SD 78) for the third awakening.

Analyzing the recurrence time as interval between the first 3 consecutive awakenings, in the 8 subjects presenting 3 or more awakenings, we found that the recurrence time for the first awakening was 94 minutes (SD 19.15), for the second awakening was 40 minutes (SD 38.68) and for the third awakening was 126 (SD 109.65). The difference was not statistically significant ($F = 3.27$; $p = 0.06$), indicating that there could be a periodicity in the appearance of awakenings.

Also, the duration of the awakenings was similar in all the first three awakenings (respectively 7.61; 7 and 6.68 minutes) considered ($F = 0.06$; $p = 0.94$).

In the eleven subjects with 1–2 awakenings the recurrence time of the first awakening was 181 minutes (SD 153.7).

Table 3. Mean (SD) recurrence time in minutes of awakenings according to part of the night

	N° of awakenings	Recurrence time
First	23	66.26 (49.76)
Second	19	123.16 (113.22)
Third	8	254.63 (137.25)
Whole night	50	118.02 (113.25)

Splitting the night sleep into three parts (1st, 2nd and 3rd of the night) we found that the mean recurrence time of awakenings showed a trend toward a progressive increase of the time between awakenings (Table 3) with a significant effect of the third part of the night vs. the first and the second part ($F = 11.91$; $p = 0.000065$).

In order to evaluate if the length of sleep stage preceding awakenings correlated with the duration of the awakening, we performed a Spearman correlation between the duration of wakefulness following awakenings and the duration of the preceding sleep stages that failed to show significant relationship ($r = 0.06$; $p = 0.64$).

Different structural characteristics of stages preceding awakenings

The analysis of the 5 minutes of stable sleep preceding the awakenings showed differences related to the preceding stage (Fig. 3): stage 2NREM were characterized by burst of phasic events (K complex+spindles or K-alpha), periodic EMG bursts or even periodic limb movements, when recorded. On the contrary no phasic activity (either EEG or EMG) were recorded from stage 4NREM or REM. Stages 1NREM preceding awakenings lasted less than 5 minutes and were therefore not considered.

Discussion

To our knowledge, our study is the first to analyse the awakenings in school-age children. Evaluating the absolute number of awakenings, our data agreed with the developmental trend of awakenings' decrease with age, as shown by studies of infants and younger children (Hoppenbrouwers et al., 1987; Louis et al., 1997 and Ficca et al., 1999). Overnight distribution of awakenings showed a peak between midnight and 1 AM and seemed to confirm the clinical impression and the parental report that first awakening often happen about 1h 30m–

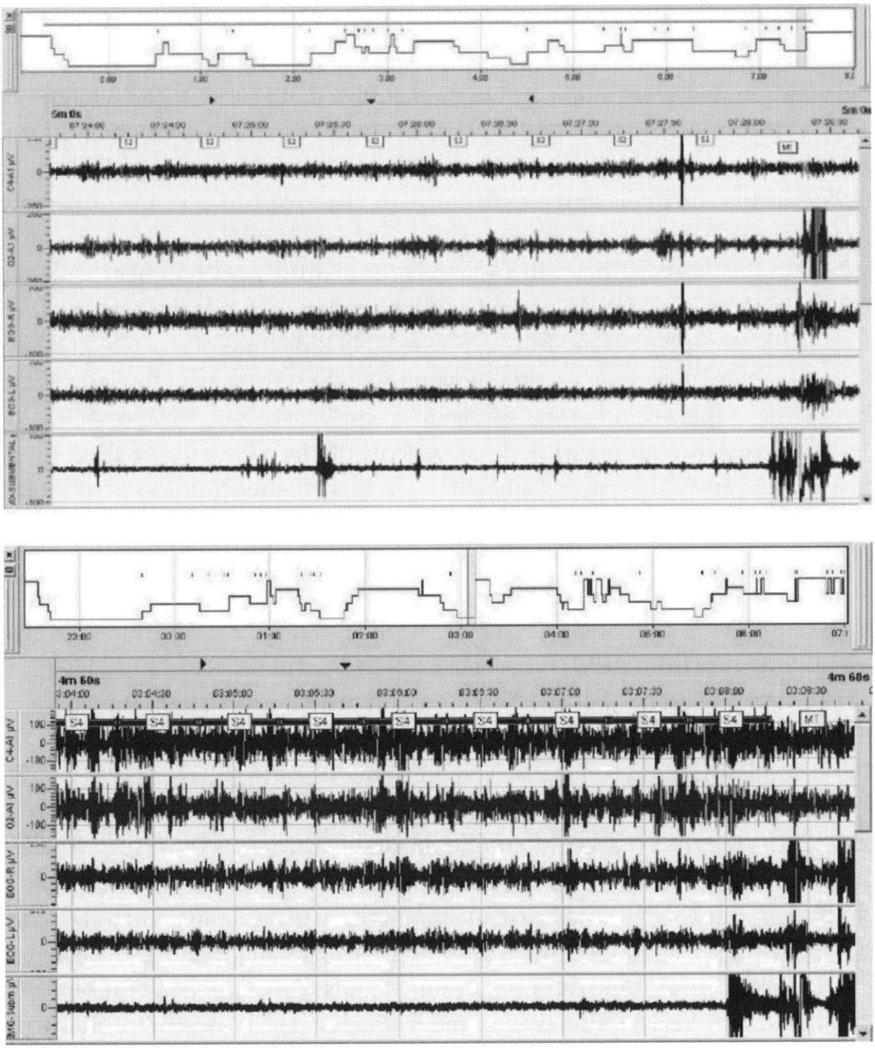

Figure 3. Example of 5 minutes recording of stage 2NREM (upper) and of stage 4NREM (lower) preceding awakenings. The stage 2NREM is characterzied by bursts of phasic events (K complex+spindles or K-alpha) and periodic EMG bursts, while stage 4NREM is more stable without phasic activity (either EEG or EMG).

2h after the sleep onset, since the bedtime in pre-school children (about 21.43 for 3–6 years old children: Ottaviano et al., 1996) and school age children in Italy (21.49 at 9–10 years; 21.53 at 11–12 years; 22.09 at 13–14 years: Bruni et al., 1994) is later than in other European countries and we can correctly assume that the timing of awakenings around 00–1AM of our sample could correspond to the timing of awakenings of normal population. Further, we can hypothesize that there is a "gate" to awakenings that is about 90–120 minutes after the sleep onset. The timing of occurrence of the first awakening in our sample could be related to the periodicity of 100 minutes found by Ficca et al. (1999) by the end of the first year of life; in our sample, however, the recurrence time of awakenings failed to show a such clear periodicity.

Since the decrease in number of awakenings during development is mainly related to those out of REM sleep, it could be expected that at this age, in which the NREM components are fully expressed, NREM could play a role in determining awakenings. Our results, showing a higher propensity to awake from NREM sleep (particularly stage 2), seems to confirm this expectation.

The transformation, with development, of the modality of sleep onset (from REM to NREM sleep) and the functional maturation of sleep leading to the maximal expression of NREM sleep in the school-age, could explain the propensity to awake spontaneously out of NREM sleep.

It should be underlined that the propensity to awake from NREM sleep was higher in middle chilhood and in elderly while infants and adults have prevalent awakenings from REM (Ficca et al., 1999; Salzarulo et al., 1999). This alternating trend could be explained with the increase of cyclic alternating pattern (CAP) rate typical of these two period of life (Parrino et al., 1998; Bruni et al., 2001) configuring an U-shaped curve from childhood to elderly. CAP is a physiological component of normal NREM sleep with maximal expression during stage 2NREM and a marker of arousal instability during NREM sleep. The increase of CAP rate (and, consequently, of arousal instability) during middle childhood and elderly could explain the higher susceptibility to awake from NREM. Unfortunately, no studies about CAP rate in infancy are available.

The mean awakening duration in our sample is shorter than that reported in infants (6.21 vs. 18 minutes reported by Ficca et al., 1999) and could correspond to the process of consolidation of sleep that lead to a global reduction in awakenings, to a shortening of the bouts of wakefulness after awakenings out of QS and to a higher propensity to sleep again after a sleep interruption.

The only factor we found to affect the mean duration of wakefulness following awakenings was the preceding sleep stage: the duration of wakefulness increased progressively with the depth of NREM sleep with lower length if awakenings followed respectively REM sleep or stage 1 or 2NREM.

Some Authors speculated that awakenings out of QS reflect an interruption of the sleep episode, before completing a sleep cycle and therefore subjects could have more difficulty in falling asleep again and present longer bouts of wakefulness after awakenings out of QS (Salzarulo & Fagioli, 1992).

Since the duration of awakenings was not affected by the third of the night considered, we can hypothesize that the longer wakefulness following awakenings out of Slow Wave Sleep, is not dependent on the homeostatic component of sleep regulation 'S process' (Dijk et al., 1999), but is stage related and other ultradian components, related to sleep microstructure, could be implicated. Moreover, the analysis of sleep microstructure could elucidate the different mechanisms leading to awakenings out of different stages; visual analysis showed some differences in the five minutes of stable stage 2NREM and stage 3–4NREM leading to awakening. The differences are in terms of phasic activity with periodic EMG bursts and K complex+spindles in stage 2 NREM while no phasic activity (either EEG or EMG) were recorded from stage 4NREM or REM. We can hypothesize that stage 2NREM "prepares" the homeostatic mechanism to the event awakening, while the exit from the stage 3–4NREM is not "prepared", it is abrupt. This could explain why the duration of wakefulness after an awakening from stage 3–4NREM is longer than after the other stages.

During development, different psychophysiological processes could determine the changes in the awakenings pattern (Ficca et al., 1999; Salzarulo et al., 1999): in infants, the high number and the short duration of awakenings could be expression of the polyphasic sleep-wake rhythm; in the elderly, instead, spontaneous awakenings seem to be the expression of a disorganization of sleep.

In school age children, the arousability changes and also the intrinsic mechanism that leads to awakenings, with a progressive change in sleep organization that modifies the propensity to the arousal and awakenings.

References

Blader, J.C., H.S. Koplewicz, H. Abikoff & C. Foley (1997). Sleep problems of elementary school children: A community survey. *Archives of Pediatric and Adolescent Medicine, 151*, 473–480.

Bruni, O., M. Romoli, M. Innocenzi, F. Cortesi, F. Giannotti & S. Ottaviano (1994). Prevalenza dei disturbi del sonno in età scolare. In Di Perri R., M. Raffaele, L. Silvestri & S. Smirne (Eds), *Il Sonno in Italia* (163–171). Poletto edizioni.

Bruni, O., R. Ferri, G. Della Marca, B. Farina, S. Miano, E. Verrillo, G. Mennuni & S. Ottaviano. Analysis of sleep microstructure through Cyclic Alternating Pattern in school age children. *Sleep, 24*: A200, 2001.

Campbell, S.S. (1985). Spontaneous termination of a libitum sleep episodes with special reference to REM sleep. *Electroenchephalography and Clinical Neurophysiology, 60,* 237–242.

Carskadon, M., S. Keenan & W.C. Dement (1987). Nighttime sleep and daytime sleep tendency in preadolescents. In Guilleminault C. (Ed.), *Sleep and its disorders in children* (43–52). New York, Raven Press.

Carskadon M. (1982). The second decade. In: Guilleminault C. (Ed.), *Sleeping and waking disorders: indications and techniques* (99–125). California: Addison-Wesley.

Coble, P.A., D.J. Kupfer, C.F. Reynolds III & P. Houck (1987). EEG sleep of healthy children 6 to 12 years of age. In C. Guilleminault (Ed.), *Sleep and its disorders in children* (29–40). New York, Raven Press.

Dijk, D.J. & J.F. Duffy (1999). Circadian regulation of human sleep and age-related changes in its timing, consolidation and EEG characteristics. *Annals of Medicine, 31*: 130–140.

Ficca, G., S. Gori, I. Fagioli & P. Salzarulo (1998). Awakenings across the life span. *Journal of Sleep Research, 7* (suppl. 2): 87.

Ficca, G., I. Fagioli, F. Giganti & P. Salzarulo (1999). Spontaneous awakening from sleep in the first year of life. *Early Human Development, 55,* 219–228.

Fisher, B.E., C. Pauley & K. McGuire (1989). Children's sleep behavior scale: normative data on 870 children in grades 1 to 6. *Perceptual Motor Skills, 68,* 227–236.

Garma, L., G. Bouard & O. Benoit (1981). Age et insomnie: parts respectives du nombre et de la durée des éveils. *Revue EEG Neurophysiologie, 11*: 96–101.

Giganti, F., G. Ficca, E. Biagioni, G. Cioni, M.T. Puliti, I. Fagioli & P. Salzarulo (1999). Awakenings in pre-term and near-term infants. *Sleep Research Online, 2*: 201.

Hoppenbrouwers, T., J. Hodgman, K. Arakawa, S.A. Geidel & M.B. Sterman (1988). Sleep and wakings states in infancy ; normative studies. *Sleep,* 11: 387–401.

Kahn, A., C. Van de Merckt, E. Rebuffat, M.J. Mozin, M. Sottiaux, D. Blum & P. Hennart (1989). Sleep problems in healthy preadolescents, *Pediatrics, 84*(3): 542–546.

Klackenberg, G. (1971). A prospective longitudinal study of children. Data on psychic health and development up to 8 years of age. *Acta Paediatrica Scandinavica, 224*: 1–239.

Louis, J., C. Cannard, H. Bastuji & M.J. Challamel (1997). Sleep ontogenesis revisited: a longitudinal 24-hour home polygraphic study on 15 normal infants during the first two years of life. *Sleep, 20*: 323–333.

Ottaviano, S., F. Giannotti, F. Cortesi , O. Bruni & C. Ottaviano (1996). Sleep characteristics in healthy children from birth to 6 years of age in the urban area of Rome. *Sleep, 19*(1): 1–3.

Owens, J.A., A. Spirito, M. McGuinn & C. Nobile (2000). Sleep habits and sleep disturbance in elementary school-aged children, *Journal of Development and Behavioral Pediatrics, 21*: 27–36.

Paavonen, E.J., E.T. Aronen, I. Moilanen, J. Piha, E. Rasanen, T. Tamminen & F. Almqvist (2000). Sleep problems of school-aged children. A complementary view, *Acta paediatrica, 89*: 223–228.

Parrino, L., M. Boselli, M.C. Spaggiari, A. Smerieri & M.G. Terzano (1998). Cyclic Alternating Pattern (CAP) in normal sleep: polysomnographic parameters in different age groups. *Electroenchephalography and Clinical Neurophysiology, 107*: 439–450.

Rona, R.J., L. Li, M.C. Guillford & S. Chinn (1998). Disturbed sleep: effects of sociocultural factors and illness, *Archives of Disease in Childhood, 78*: 20–25.

Salzarulo, P & I. Fagioli (1992). Sleep-wake rhythms and sleep structure in the first year of life. In: Stampi C. (Ed.), *Why We Nap* (50–57). Boston: Birkhauser.

Salzarulo, P. & A. Chevalier (1983). Sleep problems in children and their relationship with early disturbances of the waking-sleeping rhythms, *Sleep*, *6*: 47–51.

Salzarulo, P., I. Fagioli, P. Lombardo, S. Gori, C. Gneri, R. Chiaramonti & L. Murri (1999). Sleep stages preceding spontaneous awakenings in the elderly, *Sleep Research Online*, *2*: 73–77.

Salzarulo, Piero, Fiorenza Giganti, Gianluca Ficca, Igino Fagioli & Monica Toselli (2000). Gates to awakening in early development. *Clinical Neurophysiology, 53*, S352–S354.

Schulz, H., R. Massetani, I. Fagioli & P. Salzarulo (1985). Spontaneous awakening from sleep in infants. *Electroenchephalography and Clinical Neurophysiology*, *61*(4): 267–271.

Smedje, H., J.E. Broman & J. Hetta (2000). A short-term prospective study of five sleep disturbances in a sample of 614 latency children: sleep and behaviour at follow-up. In Smedje H. (Ed.), *Nighttime sleep and daytime behaviour in children.* Uppsala University.

Smedje, H., J.E. Broman & J. Hetta (1999). Parents report of disturbed sleep in 5–7-year-old Swedish children. *Acta Paediatrica,* 88: 858–865.

Awakenings, sleep–wake cycle and thermal environment in neonates

Véronique Bach, Frédéric Telliez, Lenzi Pierluigi, Karen Chardon, André Leke, and Jean-Pierre Libert
Faculty of Medicine, University of Picardy, Amiens, France / Department of Human and General Physiology, University of Bologna, Italy / Department of Neonatology, Pediatry II, University Hospital, Amiens, France

Arousal is considered to be an important response to a life-threatening stimulus. Less waking, more sleep, reduced motility (Schechtman et al., 1992) and an increased arousal threshold are found in victims of Sudden Infant Death Syndrome (SIDS) when compared with controls. Furthermore, during active sleep (AS), there is a temporary arousal deficit from 2 to 4 months of age, which could explain the peak incidence of SIDS observed at this age (Newman et al., 1989). As assumed by Hunt (1989) and more recently by Harper et al. (2000), an impairment in arousal responsiveness – probably as a result of deficits originating in fetal life – may be necessary (but not sufficient) for SIDS to occur. There is a need for a trigger factor – for example a respiratory challenge – which would be harmless if arousal occurs, but could be lethal otherwise. As a result, various factors likely to produce apnea or asphyxia (such as a prone position, a covered head...) superimposed on an underlying arousal deficit could cause death. The same statement may hold for the conditions likely to lead to thermal imbalance (overheating, heavy wrapping, co-sleeping, fever...). Indeed, when neonates are exposed to a warm environment, the functional interaction between respiratory and thermoregulatory processes induces more frequent and longer apneas (Bader et al., 1998), while periodic respiration is increased, especially during AS (Berterottière et al., 1990).

There is no single, widely-accepted definition of arousal. There is probably a hierarchy of arousal phenomena. For example, arousal by tactile stimulation has been described by a sequence that commences with a spinal withdrawal reflex, is followed by brain stem responses (respiratory and "startle" responses), and ends in cortical arousal (McNamara et al., 1998). Arousal can be characterized by a brief increase of the electromyographic tone, increased sympathetic activity (heart rate increase, peripheral vasoconstriction, respiratory modification etc.) and electroencephalographic modifications, until sleep stage changes to full awakening. Similarly, in adults, transient activation phases have been described as concomitant and reversible electrophysiological modifications: short replacement of usual activities by fast frequency activities on EEGs, increase of muscular tone and occurrence of bursts of muscle potentials, heart rate increase, decrease in finger pulse amplitude, all of which are often accompanied by body movements (Schieber et al., 1971).

Various studies performed first in animals (and later in adults and neonates) have pointed out that sleep and thermoregulation are linked. Thermoregulatory capabilities differ according to the sleep stage and they are impaired during desynchronized sleep (Parmeggiani & Rabini, 1970). This could result from a transient and reversible inactivation of the hypothalamic nervous structures, so that the body temperature regulation becomes inefficient during this sleep stage – in contrast to synchronized sleep (Parmeggiani, 1988). Impairment of thermoregulatory processes during synchronized sleep leads to a conflict between the need for synchronized sleep and the maintenance of homeothermia.

In humans, this impairment is not as pronounced but thermoregulatory responses measured during rapid eye movement (REM) sleep are less efficient than those measured during non-REM sleep. REM sleep is thus depressed, and wakefulness is increased when sleeping in cool or warm environments.

In contrast, the neonate's thermoregulatory centers are operative during AS (review in Bach et al., 1996): the thermoregulatory response of the neonate persists and is usually assumed to be greater than that recorded during quiet sleep (QS) in fullterm (during the first week of life: Fleming et al., 1988; Stothers & Warner, 1984; Stothers & Warner, 1978; until 3 months: Azaz et al., 1992) as in a few-week-old preterm babies (Bach et al., 1994; Bach et al., 2000a; Darnall & Ariagno, 1982). Maintenance of the efficiency of homeothermic processes during AS protects the neonate from the long periods of ectothermy that would otherwise occur (Darnall & Ariagno, 1982), and/or from AS deprivation. This is of particular relevance since AS episodes can be of long duration and this sleep stage is involved in maturational processes of the central nervous system. Energy consumption (and therefore heat production) at thermoneutrality on one hand, and the relative efficiency of the thermoregulatory responses in a cold environment on the other, are greater during wakefulness when compared with AS in preterm babies (Darnall & Ariagno, 1982).

In neonates, in contrast to adult animals (and, partly, humans), the disruption or continuation of the sleep cycle cannot be described as an alternative between an endothermic and an ectothermic state, strictly speaking. However, sleep architecture, sleep continuity parameters, body movements, apneas etc. are disturbed by a cool exposure.

The present paper aims to review the alterations of sleep continuity in neonates sleeping in non-thermoneutral environments, i.e. where thermal responses against cold or warm exposures are requested. Several parameters describing wakefulness, body movements, sleep continuity, disruption, efficiency etc. will be considered since arousals, strictly speaking, have never been scored during thermal exposure. Most of the studies of the sleep-thermoregulation interaction have been performed in adults, and so results of that work will be presented here when there is no corresponding neonate data available. Indeed, it seems reasonable to suppose that sleep would also be disrupted in neonates or children in such conditions. Modifications in sleep architecture will also be briefly described, since they can be at the origin of changes in the reactivity of sleep and the arousal ability in response to other stimuli, endogenous or exogenous. Arousals following auditory (Newman et al., 1989) or head up tilting (Galland et al., 1998) stimulation are less frequent in QS when compared with AS.

Thermal parameters of the environment likely to alter sleep

Neonates are particularly at risk of cooling or overheating since body temperature changes are greater and more rapid than in adults. This results from disadvantageous morphological and physiological parameters such as the high value of the ratio of skin surface area to body volume, strong curvatures of body surface areas which imply larger convective heat loss coefficients, low skin thermal insulation and low metabolic heat production when expressed per unit body surface area.

However, neonates are able to maintain body homeothermia with efficient thermoregulatory processes, at least during short-term exposures. The first thermoregulatory responses to cool exposure are the adoption of a crouched position (thus reducing the body surface area exposed to the environment) and peripheral vasoconstriction. Heat production (expressed by oxygen consumption, $\dot{V}_{02}$) can also be increased by non-shivering thermogenesis and/or body activity. However, the efficiency of body activity in the maintenance of body homeothermia is still under debate, since heat production of muscles would only represent a small part of total energy expenditure: body activity can therefore be considered as a criterion describing discomfort in 2- to 3-week-old preterm neonates (Bach et al., 1994; Telliez et al., 1997a).

In warm environment, increased heat loss – mainly due to evaporative skin cooling and to respiratory water loss – can balance body heat gains.

Body heat storage results from heat transfers between the neonate and his surroundings via 4 channels i.e.: conduction (between the skin surface and any material in contact), convection (between the skin surface and air), radiation (between the skin surface and the facing surfaces) and evaporation from respiratory, transepidermal water loss and sweating. A low air temperature increases convective and evaporative heat losses, as does high air velocity, if skin temperatures are greater than the air temperature. Evaporative heat losses are lowered by increasing air water vapor pressure; this could lead to increased body heat storage if the air temperature is not concomitantly reduced. Finally, wall temperatures influence radiative heat losses. These parameters can directly or indirectly modify body heat storage, and therefore the thermal inputs from the cutaneous and internal thermoreceptors to the hypothalamic structures. As a consequence, air temperature, air velocity, air humidity and radiant temperature are likely to alter sleep patterns through changes in body heat storage.

Effect of air temperature level

Amongst the ambient parameters, the effects of air temperature on sleep have been the most studied. Short term and long-term exposures have been performed.

Acute thermal load

Neonate QS appears to be particularly sensitive to cool thermal stress, which induces partial or sometimes total QS deprivation (Fleming et al., 1988). Sleeping in a cool environment decreases the total duration of QS at the benefit of AS in fullterm (Fleming et al., 1988; Azaz et al., 1992) as well as in preterm neonates (Brück et al., 1962; Bach et al., 1994; Telliez et al., 1997 b; Telliez et al., 1998 a; Bach et al., 2000 a, 2001). Thus, neonates exposed to cool environment favor AS (consequently their body temperature regulation), leading to increased metabolic energy expenditure rather than energy conservation (energy conservation being greater during QS). This modification of QS and AS is less frequent in 3-month-old infants (Azaz et al., 1992).

Cool exposure has drastic effects on sleep continuity. Karlsson et al. (1995, 1996) reported more awakenings and body activity in preterm infants when the air temperature was decreased (as much as 4°C below thermoneutrality). The lower the air temperature, the more pronounced the disruption. In preterm neonates, total sleep time is reduced (Bach et al., 1994; Telliez et al., 1997b; Bach et al., 2000a, 2001) due to earlier final awakening (Bach et al., 2000a, 2001). Similarly, 3- and 4-month-old infants woke up earlier when lightly clad in cool rooms, though their body temperatures were not low (Wailoo et al., 1990). According to Azaz et al. (1992), increased wakefulness is associated with older neonates (3-month-old) and could be related to body activity, which increases at this age. The frequency of incomplete sleep cycles (AS → awakening, in contrast to a complete sleep cycle: AS → QS episode) is increased (Bach et al., 2001).

The pattern of QS episodes is also affected. In preterm neonates, QS episodes are less frequent (Telliez et al., 1997 b; Bach et al., 2000 a) and the longer QS episode becomes shorter (Bach et al., 2000 a). The decrease in the mean duration of QS episodes (Fleming et al., 1988) and the longer AS episodes seem to be specific to 1 week-old full-term neonates (Azaz et al., 1992). In contrast, 1- to 3-month-old neonates woke up more often. Similarly, an absence of significant changes in the mean duration of QS or AS episodes was observed in 3-week-old preterm neonates (Bach et al., 2001).

It is worthwhile noting that the effects of cold exposure on AS episodes differ according to the episode outcome (towards QS episode i.e. a complete sleep cycle, or towards wakefulness i.e. an incomplete sleep cycle): AS episodes followed by QS were shortened (-17 ± 28 min) and less frequent ($-0.004 \pm 0.015\ \text{min}^{-1}$), whereas AS episodes followed by wakefulness were lengthened ($+0.010 \pm 0.035\ \text{min}^{-1}$). The outcome of AS in neonates is not related to a specific value of body temperature at the time of sleep stage transition. In contrast, low body temperature at the beginning of the AS episode and/or a progressive rise in body temperature enhance the transition towards wakefulness (Bach et al., 2001).

When examining sleep continuity parameters, males seem to exhibit lower sleep quality and greater interindividual variability. However, this gender difference is not observed with respect to thermal stress (Bach et al., 2000b).

Body movements take part in the behavioural response to cold, and participate in the maintenance of homeothermia. They also reflect discomfort upon cool exposure, interrupt sleep continuity and can induce sleep stage changes or awakenings. Perlstein et al. (1974) observed increased body activity in preterm neonates sleeping in a cool environment. Azaz et al. (1992) reported increased body activity during cool exposure which often led to the infant waking up. Fleming et al. (1988) and Azaz et al. (1992) found increases in small body movements, which were more pronounced in 1 to 3-month old full-term babies than in younger ones, whatever the sleep stages. In preterm neonates, Bach et al. (1994) reported concomitant increases of the frequency and the mean duration of body movements, but only during AS, which is already characterized at thermoneutrality by larger duration and frequency of body movements. In disagreement with the above-cited results, Hey & O'Connell (1970) did not describe increased body movements in response to cooling.

Warm exposure disturbs sleep continuity and structure less than cold one. No modification of sleep structure is observed in a mild warm condition (Brück et al., 1962; Bach et al., 1994). Data referring to changes in body movements give conflicting results: in some neonates body movements are less frequent (Bach et al., 1994) whereas others (usually older and heavier newborns) become restless. However, in general, body movements seem to be less frequent whereas apneic episodes are longer and more frequent (Bach et al., 1994).

Awakening and diet thermic effect

Physiological strain of cool exposure can be altered by passive endogenous metabolic heat resulting from diet thermic effect. This effect corresponds to the thermic response to food ingestion. It consists in an obligatory component corresponding to the energy cost of digestion and processing of nutrients, and a facultative component mainly mediated by the sympathetic nervous system. It could be involved in the sleep-wake cycle through the thermoregulatory control of feeding that may occur in neonates (Himms-Hagen, 1995). According to this hypothesis, during interfeeding episodes, body temperature decreases to a level that activates the sympathetic nervous system: brown adipose tissue thermogenesis is activated, thus inducing a transient dip in blood glucose, which is at the origin of the initiation of a feeding episode.

As the diet thermic effect is an important component of body temperature maintenance between two feeding episodes (Mestyan et al., 1968), we can assume that time to the next meal (corresponding to the duration of sustained sleep) depends both on the previous meal (in terms of quality and quantity) and the ambient thermal environment: the lower the ambient temperature and/or the lower the diet thermic effect of the previous meal, the earlier the awakening, allowing the infant to attract his mother's attention. Therefore, the reduction of sleep time by earlier awakening observed during cool exposure (previously described) could be assumed to be an integral part of the behavioural response involved in spontaneous thermoregulatory feeding. The lowering of body temperature stimulates hypothalamic thermoregulatory centers, which respond by setting in motion a series of behavioural events that include arousal, crying, a nutritive suckling reflex and the ingestion of milk.

This hypothesis is reinforced by data comparing the effects of two different formulae in lipid supply (medium vs long chain triglycerides) on neonate sleep (Telliez et al., 1998b). The group of neonates characterized by a lower diet thermic effect woke earlier and thus reduced the sleep time between feeding episodes. As suggested by Wright et al. (1983), hunger may also be a cause of awakenings during the night.

Prolonged thermal load

Prolonged exposure to cool load improve resistance to this form of stress in preterm (Glass et al., 1968) as well as in full-term neonates (Perlstein et al., 1974). To our knowledge, only one study concerns thermal adaptation and sleep in neonates (Telliez et al., 1998a): it gave evidence of persistent sleep disturbances during a 75 hr-long cool exposure (1.5°C below thermoneutrality), i.e. as long as thermoregulatory processes are activated. QS duration remains at lower levels than during the first thermoneutral condition. Moreover, sleep continuity deteriorates as indicated by increasing percentage of wakefulness after sleep onset. In contrast, adaptive cool thermal responses appear: the metabolic heat production increases from the first to the last cool exposure.

During the subsequent recovery experimental condition (at thermoneutrality), wakefulness duration decreases while QS duration increases.

Recovery from a thermal load

To our knowledge, the after-effects of a thermal exposure – i.e. effects observed after having been exposed to cool or warm air temperatures – have never been studied in neonates.

In adults, a daytime heat load has been shown to have indirect effects on subsequent nighttime sleep (Bunnell et al., 1988; Di Nisi et al., 1989; Horne & Reid, 1985; Horne & Staff, 1983; Libert et al., 1991), if the delay between daytime exposure and bedtime is not sufficient for the elimination of the accumulated body heat (Bunnel et al., 1988). Increased SWS duration and number of sleep stage changes can be observed. The higher the body temperature at sleep onset, the greater the sleep alterations.

Effects of thermal transients

Decreased air temperature from 24–27°C to 18–21°C over about 20 min during QS induced preferential switchings into AS sleep – during which the metabolic response is more effective (full-term babies: Azaz et al., 1992; Fleming et al., 1988). This switching, accompanied by an increase in $\dot{V}_{02}$, is not observed when the energy production is greatly increased during the QS episode (+41%, (Fleming et al., 1988)). When this cooling occurred during an AS episode, half of the neonates did not enter QS. Few of the older infants (3-month-old) remained in the same sleep stage before and after the cooling process (Azaz et al., 1992).

During a heating period (progressive heating to achieve an increase of 5°C after 30 min), Tirosh et al. (1996) observed a significant decrease of the AS/QS ratio, whereas during the progressive cooling period (occurring 1 hr after the start of the heating period, i.e. in the same interfeeding interval), the ratio decreased in preterm neonates but increased in fullterm neonates. These results are difficult to interpret because of the possible bias due to the interfeeding interval distribution of AS and QS (a greater AS/QS ratio during the first part of the interval, later decreasing). This could over-ride the specific temperature effect. According to these authors, the preterm neonates responded more to a change of the air temperature rather than its absolute value: this might be attributed to maturational factors.

Certain authors have described the effects of air temperature instability on apneic attacks, which become more frequent in preterm neonates (Daily et al., 1969; Perlstein et al., 1970). In a clinical setting, it is therefore strongly recommended to adequately measure and control thermal conditions in incubators, since air temperature fluctuations of as little as 2°C are sufficient to induce thermal stress.

Air humidity level

To our knowledge, only one study has been performed on the effect of humidity on sleep in neonates (Telliez et al., 2001). The experiment was performed by reducing evaporative heat losses (an increase in air humidity from about 2 000 to 4 000 Pa water vapor pressure) and increasing convective heat losses (a 1.5°C reduction in air temperature). As a result, thermal exchange modalities were modified but total heat losses were maintained constant. The results pointed out that, when thermoregulatory processes are not activated, sleep and body activity of the preterm neonates are not altered.

These results disagree with those obtained from an adult study (Okamoto-Mizuno et al., 1999). Increased wakefulness and reduced sleep efficiency, REM and non-REM sleep durations were observed with humid heat exposure. However, according to these authors, this may be attributed to the changed thermal load rather than to a specific effect of humidity level.

Air velocity and radiant temperature

Air velocity heterogeneity due to turbulences on one hand and changes in radiant temperature on the other can disturb the homeostatic mechanisms via convective and radiative body heat losses. Thermal non-uniformity induces interregional skin temperature differences, which can be related to thermal discomfort. Thermal irradiation of the face has an effect on the metabolic rate, while facial cooling increases restlessness (Mestyan et al., 1964) and may be implicated as a cause of apneic attacks. The impact of face thermal irradiation on sleep, thermoregulatory and respiratory processes remains to be explored in neonates as well as in adults.

As recommended for standing adults, the vertical asymmetry (difference between temperature measured at the head and that measured at the feet) should not exceed 3°C for air temperature and 5°C for radiant temperature to preserve thermal comfort (Fanger, 1970). These recommended conditions are rarely attained in neonates nursed under radiant warmers.

Mechanisms involved

Our analysis of the mechanisms involved in the effects of thermal environments on sleep continuity will consider almost exclusively results obtained in animal or adult studies.

However, relevant differences exist between neonates and adults concerning both sleep and thermoregulation. In particular, AS in neonates only partly corresponds to REM sleep in adults. In fact, contrary to REM sleep in adults, AS in neonates shows no muscle atonia, while thermoregulatory ability is more effective than in QS (review in Bach et al., 1996). Thus, while adult REM sleep is characterized by impaired thermoregulatory capabilities, and hence is shortened when sleeping in a non-thermoneutral environment, in neonates AS duration is increased in the cool, as shown before.

Moreover, at variance with adults, in neonates AS occurs prior to QS, which, in turn, intervenes only if thermal conditions are suitable, otherwise wake occurs instead (Bach et al., 2001).

Such differences are likely due to the fact that sleep and thermoregulatory function in the adult result from the interplay of different nervous structures hierarchically interconnected, located in different parts of central nervous system (CNS), i.e. spinal cord (for thermoregulation only), brain stem, diencephalon and telencephalon. The hierarchical dominance is diencephalon > brain stem > spinal cord for thermoregulation (Satinoff, 1978). For sleep, this hierarchical dominance changes in the different states: telencephalon > diencephalon > brain stem in W, diencephalon > brain stem > telencephalon in NREM sleep and brain stem > telencephalon > diencephalon in REM sleep (Parmeggiani, 1988).

In neonates, the higher structures are not fully mature and the resulting sleep and thermoregulation are not so finely tuned as in adults, due to the lack of higher structures function.

Sleep processes and thermal regulation interact in a complex way: on one hand, sleep modifies thermal regulation, on the other body temperature affects sleep.

As an example of the first case, the ability to respond to thermal challenges is reduced to some extend in animal QS (no behavioural thermal regulation through searching for safe environment) and even more in desynchronized sleep (DS), leading to failure to maintain proper physiological responses to thermal loads, as indicated by cessation of piloerection, shivering and peripheral vasoconstriction in cold environments and cessation of thermal tachypnea in hot environments (review in Parmeggiani, 1987). Studies of humans are characterized by a reduction of sweating rate in the presence of increased body temperatures, an increase in mean body temperature during AS and a decrease in mean body temperature in all other sleep states in humans (Sagot et al., 1987; Libert et al., 1988; Lenzi et al., 1990).

As an example of the second case, thermal loads influence the entry into sleep as well as the transition between different sleep states. In this respect, it is important to distinguish between heavy thermal loads (which exert unspecific arousal effects in every sleep state and then influencing the wake-sleep cycle independently of thermoregulatory mechanisms) and mild thermal loads within the thermoneutral zone (Parmeggiani, 1987). Mild thermal loads specifically interact with sleep processes, and may either favor or hinder the transition from wakefulness to sleep and between different sleep states: in animals, cooling the anterior hypothalamus – preoptic area (AH-PO) increases waking time, warming favors both QS and DS (Sakaguchi et al., 1979), while entry into DS is more likely to occur when thermal regulation during the preceding QS is tuned toward heat loss (Parmeggiani et al., 1975). Mild increases in skin temperature also favor cortical synchronization (Nakayama & Hardy, 1969).

The structural basis of the interaction between sleep processes and body temperature regulation relies on the presence in the CNS of neuronal populations whose firing rate changes not only in response to changes in central or peripheral body temperature, but also in the transition between different wake-sleep states. Such neurons – probably involved in both temperature regulation and sleep processes – have been found in numerous CNS regions, including Midbrain Reticular Formation (MRF), Posterior Hypothalamus, AH-PO, Diagonal Band of Broca, Midline Thalamic Nuclei (MTN) and Cerebral Cortex (review in Van Someren, 2000). In these regions – with the possible exception of MRF and MTN – the change in firing that occurs with increasing central or cutaneous temperatures is similar to that which occurs at QS onset. Thus, increasing body temperature by heating the environment favors QS onset, while cooling hinders it. Likewise, QS onset (characterized by an increased firing rate in the same neuronal population) favors heat loss and hinders heat storage.

As an example, AH-PO warm-sensitive neurons may be considered. Their firing rate increases under the effect of both central and skin warming and also increases in the transition from quiet wakefulness to QS. As a consequence of this structural arrangement, thermal conditions entailing the activation of effectors for heat loss induce the same changes in these neurons as those characterizing QS development, while QS development entails firing changes characteristic of the thermal response favoring heat loss. In conclusion, thermal conditions promoting heat loss favor QS, while QS development favors heat loss.

Entry into QS is favored by mild warming, and hindered by cooling. As Parmeggiani (1987) points out, this sleep-promoting or sleep-hindering effect of temperature is only facultative in wakefulness, since sleep may also occur in adverse thermal conditions, pressure for sleep being the main controlling factor in this case. On the contrary, during QS thermoregulatory structures participate in sleep regulation as well, and DS may develop only if heat loss response is established by thermal regulation – otherwise, waking would occur instead. In adverse thermal conditions, QS duration may increase because of the difficulty in initiating DS, while total DS time may be heavily reduced. In this case, even if pressure for DS also plays a role, the QS to DS transition is mainly controlled by the thermal regulatory response.

Circadian rhythms of body temperature also influence ultradian wake-sleep rhythms. In fact, according to the above-cited observations concerning the interaction between sleep and mild body temperature changes, the transition from QW to QS is favored during the circadian phase in which a thermoregulatory response promoting heat loss is established, i.e. when a maximum negative slope occurs in core body temperature, determined by a maximum increase in mean skin temperature. This normally occurs between 23:00 and 7:00. The opposite occurs when a thermoregulatory response promoting heat retention is established, i.e. when core body temperature increases due to the effect of a decrease in mean skin temperature. This normally occurs between 8:00 and 12:00, as well as between 16:00 and 20:00 (review in Van Someren, 2000). The transition from QS to DS is also influenced by the circadian phase of body temperature: in humans, DS preferentially occurs around the minimum core temperature (Czeisler et al., 1980; Zulley & Wever, 1982). Circadian fluctuations in body temperature are characterized by opposite changes in core temperature and mean skin (especially distal) temperatures (Krauchi and Wirz-Justice, 1994). Opposite temperature changes during short-term adjustments are an intrinsic feature of mammalian thermoregulation (Lenzi et al., 1986).

It is worth noting that the positive feedback loop existing between skin temperature and skin blood flow regulation (an increase in skin temperature favors an increase in skin blood flow, which in turn increases skin temperature) determines a tendency of thermoregulatory system to remain in the condition of heat loss or retention it is. In fact, once body temperatures balance activated heat loss effectors, among which cutaneous vessels, the increase in skin temperature further increases heat loss, until the decrease progressively produced in internal temperature will turn thermoregulation to heat retention. To the extent sleep is favored by the heat loss thermoregulatory condition, stabilizing thermoregulatory condition also stabilizes the sleep or wake condition.

Heavy thermal loads deeply affect sleep by altering its structure and even provoking selective sleep deprivation. In cats, waking time increases with thermal load, negative thermal loads being better tolerated than positive ones. With increasing thermal loads, QS time first increases (due to the difficulty in starting AS, see above) and then decreases (Parmeggiani et al., 1975). This also occurs in humans (Sewitch et al., 1986). AS time, in turn, only decreases with increasing thermal loads, thus showing opposite changes with respect to wake time (review in Parmeggiani, 1987). In humans, thermal loads reduce total sleep time, while increasing wake time and sleep instability (review in Libert et al., 1995). These effects are probably independent of thermoregulatory mechanisms i.e. induced by the amount of thermal discomfort associated with thermal loads – thermal stimuli nonspecifically affect arousal mechanisms in the CNS (Parmeggiani, 1987), just as other sensory stimuli do.

Many brain structures are involved in wake-sleep regulation and, due to the complex wiring between them, it is not possible to recognize a unique center regulating wake-sleep rhythms. However, some main structures involved in arousal control may be considered (review in Van Someren, 2000). The MRF, including locus ceruleus and raphé nuclei, activates brain activity and controls mental awareness through widespread connections to the entire forebrain (Kelly, 1985). Deactivation of the reticular formation is necessary to promote sleep (Moruzzi, 1969). The posterior hypothalamus is also involved in cortical activation. Midline, medial and intralaminar thalamic nuclei are implicated in the generation of electroencephalographic (EEG) patterns typical of wake and sleep. High input levels in these thalamic neurons provoke a tonic discharge and induce the wake cortical EEG (a high frequency-low amplitude pattern). A decreased input causes these thalamic neurons to hyperpolarize and discharge in burst mode, thus inducing sleep cortical EEG (a low frequency-high amplitude pattern). The thalamic nucleus reticularis is involved in spindle generation. Neuron populations that are typically active during sleep exist in other brain regions, for example AH-PO and the diagonal band of Broca (Szymusiak, 1991). It has been suggested that GABAergic, sleep-related neurons and cholinergic, arousal-related neurons in basal forebrain influence cortical arousal (Szymusiak, 1995). At the cortical level, the arousal condition is classified on the basis of the EEG pattern resulting from thalamocortical interactions (low amplitude and high frequency during wake, high amplitude and low frequency during QS). Regulation of wake-sleep rhythms is thus dependent on the interplay of various brain structures activated differently by sensory stimuli (both environmental and internal in origin), as well as sleep pressure and circadian rhythms. Arousal levels may increase by the effect of sensory stimuli – in particular stressful stimuli such as heavy thermal loads – but also as a consequence of decreased sleep pressure, or circadian phases favouring wake. One can consider that a variety of gradual responses provokes increasing levels of arousal, including EEG changes towards lower amplitude-higher frequency patterns, increase in muscle tone, changes in cardiac and respiratory regulation, as well as in sympathetic outflow to the skin. Full awakening may eventually ensue, but arousals without awakening are also worth considering.

The increase in arousal induced by stressful stimuli such as heavy thermal loads is teleologically significant. In fact, in stressful thermal conditions only wake allows activation of all thermal responses (including the behavioural ones) and waking from sleep improves the ability to face the environmental challenge. However, the need for sleep has to be satisfied. Thus, thermal regulation and sleep regulation finely interplay in order to satisfy the most urgent needs. The pattern of sleep structure modifications considered above is thus produced.

Conclusion

From the results reported above, the high sensitivity of neonate sleep to thermal disturbances becomes evident. Sleep continuity and body movements are very sensitive to small thermal disturbances, even though the latter do not always elicit thermal responses (for example within the range of thermoneutrality). Sleep continuity parameters could allow definition of a narrower range of thermal comfort than do thermoregulatory parameters.

Alterations of sleep continuity mainly consist in increasing wakefulness and body movements. AS sleep is also promoted. According to these observations, cold stress is preferentially countered by an increase in heat production rather than by a reduction of heat expenditure (that would promote QS), even though the thermal stress is of low magnitude. An energy conservation policy could compromise body homeothermia.

As a result, maintenance of thermoneutrality for preterm neonates via incubators not only promotes optimal body growth and health, but also preserves sleep – especially sleep continuity – a crucial function for a baby's development.

Acknowledgements

The authors wish to thank the Regional Council of Picardie and the French Ministry of Research for their support of the different research projects performed in our laboratory and presented in this manuscript.

References

Azaz, Y., P.J. Fleming, M.R. Levine, R. McCabe, A. Stewart & P. Johnson (1992). The relationship between environmental temperature, metabolic rate, sleep state, and evaporative water loss in infants from birth to three months. *Pediatric Research, 32*, 417–423.

Bach, V., B. Bouferrache, O. Kremp, Y. Maingourd & J.P. Libert (1994). Regulation of sleep and body temperature in response to exposure to cool and warm environments in neonates. *Pediatrics, 93*, 789–796.

Bach, V., F. Telliez, G. Krim & J.P. Libert (1996). Body temperature regulation in the newborn infant: interaction with sleep and clinical implications. *Neurophysiologie Clinique, 26*, 379–402.

Bach, V., F. Telliez, G. Zoccoli, P. Lenzi, A. Leke & J.P. Libert (2000 a). Interindividual differences in the thermoregulatory response to cool exposure in sleeping neonates. *European Journal of Applied Physiology and Occupational Physiology, 81*, 455–462.

Bach, V., F. Telliez, A. Leke & J.P. Libert (2000 b). Gender-related sleep differences in neonates in thermoneutral and cool environments. *Journal of Sleep Research, 9*, 249–254.

Bach, V., F. Telliez, A. Leke, C. Chiorri & J.P. Libert (2001). Interaction between body temperatures and the direction of sleep stage transition in neonates. *Sleep Research Online, 4* (2), 43–49.

Bader, D., E. Tirosh, H. Hodgins, M. Abend & A. Cohen (1998). Effect of increased environmental temperature on breathing patterns in preterm and term infants. *Journal of Perinatology, 18*, 5–8.

Berterottière, D., A.M. D'Allest, M. Dehan & C. Gaultier (1990). Effects of increase in body temperature on the breathing pattern in premature infants. *Journal of Developmental Physiology, 13*, 303–308.

Brück, K., A.H. Parmelee & M. Brück (1962). Neutral temperature range and range of "thermal comfort" in premature infants. *Biology of the Neonate, 4*, 32–51.

Bunnell, D.E., J.A. Agnew, S.M. Horvath, L. Jopson & M. Wills (1988). Passive body heating and sleep: influence of proximity to sleep. *Sleep, 11*, 210–219.

Czeisler, C.A., J.C. Zimmerman, J.M. Ronda, M.C. Moore-Ede & E.D. Weitzman (1980). Timing of REM sleep in coupled to the circadian rhythm of body temperature in man. *Sleep, 2*, 329–346.

Daily, W.J.R., M. Klaus & H.B.P. Meyer (1969). Apnea in premature infants: monitoring, incidence, heart rate changes, and an effect of environmental temperature. *Pediatrics, 43*, 510–518.

Darnall, R.A., & R.L. Ariagno (1982). The effect of sleep state on active thermoregulation in the premature infant. *Pediatric Research, 16*, 512–514.

Di Nisi, J., J. Ehrhart, M. Galeou & J.P. Libert (1989). Influence of repeated passive body heating on subsequent night sleep in humans. *European Journal of Applied Physiology and Occupational Physiology, 59*, 138–145.

Fanger P.O., *Thermal comfort*. New York: Mc Graw Hill, (1970).

Fleming, P.J., M.R. Levine, Y. Azaz & P. Johnson (1988). The effect of sleep state on the metabolic response to cold stress in newborn infants. In Jones C.T. (Ed.), *Fetal and neonatal development* (635–639). Ithaca & New York: Perinatology Press.

Galland, B.C., G. Reeves, B.J. Taylor & D.P.G. Bolton (1998). Sleep position, autonomic function, and arousal. *Archives in Disease Childhood Fetal Neonatal Ed, 78*, 189–194.

Glass, L., W.A. Silverman & J.C. Sinclair (1968). Effect of the thermal environment on cold resistance and growth of small infants after the first week of life. *Pediatrics, 41*, 1033–1046.

Harper, R.M., H.C. Kinney, P.J. Fleming & B.T. Thach (2000). Sleep influences on homeostatic functions: implications for sudden infant death syndrome. *Respiration Physiology, 119*, 123–132.

Hey, E.N., & B. O'Connell (1970). Oxygen consumption and heat balance in the cot-nursed baby. *Archives of Disease in Childhood, 45*, 335–343.

Himms-Hagen, J. (1995). Does thermoregulatory feeding occur in newborn infants? A novel view of the role of brown adipose tissue thermogenesis in control of food intake. *Obesity Research, 3*, 361–369.

Horne, J.A., & A.J. Reid (1985). Night-time sleep EEG changes following body heating in a warm bath. *Electroencephalography and Clinical Neurophysiology, 60*, 154–157.

Horne, J.A., & L.H.E. Staff (1983). Exercise and sleep: body-heating effects. *Sleep, 6*, 36–46.

Hunt, C.E. (1989). Impaired arousal from sleep: relationship to sudden infant death syndrome. *Journal of Perinatology, 9*, 184–187.

Karlsson, H., S.E. Hamel, K. Nilsson & R. Olagard (1995). Measurement of skin temperature and heat flow from skin in term newborn babies. *Acta Paediatrica, 84*, 605–612.

Karlsson, H., R. Olegard & K. Nilsson (1996). Regional skin temperature, heat flow and conductance in preterm neonates nursed in low and in neutral environmental temperature. *Acta Paediatrica, 85*, 81–87.

Kelly, J.P. (1985). Cranial nerve nuclei, the reticular formation, and biogenic amine-containing neurons. In Kandell E.R. & J.H. Schwartz (Eds), *Principles of neural science* (558–560). New York, Elsevier.

Krauchi, K., & A. Wirz-Justice (1994). Circadian rhythm of heat production, heart rate, and skin and core temperature under unmasking conditions in man. *American Journal of Physiology, 267*, R819–R829.

Lenzi, P., J. P. Libert, T. Cianci & C. Franzini (1990). Comparative aspects of the interaction between sleep and thermoregulation. In J. Horne (Ed.) *Sleep '90* (388–390). Bochum: Pontenagel Press.

Lenzi, P., J.P. Libert, C. Franzini, T. Cianci & P.L. Guidalotti (1986). Short-term thermoregulatory adjustments involving opposite regional temperature changes. *Journal of Thermal Biology, 11*, 151–156.

Libert, J.P., V. Bach, L.C. Johnson, J. Ehrhart, G. Wittersheim & D. Keller (1991). Relative and combined effects of heat and noise exposure on sleep in humans. *Sleep, 14*, 24–31.

Libert, J.P., J. Di Nisi, H. Fukuda, A. Muzet, J. Ehrhart & C. Amoros (1988). Effect of continuous heat exposure on sleep stages in humans. *Sleep, 11*, 195–209.

Libert, J.P., C. Franzini & P. Lenzi (1995). Thermorégulation et sommeil. In O. Benoit and J. Forêt (Eds), *Le sommeil humain* (39–46). Paris: Masson.

McNamara, F., H. Wulbrand & Thach Bt (1998). Characteristics of the infant arousal response. *Journal of Applied Physiology, 85*, 2314–2321.

Mestyan, J., I. Jarai, G. Bata & M. Fekete (1964). The significance of facial skin temperature in the chemical heat regulation of premature infants. *Biology of the Neonate, 7*, 243–254.

Mestyan, J., I. Jarai & M. Fekete (1968). The total energy expenditure and its components in premature infants maintained under different nursing and environmental conditions. *Pediatric Research, 2*, 161–171.

Moruzzi, G. (1969). Sleep and instinctive behavior. *Archives Italiennes de Biologie, 108*, 175–216.

Nakayama, T., & J.D. Hardy (1969). Unit responses in the rabbit's brain stem to changes in brain and cutaneous temperature. *Journal of Applied Physiology, 27*, 848–857.

Newman, N.M., J.A. Trinder, K.A. Phillips, K. Jordan & J. Cruickshank (1989). Arousal deficit: mechanism of the sudden infant death syndrome? *Australian Paediatric Journal, 25*, 196–201.

Okamoto-Mizuno, K., K. Mizuno, S. Michie, A. Maeda & S. Lizuka (1999). Effects of humid heat exposure on human sleep stages and body temperature. *Sleep, 22*, 767–773.

Parmeggiani, P.L. (1987). Interaction between sleep and thermoregulation: an aspect of the control of behavioral states. *Sleep, 10*, 426–435.

Parmeggiani, P.L. (1988). Thermoregulation during sleep from the view point of homeostasis. In Lydic R. & J.F. Biebuyck (Eds), *Clinical Physiology of Sleep, American Physiological Society* (159–169). Bethesda, Maryland.

Parmeggiani, P.L., L.F. Agnati, G. Zamboni & T. Cianci (1975). Hypothalamic temperature during the sleep cycle at different ambient temperatures. *Electroencephalography and Clinical Neurophysiology, 38*, 589–596.

Parmeggiani, P.L., & C. Rabini (1970). Sleep and environmental temperature. *Archives Italiennes de Biologie, 108*, 369–387.

Perlstein, P.H., N.K. Edwards & J.M. Sutherland (1970). Apnea in premature infants and incubator-air-temperature changes. *New England Journal of Medicine, 282*, 461–466.

Perlstein, P.H., C. Hersh, C.J. Glück & J.M. Sutherland (1974). Adaptation to cold in the first three days of life. *Pediatrics, 54*, 411–416.

Sagot, J.C., C. Amoros, V. Candas & J.P. Libert (1987). Sweating responses and body temperatures during nocturnal sleep in humans. *American Journal of Physiology, 252*, R462–R470.

Sakaguchi, S., S.F. Glotzbach & H.C. Heller (1979). Influence of hypothalamic and ambient temperatures on sleep in kangaroo rats. *American Journal of Physiology, 237*, R80–R88.

Satinoff, E. (1978). Neural organization and evolution of thermal regulation in mamals. *Science , 201,* 16–21.

Schechtman, V.L., R.M. Harper, A.J. Wilson & D.P. Southall (1992). Sleep state organization in normal infants and victims of the sudden infant death syndrome. *Pediatrics, 89*, 865–870.

Schieber, J.P., A. Muzet & P.J.R. Ferrière (1971). Les phases d'activations transitoires spontanées au cours du sommeil normal chez l'Homme. *Archives in Sciences of Physiology, 25*, 443–465.

Sewitch, D.E., M.W. Kittrell, D.J. Kupfer & C.F. Reynolds (1986). Body temperature and sleep architecture in response to a mild cold stress in women. *Physiology & Behavior, 36*, 951–957.

Stothers, J.K., & R.M. Warner (1978). Oxygen consumption and neonatal sleep states. *Journal of Physiology (London), 278*, 435–440.

Stothers, J.K., & R.M. Warner (1984). Thermal balance and sleep state in the newborn. *Early Human Development, 9*, 313–322.

Szymusiak, R. (1991). Exposure to heat restores sleep in cats with preoptic/anterior hypothalamic cell loss. *Brain Research, 541*, 134–138.

Szymusiak, R. (1995). Magnocellular nuclei of the basal forebrain: substrates of sleep and arousal regulation. *Sleep, 18*, 478–500.

Telliez, F., V. Bach, S. Delanaud, B. Bouferrache, G. Krim & J.P. Libert (1997 a). Skin derivative control of thermal environment in a closed incubator. *Medical & Biological Engineering & Computing, 35*, 521–527.

Telliez, F., V. Bach, S. Delanaud, A. Leke, M. Abdiche & K. Chardon (2001). Influence of incubator humidity on neonates' sleep and behaviour at thermoneutrality. *Acta Paediatrica, 90*, 998–1003.

Telliez, F., V. Bach, G. Dewasmes, A. Leke & J.P. Libert (1998 a). Sleep modifications during cool acclimation in human neonates. *Neuroscience Letters, 245*, 25–28.

Telliez, F., V. Bach, G. Dewasmes, A. Leke & J.P. Libert (1998 b). Effects of medium and long chain triglycerides on sleep and thermoregulatory processes in neonates. *Journal of Sleep Research, 7*, 31–39.

Telliez, F., V. Bach, G. Krim & J.P. Libert (1997 b). Consequences of a small decrease of air temperature from thermal equilibrium on thermoregulation in sleeping neonates. *Medical & Biological Engineering & Computing, 35*, 516–520.

Tirosh, E., D. Bader, H. Hodgins & A. Cohen (1996). Sleep architecture as related to temperature changes in neonates at term. *Clinical Physiology, 16*, 603–608.

Van Someren, E.J.W. (2000). More than a marker: interaction between the circadian regulation of temperature and sleep, age-related changes, and treatment possibilities. *Chronobiology International, 17*, 313–354.

Wailoo, M.P., S.A. Petersen & H. Whittaker (1990). Disturbed nights and 3–4 month old infants: the effects of feeding and thermal environment. *Archives of Disease in Childhood, 65*, 499–501.

Wright, P., H.A. Macleod & M.J. Cooper (1983). Waking at night: the effect of early feeding experience. *Child Care Health Deelopment, 9*, 309–319.

Zulley, J. & R.A. Wever (1982). Interaction between the sleep wake cycle and rhythms of rectal temperature. *Vertebrate Circadian Systems*, 253–261.

Time pattern analysis of activity–rest rhythms in families with infants using actigraphy

Katharina Wulff and Renate Siegmund
Institut für Anthropologie, Humboldt-Universität zu Berlin

1. Introduction

1.1 Rhythms and time patterns

Biological rhythms generally demonstrate a wide spectrum of recurrent cycles, which form all sorts of distinct patterns: from single peaks such as corticosteroid secretion in the early morning (Moore-Ede et al., 1983) to rectangular on/off phenomena like our most obvious daily rhythm of sleep and wakefulness. Although these cycles maintain a state of temporal relationship in the individual, the internal state of a particular variable is a far from stable equilibrium. Complex pattern formation (superimposed oscillations) requires interactive structures (interactions of activation and inhibition) between the system components. With a view to optimal coordination organisms have made use of oscillatory timing systems, e.g for signal transmission (action potentials, pulsatile hormone release), for motoric or transport mechanisms (body movement, breathing) and for "clock" functions. In mammals, the suprachiasmatic nuclei (SCN) were identified as the principal "biological clock", located in the anterior hypothalamic area and consist of neuronal pacemaker tissue (Moore & Lenn, 1972; Moore, 1973). This neuronal tissue exhibits *endogenous* rhythmicity (capable of self-sustaining oscillations) (Schwartz, 1991), while genetic control is involved in determining specific properties of the interactive structures of the oscillatory timing system (Ralph & Menaker, 1988; Vitaterna et al., 1994). A particular property is *entrainability* (coupling of a self-sustained oscillation to a zeitgeber [forcing oscillation]), which results either in both oscillations having the same frequency (*synchronisation*) or frequencies that are integral multiples (frequency-demultiplication), (Aschoff, 1965). This ability allows optimal adaptation of the organism to periodic changes in the environment. According to the periodicities that exist in the environment biological rhythms are divided into *circadian* rhythms (oscillations of approximately 24 hours, derived from day-night changes), *annual* rhythms (derived from 12 months a year), *tidal* and *lunar* rhythms (derived from the orbit of the moon). Cycles of a period length shorter than 20 hours are called *ultradian* rhythms (e.g. food-intake). Organisms do not passively follow the environmental changes. Instead, the opposite takes place: the SCN actively produce circadian rhythmicity endogenously, which synchronises with the environment when exposed to specific signals (*zeitgeber* or *time cues*). *Zeitgeber* are not only responsible for the entrainment of the organism's biological rhythms with the environment but also ensure internal synchronisation of physiological variables (neurological, hormonal and metabolic factors) transmitted through the SCN (Hastings, 1997; Haus & Touitou, 1997). As a result, the timing system exerts potent influences on human behaviour.

1.2 Non-photic entrainment and human social behaviour

A multitude of forced rhythms have been described as being circadian, whose maxima and minima map to phases of day and night. Notable examples include the activity-rest rhythm, body temperature rhythm, and rhythms in cortisol (Weitzman et al., 1975) and melatonin (Arendt, 1997). As the most prominent zeitgeber for circadian rhythmicity light mainly entrains the activity-rest rhythm but the circadian system is also very sensitive to social zeitgebers. Human behaviour is largely directed by *social* zeitgebers (defined as family life or interpersonal relationships, work or school, weekdays and -ends) and therefore internal clock time of the subject can be affected by interaction with the partner and children. Social contacts that commonly involve arousal of the subjects can shift the clock in individuals studied in both experimental or natural settings (Aschoff et al., 1971; Ehlers et al., 1988). Even an arousal that has no direct effect on the timing system is able to activate serotonergic cells of the raphe nuclei, which have an input to the SCN (Jacobs & Azmitia, 1992). If social interactions induce a direct action, e.g. wakefulness from sleep, this exerts a *masking* effect (immediate temporary synchronisation, opposite to a permanent phase-shifting effect, [Waterhouse & Minors, 1988]). But if this interaction is applied regularly it may alter the timing of wakefulness in the long term. During infant development, mother-infant interaction can exert an exogenous force on the circadian system, whose functioning matures during the postnatal period.

Characterisation of activity-rest time patterns among family members and families with a different cultural background (e.g. industrialised vs. traditional cultures) reveal insights into the influence of social zeitgebers. In a young family there is a particularly tight bonding between the infant and the mother that makes it ideal to diagnose pattern changes for both subjects. Activity-rest patterns of young infants differ greatly from those of their parents. Time patterns of both parents are adapted to the diurnal life dominated by more or less stable circadian rhythms. In contrast, activity-rest patterns of young infants are divided into many short phases of rest and activity that can interfere with the well-established diurnal pattern of their parents. Recurrent behavioural patterns may have considerable impact as modulators on infant entrainment and development. A priority to assess non-photic zeitgeber functions in natural settings is the ability to collect activity information for extended periods. Continuous and accurate data of activity are useful to detect modulatory influences between family members, which may denote deviations from regular patterns. To date, activity monitoring using actigraphy allows non-supervised continuous recordings of an individual's activity-rest time pattern by measuring arm or leg movements across many days and nights. Long-term measurements form the basis on which time patterns can be analysed for their alterations in the pattern formation, their cyclicity and sleep-related parameters such as sleep interruptions, going-to-bed time and get-up time. When non-photic zeitgeber functions during ontogeny are questioned, it is of particular interest to investigate the time course of the infant's adaptation to his/her environment, and thereby, how activity patterns of parents and infants agree or disagree with each other. This chapter addresses the application of actigraphy and time series analysis, giving particular attention to parallel recordings of father, mother and infant and to aspects related to corresponding activity timing, entrainment, ultradian and circadian rhythms, and adds examples of intercultural comparison. Since biological rhythmicity and parent-infant synchronisation is central to the timing of wakefulness in infants, actigraphic time series provide a tool for the evaluation of cyclic response patterns among family members. This will become increasingly important in the choice of criteria concerning what is normal and problematic behaviour in infants.

1.3 Actigraphic time series – the search for patterns and cycles

Actigraphy is a non-invasive method of recording time patterns of activity and rest in different age groups, including pre-term and full-term neonates, infants, children, adults and the elderly. There are several strategies to monitor activity: sleep logs, sensitive mattresses, pad sensors, actigraphy and videography. The search for activity-rest cycles in newborn infants using actigraphy began about 85 years ago. Szymanski (1918) invented a free-swinging crib, whose oscillations, derived from the infant's movements, were marked directly on a rotating cylinder with a period of 24 hours. Recent experiments using sensitive mattresses or pad sensors to monitor activity have to deal with the same problems that Szymanski faced: (a) the apparatuses are fixed and the recorded periods are therefore restricted to the time when the infant is in bed and social or caretaking periods (cuddling, nursing/feeding) are left out, and (b) recording techniques inhibit longitudinal long-term measurements. In addition to these approaches, activity-rest cycles were recorded by using observation protocols, which allow the identification of rhythms and phase shifts. Long-term observations of the sleep-wake process in infants from birth to six months using sleep logs showed that this type of monitoring produces largely spaced recordings, which depend heavily on an individual's accuracy. This unsatisfactory situation was dramatically improved by the flexible actigraphic approach used in recent years. This approach was opened by the invention of actigraphic monitors (actometers or actigraphs), which resemble wrist-watches. The great advantage of using small actometers lies in their independency from a certain place or clinical setting and their ability to be worn continuously over many days, weeks and months. Actometers, therefore, are equally well-suited for measurements at the subjects' home, in rural and urban regions and in industrialised and traditional cultures (Figure 1).

As a result of 10 years of human studies in biological rhythm research, it became clear that environmental conditions affect the daily rhythm of activity and rest in man. Hospitals and sleep laboratories are necessary institutions of a modern health care service but measurements may capture side effects in response to the unfamiliar environment for the patient. Continuous monitoring of activity and physiological functions being made at home under real living conditions ensures physiological accuracy and makes it possible to investigate the influence of social time cues and other parent-infant behaviour on entrainment, in particular during postnatal development in infants.

Actigraphy meets an increasing demand to quantify patterns of sleep, arousal and awakening in a long-term approach. Mullaney et al. (1980) demon-

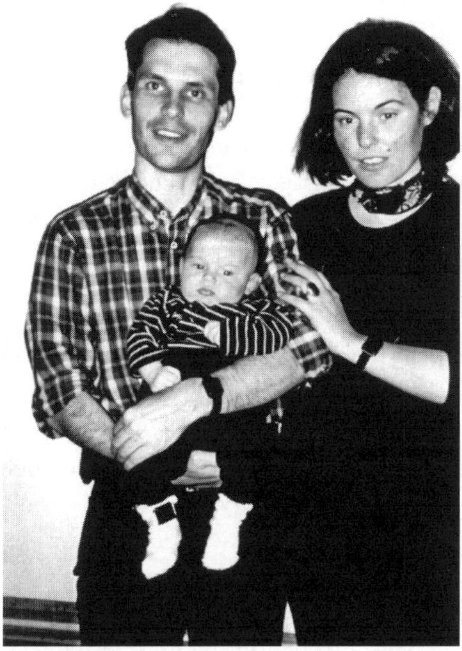

Figure 1. Family from Berlin (Germany) with a three month old boy, all of them wearing an actometer (Actiwatch®, Cambridge Neurotechnology Ltd, UK). Photo K.W.

strated that sleep and wakefulness could be estimated using wrist movements detected by actigraphy. 85.3% agreement between movements registered on infants' legs through actigraphs and wakefulness measured by polysomnograph was found by Sadeh et al. (1991). Progress in actigraphic modalities led to diverse systems of monitors with differences in motion sensor, directional sensitivity, filter settings and modalities of quantification algorithms (Jean-Louis et al., 2001, Van Someren et al., 1996). Among different activity monitors reliable sleep estimates relative to polysomnographic estimates could be found with correlations of 0.79 to 0.94 for sleep duration and 0.55 to 0.87 for sleep efficiency (Jean-Louis et al., 2001). This means, activity-rest behaviour is not always identical to sleep-wake behaviour. When using actigraphy, the actometer actually measures exactly whether a subject is moving or not and it does not measure wakefulness and sleep. It cannot distinguish between sleep and calm activities like dozing or reading. To overcome this problem it is advisable to let people always keep a diary of their activities.

In particular the different features of polysomnography and actigraphy enable them to complement each other in a series of analyses, e.i. the endogenous ultradian rhythm during sleep and the circadian rhyhtm in activity and rest. Activity monitors are equipped with a piezoelectric sensor that detects the acceleration of a movement and its output is quantified by using a series of linked algorithms. Activity counts acquired at equidistant intervals of a preset length are stored in the actometer's memory, which is read out by a computer after completion of the recording. From the continuous record of people's movements one needs to extract phases of rest and activity. This is achieved through mathematical algorithms which can search digital time series for subtle but critical signal content. For many analyses, essential requirements are equally spaced data points and no missing data. To avoid false results caused by incorrect data sequences, e.g. zero values produced when taking the actometer off while having a shower, these incorrect values have to be edited with an adequate sequence of activity values, which should be taken from the same person. Given that these purification criteria have been met, various time series analysis can be applied, including spectral analysis, maximum entropy spectrum, various periodogram analyses, auto-correlation, cross-correlation etc. Spectral analysis seeks to identify hidden periodicities in the data. This is particularly useful to determine ultradian rhythms that commonly exist in activity patterns of infants. Results of spectral analysis are displayed as spectral density distribution (Figure 6, lower panel). The spectral density distribution indicates the amount of variance attributable to various cycle frequencies. Time-ordered relationships of paired time series, such as mother-infant, father-infant and mother-father, can be detected using cross-correlation analysis. This analytical approach examines, whether both series are synchronised (simultaneous activity) or whether one time series starts before another time series (desynchronous activity, e.g. the infant's activity starts before the activity of mother).

2. Patterns and cycles during and after pregnancy

During the third trimester, awakenings after sleep onset are reported to disrupt the habitual sleep behaviour of pregnant women (Brunner et al., 1994). We made a longitudinal analysis of the activity-rest behaviour in 12 couples from late pregnancy until birth, and continued with the same couples and their infants from the third postnatal day until four months after birth (Wulff & Siegmund, 2000). Activity plots reveal that pregnant women clearly show significantly more activity at night than non-pregnant women. Contrary to expectations, this does not result in a longer nocturnal rest phase compared with their partners or non-pregnant women but onsets of nocturnal rest and onsets of daytime activity are often shifted and subsequently resetted, which explains transient period lengthening and shortening seen in the circadian range during late pregnancy. Guilleminault et al. (2000) studied sleep architecture, respiratory patterns and the 24-hour blood pressure profile of women in which pregnancy was associated with chronic snoring. He found that at six months prenatal chronic snorers showed an increase in respiratory effort and a higher blood pressure, as compared to pregnant women with normal breathing patterns. There was no significant difference in mean total sleep time and total number of arousals between the two pregnant groups and the observed abnormal respiratory patterns were restricted to the period of pregnancy. In our study, the partners of pregnant women exhibit activity-rest patterns that are clearly structured into blocks of sustained rest at night and activity by day. When the child is born, the average day-to-night ratio of activity decreases and disruptions and dislocations of the nocturnal rest phase are observed in both parents, albeit that this is most marked in the mothers. The fathers' level of activity at night is increased during the first three weeks after birth when compared with the period before birth. Fluctuations of the circadian period length from prenatal to postnatal can be seen in a few cases. However, there is no postnatal-related reduction in the amplitude of the overt circadian activity-rest rhythm in the fathers as is evident in the mothers (Figure 6C, B respectively, lower panel).

Newborn infants show marked interindividual differences in their activity-rest patterns (Fukuda & Ishihara, 1997; Löhr & Siegmund, 1999; Shimada et al., 1999). It emerged that different types of entraining patterns exist, which can be modulated by external time cues. Activity-rest data obtained from newborn infants who were fed on demand, can be described in terms of a pattern as monophasic, biphasic, polyphasic and in the frequency domain as ultradian, circadian, entrained or free-running. Monophasic and biphasic patterns can either be entrained (Figure 2A, B; cycles in phase with the environment) or free-running (cycles phase-shifting with respect to the 24h-time scale), while monophasic is considered as circadian rhythm and biphasic as 12h-rhythm. Polyphasic patterns are characterised by short phases of activity and rest throughout day and night which exhibit considerable periodicities in the ultradian frequency domain (Figure 2C, D). Infants with highly regular, non free-running patterns during early development were perceived as more predictable than those with irregular polyphasic patterns, reported by

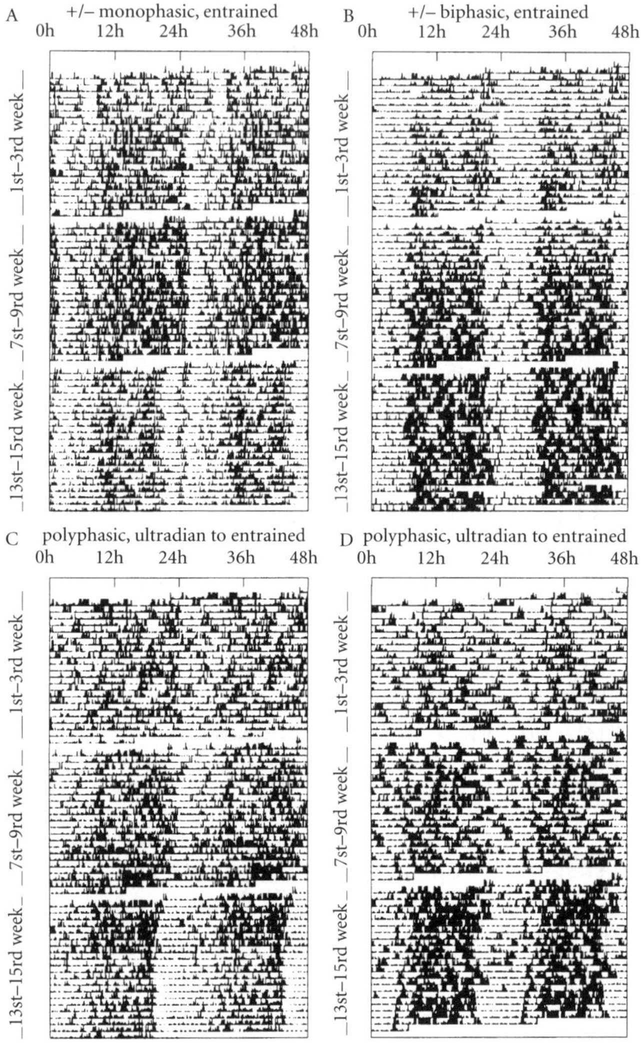

Figure 2. Activity-rest patterns of four infants showing normal variation in entrainment during the first four months after birth. Double plotted actograms, with activity as black spikes, consist of 3 series of 21 days each: During the first three weeks infants exhibit monophasic patterns (A), biphasic pattern (B), polyphasic patterns less free-running (C) and more free-running (D). During the fourth month infants comprise an early sleep onset (before 21.00) (A, C, D) or a late sleep onset (after 21.00) (B). Note entrainment in feeding habit at night in (A, last series).

the mothers during the interview after the recordings. During the later course of development, by three months after birth, two different trends become apparent according to the distribution of the nocturnal rest phase: some infants show a late onset of nocturnal rest (see Figure 2B) that is related to the tendency to prolong the circadian frequency length, while other infants show an early onset (see Figure 2A, C, D) and a circadian frequency length of exactly 24h. Infants whose onset of nocturnal rest started late had a shorter main sleep span than infants with an early onset. This significant difference of nocturnal rest period leads to the concept of "short-sleepers" and "long-sleepers" due to sleep organisation and innate circadian oscillation. Intraindividual stability of sleep duration is reported to be in part influenced by genetic factors (Benoit, 1984). Interindividual differences in the duration of sleep and wakefulness and in their phase correlation to the environment could be found for industrialised and traditional cultures (Siegmund et al., 1998).

Immediately after birth, infants start to adjust sleep to a circadian activity-rest rhythm, a process which has not been explained. The observation of fluctuations in interfeeding intervals of newborn infants on self-demand schedule and in attention during wakefulness in adults (Kleitman, 1982 and references therein) lead to the assumption that, in addition to the circadian rhythm, another rhythm with a shorter period length should exist. Long before the discovery of the non-REM/REM cycle during sleep (REMs, *rapid eye movements*), Kleitman therefore proposed the concept of a basic rest/activity cycle (BRAC) with intervals between 45 and 90 minutes. The discovery of the endogenous ultradian rhythm of non-REM/REM sleep cycles with period lengths of 90 to 100 minutes in adults confirm this concept – as far as sleep is concerned. The exact nature of the pathways combining both ultradian sleep cycles and the circadian rest-activity rhythm has yet to be analysed (Novak et al., 2000). The infants' early fluctuations of sleep-wakefulness and feeding rhythm has a strong impact on the mothers. For instance, activity at night is significantly reinforced after birth and coincides with that of their infants' activity (Wulff & Siegmund, 2000). An immediate alteration in circadian rhythmicity is evident in all mothers, expressed in a lowered circadian amplitude during the first four weeks after birth (Figure 6B, lower panel). Physical contact between mother and infant is likely to force activity phases. This could be demonstrated in postnatal frequency spectra of mothers and infants, who always have some ultradian components in common. In a few mother-infant pairs, both subjects show a circadian frequency with the same cycle length that can be prolonged by up to 25 hours. This circadian lengthening may be unusual under naturally synchronising environmental conditions but would be possible in mother-infant pairs, because infants are out of phase with the 24-hour day (Wulff et al., 2001). Close social and physical contact may couple the mother to her infant.

Pinilla & Birch (1993) showed experimentally that parents, as the closest social interaction partners of the infant, are able to actively shape their infants' patterns of nocturnal rest during the early postnatal period. Mothers, who were instructed to stretch nightly feeding intervals and to maximise the differences between day and night (e.g. level of noise, light) in order to break the association between awakening at night and being fed, facilitated long sustaining nocturnal rest phases in infants. Because analysis was based on dietary-activity diaries kept by the mothers, assessment of nocturnal activity-rest patterns is of limited accuracy, since we observed through actigraphic monitoring that infants of industrialised and traditional cultures are still active during the night without being fed and without waking up the parents (Siegmund et al., 1996). Motor activity and awakenings during the nocturnal rest phase when we usually sleep arise from periodic endogenous activation of the brain (Hobson, 1990). Entrainment in the feeding habit as shown by Pinilla & Birch (1993) or in demand for food at night by three months as illustrated in Figure 2A establishes independently of the activity-rest pattern (see also Salzarulo et al., 1979).

3. Cross-correlations of time series

Cross-correlations maintain the temporal order of time series data (termed time-domain approach, Gottman, 1981). This analytical method was used in our study to uncover corresponding activity patterns of parents and infants collected under home conditions. Parallel actigraphic time series of father, mother and infant starting with the same day and at the same time are ideal to detect simultaneous activity among them. In order to test who initiates the activity epochs an assumed reaction time of one minute seems acceptable. A one-minute activity logging interval or shorter is therefore preferred during data collection. Figure 3 represents a detail out of a long series of data analyses. It illustrates original activity data of infant, mother and father that are single-plotted across three consecutive days and arranged beneath each other (left panel). This allows the data for corresponding patterns to be inspected, e.g. events of bed time, get-up time or similar activity epochs between family members. To quantify corresponding activity patterns between all family members, only periods during which all family members are at home and, in principle, able to interact should be included. This can be done by extracting

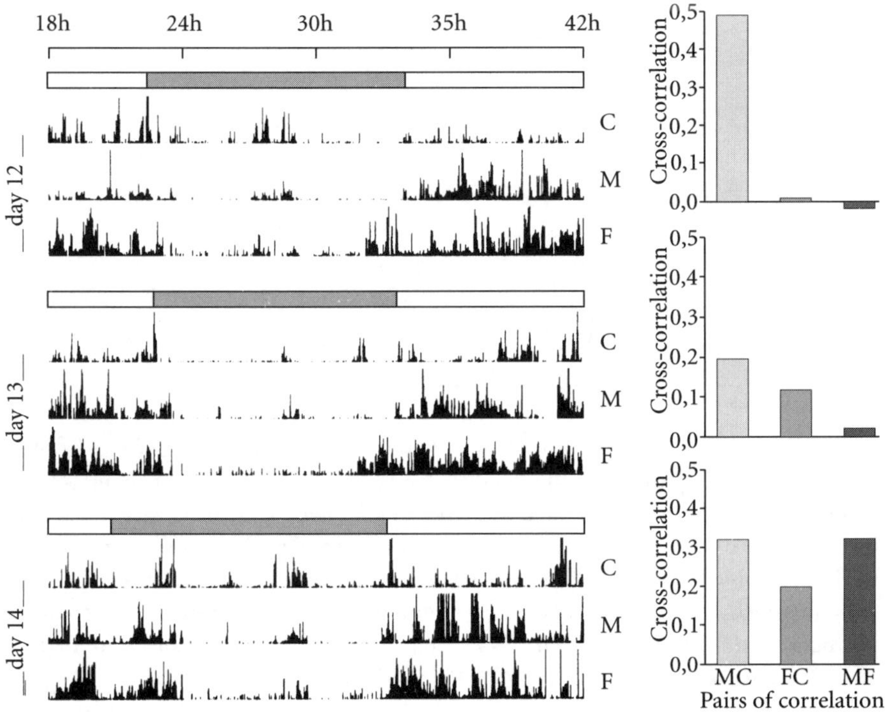

Figure 3. Single plotted actograms consisting of 3 days derived from parallel recordings of a representative family living in Berlin, Germany (left panel): C = child, M = mother, F = father. For easy viewing the actograms were timed from 18.00 to 18.00. Cross-correlations (right panel) were performed for selected times (shaded areas above actograms = infant's nocturnal rest phase) derived from the actigraphic data on the left. Pairs of cross-correlation: MC = mother-infant, FC = father-infant, MF = mother-father. See text for detailed explanation.

phases from the original data, which must be of same length among each pair. For instance, phase length may be restricted to the infant's nocturnal rest phase (shaded area). From this data, the cross-correlation coefficient can be calculated, which is a measure for the level of simultaneous movements in case of zero time shift between two paired time series. The diagrams (right panel) show cross-correlations analysed separately for each night from the activity data on the left. Each bar shows the correlation of a particular pair of time series at zero time shift, e.g. mother-child (MC). During the first night, simultaneous activity is high only between mother and infant but absent in relation to the father. During the third night, however, the mother had a similarly high cor-

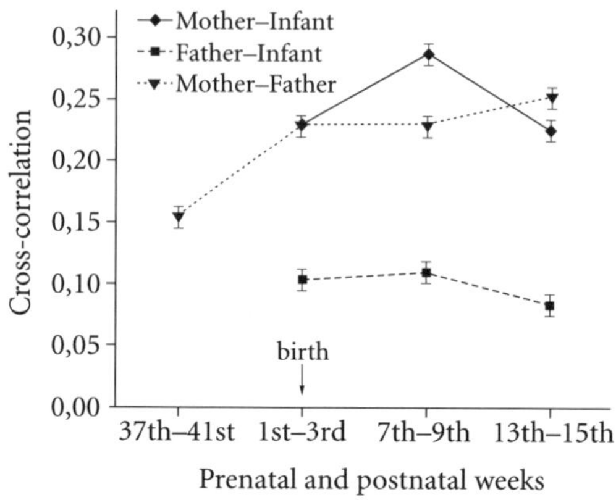

Figure 4. Mean cross-correlation values and standard errors of paired times series of 11 families from Berlin, Germany, showing the level of simultaneous parent-infant activity before and after birth. Analyses are restricted to the infants' nocturnal rest phases that includes time during the evening, night and morning and are based on recordings two weeks before birth (between 37th and 41st gestational week) and three series of 21 days each after birth. Note the increase in corresponding parental activity from prenatal to postnatal, the high level between mother and infant during the second month after birth and the overall low level between father and infant.

relation with both infant and father. From these examples, one can recognise the high day-to-day variation of concurrent activity between family members. Results on which we will focus here come from this type of analysis on a large scale (Wulff et al., 2001). It could be shown that simultaneous activity between the partners increased markedly from prenatal to postnatal and remained high throughout a four month period (Figure 4). During the first three weeks after birth the mother had a similarly strong correlation with the time patterns of the infant as with the father suggesting a direct involvement of the father by social interaction, who synchronised his get-up times and bed times with those of the mother. However, the level of simultaneous activity shared by mother and infant was always significantly higher than between father and infant. Detailed analysis of the phase relationship (lag relationship)[1] of paired time series of

1. In order to determine the lag relationship by cross-correlation the mother's time series is determined "dependent variable" and has to be shifted along the time series of her infant "independent variable" in a certain number of one-minute steps (lags). A maximum cross-correlation coefficient at a certain lag position indicates the direction of influence. Maximum correlation at zero time shift means simultaneous activity, a maximum correlation

mother and infant revealed that cross-correlations can reflect the development of mono-, bi- or polyphasic time patterns in the infant. Infants with a regular diurnal (mono-, or biphasic) activity-rest pattern from birth (see Figure 2A, B) engaged in a high degree of simultaneous activity with their mothers. Concomitantly, mother and infant were in phase with each other soon after birth. In contrast, almost all infants with an initially polyphasic pattern correlated at a comparatively low level with their mothers during the first three weeks of life. This shows that mother and infant were not fully synchronised immediately after birth but needed time to adapt. The process of adaptation reached its peak around two months after birth (see Figure 4). By that time, different strategies could be found among these mother-infant pairs. Some mother-infant pairs increased the level of simultaneous activity with the mother partly leading the infant's activity and thereby probably entraining the infant. These infants achieved a diurnal pattern very quickly after seven weeks of life (Figure 2C). Other mother-infant pairs continued with the low level of simultaneous

at a negative lag position means that the mother was active before the infant. A maximum correlation at a positive lag position means that the infant was active before the mother.

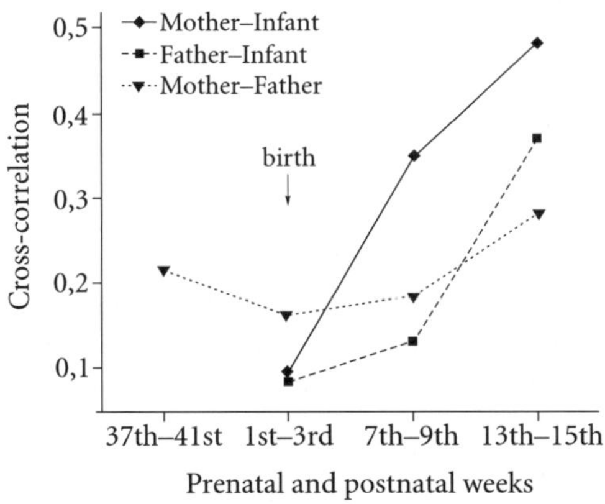

Figure 5. Mean cross-correlation values of a family with an infant having a chaotic activity pattern during the first three weeks after birth but which rapidly entrains during the further time course. Analyses are restricted to the infant's nocturnal rest phases that includes time during the evening, night and morning. Note the low correlation level between mother and infant in the first three weeks after birth and the marked increase from that time until the second month, which continued to the fourth month. At this time correlation level between father and infant is also high.

activity that was associated with the infant leading the mother's activity while the mother responded to the infant. These infants kept a polyphasic pattern beyond seven weeks of life (Figure 2D). During the further course of development, all infants expressed a circadian rhythm. Since the analysis window in cross correlation was set to the infants' nocturnal rest phase, the low correlation level at three months between mother and infant reflects different phase positions due to the earlier bed time of the infant in most families when compared with the parental bed times.

Apart from these patterns there is evidence that some infants have a chaotic time pattern at birth, which was reported by one of our families. It could be confirmed through actigraphic monitoring and indirectly deduced from cross-correlations that revealed almost no simultaneous activity between mother and infant after birth (Figure 5). This difficult period was followed by a rapid emergence of a diurnal pattern in the infant that coincided with a remarkable increase in simultaneous activity between mother and infant. The beneficial effect of a strong synchronisation between mother's and infant's activity extended beyond the third month after birth.

4. An intercultural approach to zeitgeber influences during infancy

As mentioned above, periodicities in mother-infant relationships seem to tune to each other. In humans, social interaction can be an important stimulus to change rhythmic behaviour and so it provides a potentially important time cue to mutual mother-infant synchronisation. For example, during establishment of a mother-infant bond when the child is born, the mother exhibits phase shifts in activity with desynchronisation up to a forced 25-hour rhythm in activity. The infant's early activity-rest pattern, which predominantly expresses ultradian rhythms masks the mother's rhythm, although she bears a predominant diurnal activity. In view of mother-infant attachment and the infant's adaptive capacities (Grossmann et al., 1999; Grossmann & Grossmann, 2000) the mother's close proximity to the infant may change the infant's spontaneously timed activity into a diurnal activity pattern, thus giving rise to overt circadian cycles. The presence of weak circadian cycles and the same 25-hour frequency detected concurrently with the mother support such a role (Figure 6A, B). This high concordance in periodic alteration could only be found in newborn infants and their mothers until two months after birth. The fathers, who slept in the same room and thereby close to mother and infant, never exhibited a prolonged circadian frequency in accord with their infant (Fig-

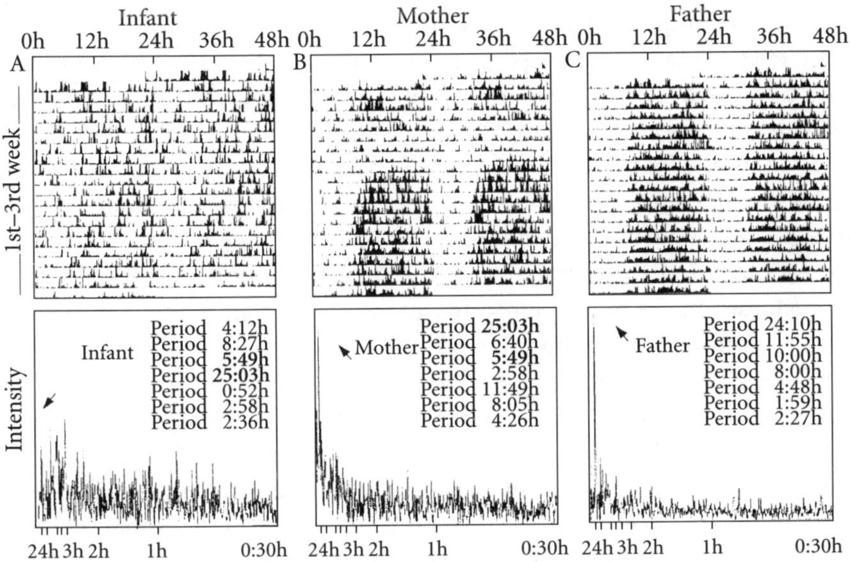

Figure 6. Double plotted actograms consisting of 21 days each derived from parallel recordings of one representative family (upper panel). Abscissa: clock time, Ordinate: days of measurements starting with the 3rd day after birth. Note the polyphasic pattern in the infant (A) and the corresponding activity epochs in the mother (B). Power spectra (fast Fourier transformation) in semi-logarithmic presentation of activity data from the same family (lower panel): intensity (amplitude) over frequency (per hour). Analyses include 11,4 consecutive days, starting with the 4th day after birth. Corresponding periods in bold print. Arrows point to circadian periods. Note corresponding periods of mother and infant and the lower circadian amplitude in the mother compared with the father (C).

ure 6C). These findings were obtained from families living in Berlin, Germany, which were adapted to western industrialised culture. Interestingly, similar results were found for families, who live on the Trobriand Islands (Papua New Guinea) (Siegmund et al., 1994). The families were adapted to a traditional culture and lived in a village, Tauwema, in which the houses had no electric light, radio or watches. Actigraphic 7-day recordings, analysed for the spectral composition of individuals, showed a corresponding 25-hour component of the rest-activity rhythm between a mother and her two months old infant. Again, the father, although sleeping in close proximity to the infant, did not show any change of his rest-activity rhythm. When the activity-rest patterns of these two families were cross-correlated for the entire length of three consecutive days (72 hours), corresponding patterns of both families were stronger between mother and infant when compared with the father. However, differences between the families exist regarding parental activity. In Tauwema, correlation was strongest between mother and infant, while in Berlin correlation was strongest between parents (Wulff et al., 2001).

The existence of corresponding activity patterns, including ultradian cycles and the simultaneous adjustment of the circadian cycle length among mother-infant pairs of industrialised and traditional cultures suggests that the entrainment of biological rhythms during early infancy is a general chronobiological phenomenon. From the perspective of the mother, she mediates – through mutual commuting – her diurnal daily rhythm to her infant, who depends on zeitgeber signals in order to adapt adequately to his/her environment. From the perspective of the infant, he/she perceives the mother's strong daily rhythm – entraining signal – which "manipulates" independent overt ultradian cycles to cluster diurnally. Given that mother-infant synchronisation occurs across cultural borders it is likely to be a universal behaviour in humans that has been tuned through a long evolutionary adaptation process (Eibl-Eibesfeld, 1995).

5. Application of actigraphy in maternal infant care

Since there is potential evidence that the circadian timing system develops prenatally (Reppert et al., 1988; Rivkees, 1997) chronobiological rhythm research becomes increasingly important in neonatal care. Rhythmicity is a property of regulatory mechanisms from which the resonance frequency plays an important role: the cycle length of a variable, e.g. activity, and its actual states, such as the time being "moving" or "immobile". Difficulties appear in determining the mean value (base-line level) for a periodic function that arises from overlapping (superimposed) oscillations through environmental influences and the organism's internal state itself (noise). In infants, age-related rapid changes in the rest-acivity distribution across day and night make it even more difficult, maybe impossible, to disentangle base-line levels (normative values) and abnormal values (see Figure 2). For instance, the emergence of a detectable circadian frequency in activity is delayed in healthy pre-term infants compared with healthy full-term infants (Korte et al., 2001). Various prominent ultradian components derived from actigraphic data occur simultaneously in the spectra. Thus, a base-line level for rhythmicity in pre-term infants is difficult to determine because there is no constant dominant ultradian period. In general, actigraphy is an appropriate method to discover patterns and rhythms in individual cases, which can, by always using the same procedure, be compared with historical data, possibly by documentation in a network's global data bank. The advantage of actigraphy is that the data collection does not depend on the maternal perceptions of their infants' sleep pattern and that the instruments are easy to wear in long-term measurements under home conditions, which is especially important for mothers with children.

There has been increased recognition that desynchronisation between coupled periodic functions, possibly caused by a weak zeitgeber, result in phase differences that trigger reactions which can be observed at times of crisis or illness: elevated restlessness, sleep disturbances, elevation of the pulse frequency, shortening of the sleep-wake cycle (Hildebrandt, 1988). Insomnia in children involves sleeplessness which may have various causes. To assess sleep disorders, infants can be diagnosed with EEG or polysomnography. Desynchronisation of parental and infant nocturnal rest patterns or parental response to the infant's changing rest-activity rhythm may also lead to disharmony and result in complaints of sleeplessness. This can be detected through parallel actigraphic monitoring. However, insomnia in infants can also result from circadian abnormalities. In this case, maxima and minima of activity should not correspond with daytime and night-time, respectively. If this is true, late evening activity, detected through activity monitoring, may reflect a phase delay of the underlying circadian pacemaker, either with respect to environmental time or to the timing of sleep onset. Indeed, an infant, previously diagnosed for attention deficit hyperactive disorder (ADHD) was monitored actigraphically for about two weeks and was found to suffer from delayed-sleep-phase syndrome. When this child was treated with light therapy every day in the early morning, the child recovered from daytime attention deficit and hyperactivity.

Actigraphy also appears to be a useful non-invasive method to study the activity-rest patterns in children with episodic illness of the central nervous system (CNS). Children suffering from West-Syndrome are mentally retarded and need supervision all day and night. When those children were monitored simultaneously with their mothers for several consecutive days and nights, the mothers' activity showed a strong correlation with their infants' patterns. Each pattern revealed seizure occurrence predominantly at night that provoked extremely short nocturnal sleep episodes, these highlight the severity of this illness, which includes marked disturbances of the patients' rhythms and the enormous efforts of the mothers (Table 1). Responses of timed administration of anti-epileptic drugs on seizure were investigated during activity monitoring (Ruiz-Miyares et al., 2000).

Application of actigraphy provides information for research, diagnosis and therapy in a multitude of disorders related to activity rhythms: e.g. in mother-

Table 1. Sleep parameters in Cuban families with children suffering from West-Syndrom derived from actigraphic recordings of 7 consecutive days in two families. Mother-child pair 1 was recorded twice. Data were obtained in 1996.

	mean sleep duration per 24 hrs. (h)	maximum duration of a sleep epoch (h)	mean duration of a sleep epoch (h)	cross-correlation of mother and child at night
mother 1 series 1	8,1	8,2	3,1	0,3
child 1, 4yrs.	11,7	5,4	1,7	
mother 1 series 2	8,4	8,3	4,4	0,34
child 1, 4yrs.	13,7	5,9	2,2	
mother 2	7,7	4,4	2	0,51
child 2, 2yrs.	8,9	5,6	1,6	

infant relationship with mothers having depression (maternity blues, postnatal depression), affective behaviour (mood, stress, aggression) or disabilities (chronic illness); in infants for physical impairment, irritability or desynchronisation.

6. Conclusion

Actigraphic monitoring allows a continuous and unbiased record of the activity-rest behaviour for entire families. When actigraphy is applied to young families, this approach contributes to the understanding of the adaptational process of the infant's biological rhythms to the daily rhythm of the family's life. We have addressed three major topics on the basis of long-term studies using time pattern analysis: (1) the parental activity-rest patterns before and after birth, (2) the entraining patterns of newborn infants after birth, and (3) the consequences of parent-infant synchronisation for the infant's development of a daily rhythm during the first four months. The timing of activity and rest is a basic feature of our daily life. In the course of life, the proportion of rest and activity changes with age and with respect to the 24-hour day. Ultradian and circadian rhythmicity in motor activity starts during fetal life; this is probably driven by the fetal SCN and to a large extent coordinated by the mother (Shibata & Moore, 1988). After birth, activity-rest behaviour of infants develops dramatically during the first few months, which is characterised by either a rapid or a gradual emergence of a diurnal time pattern. There is considerable evidence that phase synchronisation of the onset of daytime activity between mother and infant modulates the entrainment of the infant's daily rhythm to its environment, particularily through social behavioural activities. The quality of early parent-infant interaction is crucial for the future attachment quality of the infant to its social environment (Grossmann et al., 1999). Achieving early synchronisation in the timing of activity-rest patterns between parents and their infant is an important factor in stabilising the social competence of the parents, thereby supporting the optimal physical and mental maturation of the infant.

References

Arendt, J. (1997). The Pineal Gland, Circadian Rhythms and Photoperiodism. In Redfern, P.H. & B. Lemmer (Eds), *Physiology and Pharmacology of Biological Rhythms* (pp. 375–414). Berlin Heidelberg: Springer-Verlag.

Aschoff, J. (1965). *Circadian Clocks*. Amsterdam. North-Holland.

Aschoff, J., M. Fatranska, H. Giedke, P. Doerr, D. Stamm, & H. Wisser (1971). Human circadian rhythms in continuous darkness: entrainment by social cues. *Science, 171*, 213–215.

Benoit, O. (1984). Homeostatic and adaptive roles of human sleep. *Experientia, 40*, 437–440.

Brunner, D.P., M. Munch, K. Biedermann, R. Huch, A. Huch, & A.A. Borbely (1994). Changes in sleep and sleep electroencephalogram during pregnancy. *Sleep, 17*, 576–582.

Ehlers, C.L., E. Frank, & D.J. Kupfer (1988). Social zeitgebers and biological rhythms. A unified approach to understanding the etiology of depression. *Archives of general psychiatry 45*, 948–952.

Eibl-Eibesfeldt, I. (1995). *Die Biologie des menschlichen Verhaltens*. München Zürich. Piper.

Fukuda, K., & K. Ishihara (1997). Development of human sleep and wakefulness rhythm during the first six months of life: discontinuous changes at the 7th and 12th week after birth. *Biological Rhythm Research, 28*, 94–103.

Gottman, J.M. (1981). *Time series analysis*. Cambridge. Cambridge University Press.

Grossmann, K., Grossmann, K., & P. Zimmermann (1999). A wider view of attachment and exploration: Stability and change during the years of immaturity. In J. Cassidy, & P.R. Shaver (Eds), *Handbook of attachment: Theory, research and clinical applications* (pp. 760–786). New York London: The Guilford Press.

Grossmann, K., & K. Grossmann (2000). Bindung, Exploration und internale Arbeitsmodelle – der Stand der Forschung. In E. Parfy, H. Redtenbacher, R. Sigmund, R. Schoberberger & Ch. Butschek, (Eds), *Bindung und Interaktion: Dimensionen der professionellen Beziehungsgestaltung* (pp. 13–38). Wien: Facultas Universitätsverlag.

Guilleminault, C., M. Querra-Salva, S. Chowdhuri, & D. Poyares (2000). Normal pregnancy, daytime sleeping, snoring and blood pressure. *Sleep Medicine 1*, 289–297.

Hastings, M.H. (1997). The Vertebrate Clock: Localisation, Conection and Entrainment. In Redfern, P.H. & B. Lemmer, (Eds), *Physiology and Pharmacology of Biological Rhythms* (pp. 1–28). Berlin Heidelberg: Springer-Verlag.

Haus, E., & Y. Touitou (1997). Chronobiology of Development and Aging. In Redfern, P.H. & B. Lemmer (Eds), *Physiology and Pharmacology of Biological Rhythms* (pp. 95–134). Berlin Heidelberg: Springer-Verlag.

Hildebrandt, G. (1988). Temporal order of ultradian rhythms in man. In Hekkens, W.Th.J.M., G.A. Kerkhof, & W.J. Rietfeld (Eds), *Trends in Chronobiology* (pp. 107–122). Oxford: Pergamon press.

Hobson, J.A. (1990). *Schlaf: Gehirnaktivität im Ruhezustand.* Heidelberg: Spektrum der Wissenschaft Verlagsgesellschaft.

Jacobs, B.L., & E.C. Azmitia (1992). Structure and function of the brain serotonin system. *Physiological reviews, 72*, 165–229.

Jean-Louis, G., D.F. Kripke, W.J. Mason, J.A. Elliott & S.D. Youngstedt (2001). Sleep estimation from wrist movement quantified by different actigraphic modalities. *Journal of Neuroscience Methods, 105*, 185–191.

Kleitman, N. (1982). Basic rest-activity cycle – 22 years later. *Sleep, 5*(4), 311–317.

Korte, J., K. Wulff, C. Oppe, & R. Siegmund (2001). Ultradian and circadian activity-rest rhythms of pre-term neonates compared to full-term neonates using actigraphy. *Chronobiology International, 18(4)*, 697–708.

Löhr, B., & R. Siegmund (1999). Ultradian and circadian rhythms of sleep-wake and food-intake behavior during early infancy. *Chronobiology International, 16*, 129–148.

Moore, R.Y., & N.J. Lenn (1972). A retinohypothalamic projection in the rat. *The Journal of comparative neurology, 146*, 1–14.

Moore, R.Y. (1973). Retinohypothalamic projection in mammals: a comparative study. *Brain Research, 49*, 403–409.

Moore-Ede, M.C., C.A. Czeisler, & G.S. Richardson (1983). Circadian timekeeping in health and disease. Part 1. Basic properties of circadian pacemakers. *New England Journal of Medicine, 309*, 469–476.

Mullaney, D.J., D.F. Kripke, & S. Messin (1980). Wrist-actigraphic estimation of sleep time. *Sleep, 3*, 83–92.

Novak, C.M., L. Smale, & A.A. Nunez (2000). Rhythms in Fos expression in brain areas related to the sleep-wake cycle in the diurnal *Arvicanthis niloticus. Am J Physiol Regulatory Integrative Comp Physiol, 278*, R1267–R1274.

Pinilla, T., & L.L. Birch (1993). Help me make it through the night: Behavioural entrainment of breast-fed infants' sleep patterns. *Pediatrics, 91*, 436–444.

Ralph, M.R., & M. Menaker (1988). A mutation of the circadian system in golden hamsters. *Science, 241*, 1225–1227.

Reppert, S.M., D.R. Weaver, S.A. Rivkees, & E.G. Stopa (1988). Putative melatonin receptors in a human biological clock. *Science, 242*, 78–81.

Rivkees, S.A. (1997). Developing circadian rhythmicity. *Pediatric Endocrinology, 44*, 467–487.

Ruiz-Miyares, F., R. Siegmund, K. Wermke, J. Dorado-Gallego, & D.I. Escobedo-Beceiro (2000). Síndrome de West: una aproximación cronobiológica. *Revista de neurologia, 30*, 925–928.

Sadeh, A., P. Lavie, A. Scher, E. Tirosh, & R. Epstein (1991). Actigraphic home-monitoring sleep-disturbed and control infants and young children: a new method for pediatric assessment of sleep-wake patterns. *Pediatrics, 87*, 494–499.

Salzarulo, Piero, Igino Fagioli, Frančoise Salomon, Jean-Frančoise Duhamel & Claude Ricour (1979). Alimentation continue et rhytme veille-sommeil chez l'enfant. *Arch. Franc. Pediatr., 36*, 26–32.

Schwartz, W.J. (1991). SCN metabolic activity in vivo. In Klein, D.C., R.Y. Moore, & S.M. Reppert (Eds), *The suprachiasmatic nucleus: the mind's clock* (pp. 144–156). New York: Oxford University Press.

Shibata, S., & R.Y. Moore (1988). Development of a fetal circadian rhythm after disruption of the maternal circadian system. *Developmental Brain Research, 41*, 313–317.

Shimada, M., K. Takahashi, M. Segawa, M. Higurashi, M. Samejim, & K. Horiuchi (1999). Emerging and entraining patterns of the sleep-wake rhythm in pre-term and term infants. *Brain & development, 21*, 468–473.

Siegmund, R., M. Tittel, & W. Schiefenhövel (1994). Time Patterns in Parent-Child Interactions in a Trobriand Village (Papua New Guinea). *Biological Rhythm Research, 25*, 241–251.

Siegmund, R., W. Schiefenhövel, & M. Tittel (1996). Time Patterns in Infants – Activity, Rest and Mother-Child Interactions in Crosscultural Comparison. In Gottschalk-Batschkus, C.E. & J. Schuler (Eds), *Ethnomedical Perspectives on Early Childhood* (pp. 293–299). Berlin: Verlag für Wissenschaft und Bildung.

Siegmund, R., M. Tittel, & W. Schiefenhövel (1998). Activity Monitoring of the Inhabitants in Tauwema, a Traditional Melanesian Village: Rest/Activity Behaviour of Trobriand Islanders (Papua New Guinea). *Biological Rhythm Research, 29*, 49–59.

Szymanski, J.S. (1918). Versuche über Aktivität und Ruhe bei Säuglingen. *Pflügers Archiv, 178*, 424–429.

Van Someren, E.J.W., R.H.C. Lazeron, B.F.M. Vonk, M. Mirmiran, & D.F. Swaab (1996). Gravitational artefact in frequency spectra of movement acceleration: implications for actigraphy in young and elderly subjects. *Journal of Neuroscience Methods, 65*, 55–62.

Vitaterna, M.H., D.P. King, A.M. Chang, J.M. Kornhauser, P.L. Lowrey, J.D. McDonald, W.F. Dove, L.H. Pinto, F.W. Turek, & J.S. Takahashi (1994). Mutagenesis and mapping of a mouse gene, Clock, essential for circadian behavior. *Science, 264*, 719–725.

Waterhouse, J., & D. Minors (1988). Masking and Entrainment. In Hekkens, W.Th.J.M., G.A. Kerkhof, & W.J. Rietveld (Eds), *Trends in Chronobiology, Advances in the Biosciences*, Vol 73 (pp. 163–171). Oxford, New York: Pergamon Press.

Weitzman, E.D., R.M. Boyar, S. Kapen, & L. Hellman (1975). The relationship of sleep and sleep stages to neuroendocrine secretion and biological rhythms in man. *Recent progress in hormone research, 31*, 399–446.

Wulff, K., & R. Siegmund (2000). Circadian and ultradian time patterns in human behaviour: Part 1: Activity monitoring of families from prepartum to postpartum. *Biological Rhythm Research, 31*(5), 581–602.

Wulff, K., A. Dedek, & R. Siegmund (2001). Circadian and ultradian time patterns in human behaviour: Part 2: Social synchronisation during the development of the infant's diurnal activity-rest pattern. *Biological Rhythm Research, 5*, 529–546.

The eyes of parents on infants awakening

Fiorenza Giganti and Monica Toselli
Department of Psychology, University of Florence

Spontaneous awakening during nocturnal sleep is a frequent event in early development, linked to a polyphasic sleep-wake rhythm. The number of spontaneous nocturnal awakenings tends to decrease with age, together with a "less polyphasic" sleep-wake rhythm (Navelet, Benoit, & Bouard, 1982; Louis, Cannard, Bastuji, & Challamel, 1997; Ficca, Fagioli, Giganti & Salzarulo, 1999).

Parents, for their part, wish to train their child to reach an adult-like sleep organization with a continuous nocturnal sleep, and the presence and frequency of night-awakenings could become troublesome during this training. Indeed, the role of parental intervention is particularly relevant in the very early period of development when the organization of sleep-wake rhythm is being crucially modified. On the other hand, the presence of frequent nocturnal awakenings is a physiological event which can somehow influence the parent-child relationship.

If awakenings are linked to the physiological and psychological variables of infants, their detection depends on the signs used by parents to detect them. The frequency of awakenings, reported by parents, depends on their ability to perceive them as well as on their intervention usually performed to reduce them. In fact, parents may or may not notice awakenings, and when they do, they can either simply observe their infants' awakenings or intervene in order to get them to fall asleep again. These choices and the type of possible intervention are tied to the cultural setting surrounding parents, to their beliefs and to personal characteristics.

Among the child-related variables connected to awakenings, gender, temperament and tendency to signal one's own awakening will be specifically discussed.

The most relevant signs of awakening noticed by parents in the home environment will be compared with the behavioural signs used by scientists in the experimental context.

Finally, the individual and intercultural differences in caregiving practices during awakenings will be addressed.

Infant variables related to awakenings

The frequency of night awakenings is influenced by infant intrinic variables. Indeed, many aspects of growth, such as new motor skills, teething (Paret, 1983) locomotion (Scher, 2000, personal communication), as well as weaning (Wright, MacLeod, & Cooper, 1983), were shown to influence sleep-wake rhythm.

Other intrinsic variables of the infant, like gender or temperament, can be involved in the frequency of nocturnal awakenings. Gender, for instance, can prompt different forms of intervention by caregivers. Differences in awakenings between males and females were observed by Anders (1978) in two and nine months old infants. Awakenings of males are reported by parents as more frequent than awakenings of females; there is also a greater number of checking interventions by parents. Further differences were identified by Harkins and Wolff (personal communication). Male subjects took longer to shift from sleep to waking and cried and fussed more during the transitional states.

This behaviour creates a loop with parents' behaviour: mothers spend more time holding and otherwise soothing males.

Temperament also, in particular a difficult one, would seem to be related to night-waking. In an epidemiological study on 100 young children referred to a Crying Baby Clinic because of repeated waking at night, Schaefer (1990) found a great number of "difficult" temperaments (assessed through The Revised Infant Temperament Questionnaire by Carey & McDevitt, 1978 and through the Toddler Temperament Scale by Fullard, McDevitt & Carey, 1984). Likewise, Keener, Zeanah and Anders (1988) reported that infants who require frequent caregiving during the night are rated, above all by their fathers, as more difficult.

To classify infants temperament as "difficult", "easy", or "slow to warm" many scales are commonly used, with categories such as rhythmicity, activity, sensory threshold and others. Then, when more specific temperamental categories are considered, as done by Halpern, Anders, Garcia Coll and Hua (1994), relations were reported between behavioural temperament scores (irritability and lesser sociability) and night awakenings. Carey (1974) as well stressed the relationship between night waking and specific temperament categories like sensory threshold; the general pattern of easy or difficult temperament on the other hand was not related. It is noteworthy that none of the items defining sensory threshold made any reference to sleep behaviour. Therefore, it seems that night-wakings are not essential criteria to assess a difficult temperament, that is there is not a direct relationship between temperament as an intrinsic infant characteristic and night-wakings.

Negative attributes of temperament assessed by mothers (fussiness, inadequacy, unpredictability) were correlated "with greater maternal depression, higher levels of psychological distress, less perceived self-efficacy as a parent and less perceived value in the parenting role" (Anders, 1994: 18). The relationship has not yet been clarified among psychological characteristics and behaviour of mothers, their perception of infant temperament, and infant sleep-wake organization. For example, it remains an open question whether a specific temperament induces more interventions. Halpern et al. (1994) reported that maternal night-time interventions generally were unrelated to infant temperament. Further investigation is necessary to shed light on these aspects.

Some infants are frequently accustomed to signaling their awakenings during the night, mainly by crying (Anders, 1978; Paret, 1983). In particular, Anders (1978) identified signalers and non-signalers (2 and 9 months old) using a time lapse video-system: while some infants signal their awakening by crying or calling, some infants seem to be self-soothers during night awakenings. Self-soothing behaviour does not induce parental intervention and leads to underevaluating the frequency and length of infant's spontaneous awakenings. This behaviour seems to be a form of early learning in the framework of the parent-child relationship. In fact Paret reported that non-signalers are infants who had "learned" not to need to be nursed or rocked to fall asleep and who, in turn, spontaneously use thumb-sucking and transitional objects. These two behaviours are strictly linked to the attachment bond; indeed the non-signalers are infants who have less daytime separation, are further along in the total weaning process, and probably don't require the physical presence or even the breast of the mother to fall asleep again because they have acquired the representation of the maternal figure. The use of transitional objects was more frequent in children who fell asleep alone (57%) compared to children who fell asleep accompanied by the caregiver (30%) (Wolf & Lozoff, 1989).

The tendency of the infant to signal his awakenings can be influenced by parents' behaviour. Recurrent forms of behaviour by the parents act as training for the infants. Adair, Bauchner, Philipp, Levenson & Zuckerman (1991) have shown that 9-month-old infants whose parents were present at bedtime were significantly more likely to wake at night (according to parents' reports) than infants whose parents were not present. Johnson (1991) also, in a telephone survey, stressed meaningful differences in bedtime routines between night-wakers and good sleepers 12 to 35 months old. Infants who were nursed, rocked or comforted by their parents during bed-time, were more likely to be night-wakers. The majority of infants who fell asleep alone were sleeping throughout the night, whereas less than one third of the infants who fell asleep with the help of their parents were able to sleep through the night.

The parenting intervention of putting children to bed alone can develop soothing abilities in the child, but also, teach him not to rely on parents for help (Salzarulo, Giganti, Ficca, Fagioli & Toselli, 2000). Teaching not to rely on parents for help could be negative for the child if it happens too early during infant development, before the settlement of the attachment bond relationship and some first kind of autonomous Self.

Scientists and parents looking at infants' awakening

Not only the child's behaviour but also parental responsiveness could influence what happens during awakening. In fact parents, in order to detect awakenings, can use behavioural clues which, however, have not yet been systematically investigated.

In the scientific context, instead, the criteria of awakenings during the first year of life have been systematically investigated with the awakenings being detected both by physiological indices and behavioural signs. Among the most relevant behavioural signs of awakenings described in the literature, there are: eyes open, general motor activity, irregular respiration (Prechtl, 1974; Parmelee & Stern 1972; Wolff 1987), plus crying (Curzi-Dascalova, Monod, Guidasci & Korn, 1981).

In a preliminary study about parents looking at infants' awakenings, we have been able to acquire some information about mothers' ideas about the signs of awakening (Toselli, Schiano & Salzarulo, unpublished data).

The study was performed during the first two months of the mother-infant relationship, among mothers of low-risk preterm infants. Thirty-seven mothers of low risk preterm infants were interviewed, at three different times: (1) the first interview was performed 20 days after delivery; (2) the second interview was performed just after the infants were discharged from the intensive

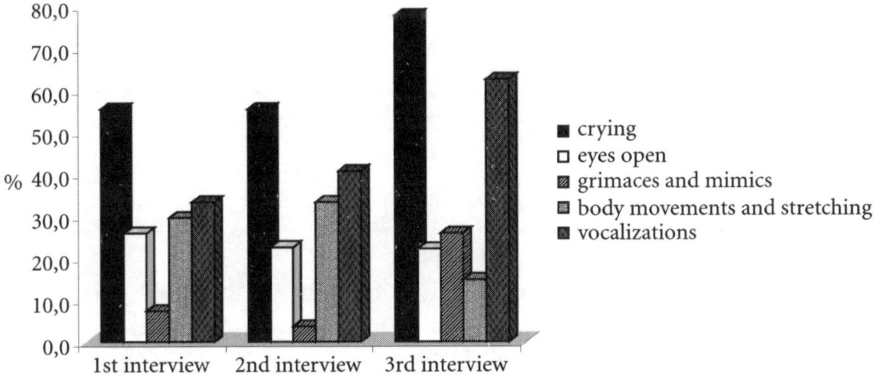

Figure 1. Signs of awakenings mentioned by mothers of preterm infants.

care unit; (3) the third interview was performed two months after the infants' discharge from the hospital.

As a whole, the most frequent sign of awakening reported by mothers was crying (see Fig. 1), other signs were also vocal, like calling and whimpering, then there were signs which must be caught by sight, like body movements, eyes open, and facial expressions.

During the course of the three interviews, as the mothers gained more and more direct experience of their infant, vocal signs were reported with an increasing frequency (crying remained the most frequent sign) while "eyes open" remained quite stable. Body movements were reported with a decreasing frequency, especially when the infants had been at home for two months. It is interesting to underscore that in the first interview the mothers' answers are based on an image of their infant and of their signs of awakenings coming from vague and general beliefs which are not linked to the current experience with that baby (although some mothers had some previous child experience as they were multiparous).

In the third interview, the mothers' answers seem to be linked to the observation of the child and of its growth. Crying is reported with an increasing frequency, as well as vocal signs and facial expressions, while some signs like body movements are reported with a decreasing frequency, due also, maybe, to the developmental trend towards a decrease in global body motility, which has been shown by several authors (Peirano, Curzi-Dascalova, & Korn, 1986; Vecchierini-Blineau, Nogues, Louvet & Desfontaines, 1994).

Table 1. Behavioural signs detected in different contexts

Scientific context	Naturalistic context (mothers' eyes)
Eyes open	Eyes open
General motor activity	Body movements
Irregular respiration	Vocal signs
Crying	Crying

Similar data concerning mothers of full-term infants in their first year of life, as well as mothers of pre-term infants at a lower post-conceptional age, would be necessary to complete the picture.

It is noteworthy that there is not a great difference between awakening signs described in the scientific context (eyes open, general motor activity, irregular respiration and crying) and the ones reported by the mothers in a naturalistic context (eyes open, body movements, vocal signs and crying). We can stress that the only difference between the two contexts is the relevance given by scientists to irregular respiration and by parents to vocal signs (see Table 1). Irregular respiration, an index of both physiological activity and object of behavioural observation, is mainly detected by scientists, while whimpers are preferentially noticed by parents as a sign of awakening. The parents' attention is attracted by whimpering, attributing it a generic communicating role. Parents in fact always tend to attribute a communicative meaning to behavioural and vocal expressions by their child (Camaioni, Volterra & Bates, 1976), also considering them to be expressions of mental activity. Moreover, we have noticed (Salzarulo & Toselli, 1997) that the smiles and grimaces during sleep of even one-month-old infants are interpreted by parents as expressing some kind of mental activity of the infants, that is oneiric activity.

However, when the infant is not sleeping in the same room as the parents, crying becomes the most frequent sign of the infant's spontaneous awakenings noticed by parents, because they are able to perceive only acoustic stimuli coming from their infants.

Nevertheless, infants show episodic crying during active sleep unrelated to environmental events or to identifiable organismic conditions or to awakenings (Wolff, 1987). Even more so in pre-term infants, Dreyfus-Brisac (1974: 131) has found that most of the periods of crying occur "simultaneously with two criteria [Rapid Eye Movements, continuous EEG] belonging to active sleep". We can suppose that if crying is such a relevant sign for parents' intervention, then some parents may interrupt their infant's sleep considering the infant awake. These interventions, when repeated, could contribute to the disorganization of the natural structure of infants' sleep.

On the other hand, Wolff (1987) has reported that most mothers are able to distinguish different kinds of crying when the child is awake (for example hunger crying from "mad" crying or "pain" crying). Wolff (1987) also reported different spectrographic characteristics. Nevertheless data is lacking about spectrographic comparisons among crying at awakening, crying during sleep (in particular active sleep) and other kinds of crying. We can anyhow place in doubt the mothers' ability to detect differences in crying during different behavioural states (in particular wakefulness vs. sleep).

Parents thus use quite macroscopic signs which can lead them to intervene when the child is still sleeping or to ignore awakenings which are instead picked up on by scientists through their more fine-grained means of detection.

Parents' interventions and beliefs: cultural background

Parents' interventions with regard to the awakening of infants are not only affected by child-related variables but also by parental variables such as their personal and emotional condition, their beliefs, as well as by the cultural background of the family. It is noteworthy to consider how infant crying (which, as we have shown, is a very common sign of awakening noticed by parents) induces different intervention policies, according to the culture.

For instance, Stork (1993) stresses that in non-Western cultures (Tunisia and many African countries) infant crying cannot be ignored as it expresses some infant need and it induces an immediate intervention by caregivers by day as well as by night. The wide number of surrogate caregivers (grandmothers, aunts) facilitates the tendency to intervene in a contingent way for the infant's cries.

In Western cultures, on the contrary, educational rules sometimes do not permit parents to answer to the infant crying, maintaining instead that not providing any contingent intervention can be an effective means for developing the infant's autonomy. In turn, sleep researchers have applied this approach, prompting parents to ignore systematically their infant's crying during the night in order to reduce night-awakenings (Rickert & Johnson, 1988; Sadeh, 1994).

Among parental interventions undertaken during the transition from wakefulness to sleep, bedtime interaction was particularly investigated, among others by Van Tassel (1985) and, as previously mentioned, by Adair and colleagues (1991) and by Johnson (1991), whereas the role in falling asleep of sleep aids, like transitional objects – such meaningful tokens of the parent-infant relationship – was stressed by Wolf and Lozoff (1989). Fewer investigations have been performed about parental care given during the transitions from sleep to waking states, that is at the time of awakening.

Nevertheless, in an African culture, that of the Soninké of Mali, E. Razy (quoted by Salzarulo, 1999) noticed that each awakening, during the day and the night, is watched and always "accompanied" by someone, the mother or another member of the family, and is generally followed by feeding. The infant never has to face being alone when entering or coming out of sleep. It seems that this culture is particularly sensitive to the need for someone's presence during the transitional phases. In any case, no specific intervention is performed at awakening, not even during the night, in order to compel the child to fall asleep again.

Parental intervention policy with regard to awakenings has emerged as a relevant variable affecting infant-caregiver attachment. The link between interventions regarding sleep and attachment was especially stressed by Anders (1994) who observed that parent's intervention affects the organization of sleep itself and the quality of the attachment. The first year of life is crucial for the reorganization of sleep-wake rhythm as well as for the development of an autonomous Self. In fact, "separation and reunion experiences remain the hallmark of attachment research... [and] ... night-time experiences early in life most certainly influence the emergence of the developing attachment system" (Anders, 1994: 14).

The attachment bond joins the child and the caregiver (generally the mother). Scher and Blumberg (1999) showed that night-wakings were more common among children whose mothers were rated high in maternal separation anxiety measured by the Emotional Status Index by Hock, McBride & Gnezda (1989).

Equalizing all other variables (infants' temperament, early life events, quality of infants' daytime environments), Sagi, Van Ijzendoorn, Aviezer, Donnell & Mayseless (1994) found that sleep arrangements, involving or not parents' nocturnal interventions during infants' awakenings, were crucial in determining the infants' security of attachment. Indeed, the kibbutz in which communal sleeping arrangements did not assure the presence of the attachment figure during the night, and then at awakenings, had more insecurely attached 14–22-month-old infants, than the kibbutz with home-based sleeping arrangements.

Sleeping arrangements are also studied as affecting the frequency of awakenings. The practice of co-sleeping – defined as parents and children sleeping in body contact with each other for all or part of the night (Lozoff, Askew & Wolf, 1996) – was associated with a greater number of nocturnal awakenings both in black and white families of both lower and higher socio-economic status (Lozoff et al., 1996). Generally, regular co-sleeping was common among black families independently of socio-economic status, but among white families co-sleeping was more common among lower socio-economic status families (Lozoff et al., 1996), showing that sleeping arrangements depend in turn on social and cultural variables of the family.

The role of historical and cultural influences in considering disrupted night sleep as a problem was stressed, among others, by Salzarulo & Chevalier (1983) and Richman (1987).

Parents' interventions and kinds of responses to awakening signs appears to be guided not only by infant behaviour but also by parents' beliefs. Parents' beliefs about awakenings pertain to how to intervene when the child wakes, to the evaluation of awakenings as stressful life events and to the reasons why the child wakes up.

Cultural differences affect, for instance, black/white families' evaluations of nocturnal awakenings as a stressful sleep problem. In the previously mentioned research, Lozoff et al. (1996) showed that among co-sleeping families, white families complain more about stressful sleep problems, such as night-waking, than black families. Lozoff and colleagues consider that black parents are more able to accept their children's sleep behaviour.

Considering parents' beliefs about the reasons why infants wake up, Toselli, Farneti & Salzarulo (1995) found that pregnant women believed hunger to be the most frequent reason for children's awakening. Hunger is the most cited reason for awakening by mothers of one-month-old fullterm (88%) and preterm (mean post-conceptional age: 34 weeks) (94%) infants (see Fig. 2; Primi, Puliti, Toselli, Cioni & Salzarulo, 1996).

Hunger remains the prevailing reason for the awakenings of one-month-old infants according to mothers recently interviewed by our group (Costabile, Toselli, Genta & Salzarulo, unpublished data) in two different Italian cultural contexts (Fig. 3), Ferrara (Northern Italy) (84%) and Cosenza (Southern Italy) (85%). The other reasons for awakening, while presenting hunger as the main one during the first month of infant life, change according to infant condition (pre-term vs. full-term) and to parental cultural context, and change even more during infant development.

In the full-term follow-up study, the same mothers who, when interviewed, cited hunger (95%) as the main reason for awakening when their infants were one month old, cited instead sufficient sleep (89%), when their infants were

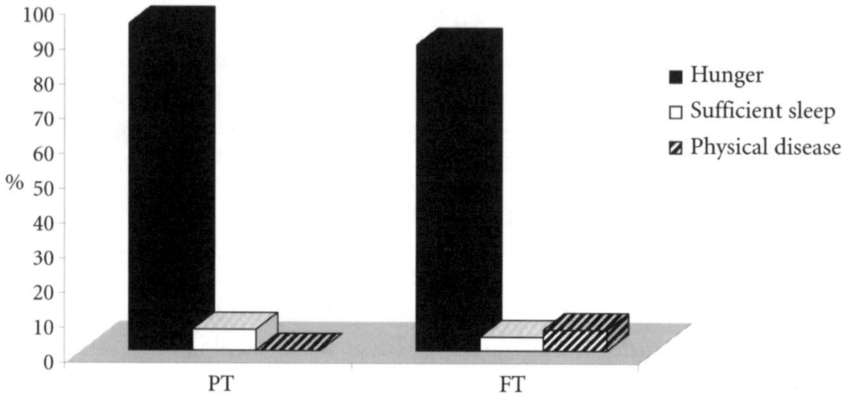

Figure 2. Causes of awakening reported by mothers for 1 month preterm (PT) and fullterm (FT) old infants.

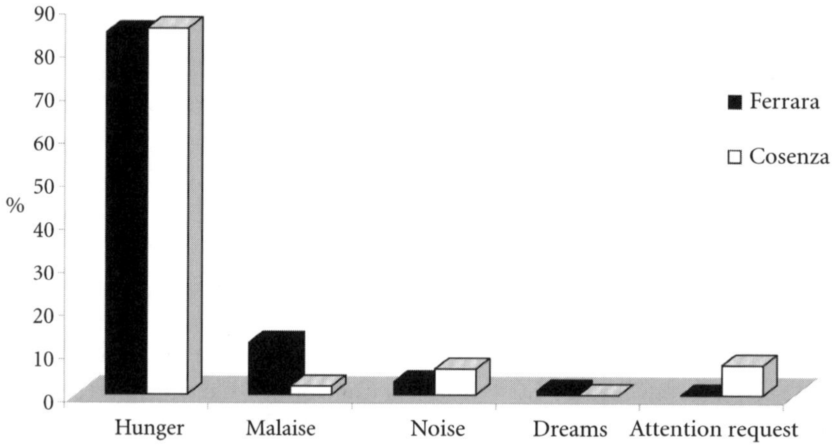

Figure 3. Causes of awakening reported by 1 month old infants' mothers in two Italian cultural contexts.

one year old (Toselli, Farneti & Salzarulo, 1998). The reasons reported for awakenings at one year of age also change according to the time of day. The same mothers who attribute nocturnal awakenings mainly to sufficient sleep believe that awakenings during the day-time naps of their one-year-old infants are linked to physical discomfort (18%), nightmares (17%), or the "wish to be taken into account" (17%) (Toselli, Farneti & Salzarulo, unpublished data).

The relationship between ideas and parents' interventions is a very complicated one. There are three different aspects involved: first the perception of the awakening, second the ideas about the cause of awakening; third the kinds of intervention. The link between these three aspects may show some contradiction, as in other domains pertaining to the relation between belief and parental behaviour (Goodnow & Collins, 1990). Indeed, although hunger was considered by mothers as the most relevant reason for awakening in the first month of life, feeding is not a common way of intervention to induce sleep in the infant (Toselli et al., 1998).

The choice of the way of feeding (breast/bottle) and the time of weaning also seem to affect the presence of night-wakings. Differences between breast-fed and bottle-fed infants were found by Wright and colleagues (1983). Breast-fed infants showed a higher frequency of awakenings than bottle-fed infants at the same age. However, the explanation for this finding may not be related to the different modalities of feeding, but rather to the parents' perception of the awakening. Wright et al. (1983) suggested that mothers of bottle-fed infants may consider awakenings as a problem to be solved and act more effectively to negatively reinforce awakenings, while mothers of breast-fed infants have "a more liberal and permissive attitude" (p. 318), and better tolerate the spontaneous awakenings of the child.

Links between feeding styles (demand vs. schedule; continuous vs. discontinuous feeding) and night-time awakenings were not found (Anders, 1994; Salzarulo, Fagioli, Salomon, Duhamel & Ricour, 1979; Schulz, Massetani, Fagioli & Salzarulo, 1985). It is hypothesised by Anders (1994:17) that "it is the pattern of inconsistent and difficult feeding interactions, rather than nutritional factors affecting the relationship, which in turn may influence the consolidation of sleep-wake patterns".

Conclusions

Frequent awakenings are usually observed during the first year of life and parents are witnesses as well as shapers of their infants' awakenings.

We believe that parents have a crucial role. Their first role is just the one of perceiving or not what is going on in the crib. Parents notice that their infants wake up, mostly from vocal signs coming from the infant; nevertheless the other signs noticed by parents do not greatly differ from those detected by scientists.

Subsequently, parents can intervene during awakenings, whenever they notice them, according to the meaning that they attribute to them. Parents, in fact, can be distressed by frequent awakenings and use every strategy available in or-

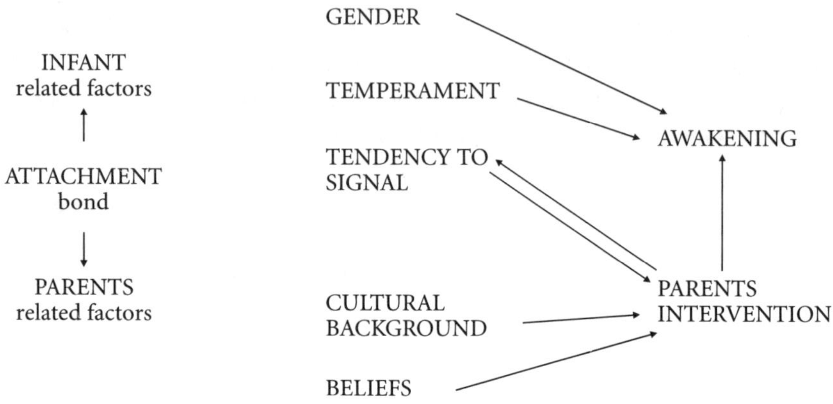

Figure 4. Factors modulating awakening.

der to reduce them, or they can judge them as not requiring their intervention: cultural backgrounds influence these choices.

Parents' interventions or lack of interventions tend to become a habit, inducing learning processes in the child and in this way shaping his behaviour at night.

The awakening and the related behaviour are, then, modulated by different factors (see Fig. 4) related both to infants and to parents, and the attachment bond is a crucial framework for understanding what happens during infant awakening. Taking into account some of the infant variables, gender and temperament – or some specific temperamental categories like sensory threshold – have been shown to be related to awakenings. Linked instead to the occurrence of parental interventions is the tendency by the infant to signal his awakening, as well as all the parent-related factors such as their beliefs and cultural constraints.

Attachment and sleep policy, including awakening interventions, develop, during the first year of the child, following two different, not always convergent, paths. While some strategies used to reduce awakenings or lack of any kind of intervention, at very early ages, may be helpful for getting a good night-long-sleeping baby, at the same time, they can negatively affect attachment.

References

Adair, R., H. Bauchner, B. Philipp, S. Levenson & B. Zuckerman (1991). Night waking during infancy: role of parental presence at bedtime. *Pediatrics, 87*, 500–504.

Anders, T. (1978). Home-recorded sleep in 2- and 9-months-old infants. *American Academy of Child Psychiatry, 17*, 421–432.

Anders, T. (1979). Night-waking in infants during the first year of life. *Pediatrics, 63*, 860–864.

Anders, T. (1994). Infant sleep, nighttime relationships, and attachment. *Psychiatry, 57*, 11–21.

Camaioni, L., V. Volterra & E. Bates (1976). La comunicazione nel primo anno di vita. *Torino: Boringhieri.*

Carey, W. (1974). Night-waking and temperament in infancy. *Behavioral Pediatrics, 84*, 756–758.

Carey, W., & S. McDevitt (1978). Revision of the infant temperament questionnaire. *Pediatrics, 61*, 735–739.

Curzi-Dascalova, L., N. Monod, S. Guidasci & G. Korn (1981). Transition veille-sommeil chez les nouveau-nés et les nourrissons avant l'âge de 3 mois. *Revue EEG Neurophysiologie, 11*, 1–10.

Dreyfus-Brisac, C. (1974). Organization of Sleep in Prematures: Implications for Caregiving. In M. Lewis & L.A. Rosenblum (Eds), *The Effect of the Infant on Its Caregiver* (123–140), New York: John Wiley and Sons.

Ficca, G., I. Fagioli, F. Giganti & P. Salzarulo (1999). Spontaneous awakening from sleep across the first year of life. *Early Human Development, 55*, 219–228.

Fullard, W., S. McDevitt & W. Carey (1984). Assessing temperament in one-to-three year old children. *Journal of Pediatric Psychology, 9*, 205–217.

Goodnow, J., & A. Collins (1990). *Development according to parents. The nature, sources and consequences of parent's ideas.* Hove, East Sussex: Lawrence Erlbaum.

Johnson, M. (1991). Infant and toddler sleep: a telephone survey of parents in one community. *Journal of Developmental and Behavioral Pediatrics, 12*, 108–114.

Halpern, L., T. Anders, C. Garcia Coll & J. Hua (1994). Infant temperament: is there a relation to sleep-wake states and maternal nighttime behaviour? *Infant Behavior and Development, 17*, 255–263.

Harkins, C., & P. Wolff (1998). Personal communication.

Hock, E., S. McBride & M.T. Gnezda (1989). Maternal separation anxiety: mother-infant separation from the maternal perspective. *Child Development, 60*, 793–802.

Keener, M., C. Zeanah & T. Anders (1988). Infant temperament, sleep organization, and nighttime parental interventions. *Pediatrics, 81*, 762–771.

Louis, J., C. Cannard, H. Bastuji & MJ. Challamel. (1997). Sleep ontogenesis revisited: a longitudinal 24-hour home polygraphic study on 15 normal infants during the first two years of life. *Sleep, 20*, 323–333.

Lozoff, B., G. Askew & A. Wolf (1996). Cosleeping and early childhood sleep problems: effects of ethnicity and socioeconomic status. *Developmental and Behavioural Pediatrics, 17*, 9–15.

Navelet, Y., O. Benoit, & G. Bouard (1982). Nocturnal sleep organization during the first months of life. *Electroencephalographic Clinical Neurophysiology, 54*, 71–78.

Paret, I. (1983). Night waking and its relation to mother-infant interaction in nine-month-old infants. In J. Cale, E. Galinsan & R.L. Tyson (Eds), *Frontiers of infant Psychiatry*, New York: Basic Books.

Parmelee, A., & E. Stern (1972). Development of states in infants. In C.D. Clemente, D.P. Purpura, & F.E. Meyer (Eds), *Sleep and maturing nervous system* (199–228). New York: Academic Press.

Peirano, P., L. Curzi-Dascalova & G. Korn (1986). Influence of sleep state and age on body motility in normal premature and fullterm neonates. *Neuropediatrics, 17,* 186–190.

Prechtl, H. (1974). The behavioural states of the newborn infant (a review). *Brain Research, 76,* 185–212.

Primi, C., MT. Puliti, M. Toselli, G. Cioni & P. Salzarulo (1996). Awakening and falling asleep in preterm infants: Mother's ideas. *Journal of Sleep Research, 5,* 373.

Rickert, V., & M. Johnson (1988). Reducing nocturnal awakening and crying episodes in infants and young children: a comparison between scheduled awakenings and systematic ignoring. *Pediatrics, 81,* 203–212.

Richman, N. (1987). Surveys of sleep disorders in children in a general population. In Ch. Guilleminault (Ed.), *Sleep and its disorders in children* (115–127). New York: Raven Press.

Sadeh, A.(1994). Assesment of intervention for infant night waking: parental reports and activity-based home monitoring. *Journal of Consulting and Clinical Psychology 62,* 63–68.

Sagi, A., M. Van Ijzendoorn, O. Aviezer, F. Donnel & O. Mayseless (1994). Sleeping out of home in a Kibbutz Communal arrangement: it makes a difference for infant-mother attachment. *Child Development, 65,* 992–1004.

Salzarulo, P. (1999). *La fine del sonno.* Torino: Bollati Boringhieri.

Salzarulo P., I. Fagioli, F. Salomon, J.-F. Duhamel & R. Ricour (1979) Alimentation continue et rythme veille-sommeil chez l'enfant. *Archives Française Pediatrie (Suppl), 36*: 26–32.

Salzarulo, P., & A. Chevalier (1983). Sleep problems in chlidren and their relationship with early disturbances of the waking-sleeping rhythm. *Sleep, 6,* 47–51.

Salzarulo, P., & M. Toselli (1997). The "motoric" dream: where mother's eye and scientist meet. 7° meeting of the European sleep club, Lyon, 12–13 September.

Salzarulo, P., F. Giganti, G. Ficca, I. Fagioli, & M. Toselli (2000). Gates to awakening in early development. *Clinical Neurophysiology at the beginning of 21st Century (Supplement to Clinical Neurophysiology), 53,* 352–354.

Schaefer, C. (1990). Nightwaking and temperament in early childhood. *Psychological Reports, 67,* 192–194.

Scher, A.(2000). Personal communication.

Scher, A., & O. Blumberg (1999). Night waking among 1-year olds: a study of maternal separation anxiety. *Child: Care, Health and Development, 25,* 323–334.

Schulz H., R. Massetani, I. Fagioli & P. Salzarulo (1985). Spontaneous awakening from sleep in infants. *Electroencephology and Clinical Neurophysiology, 61,* 267–271.

Stork, H. (1993). *Les rituels du coucher de l'enfant. Variation culturelles.* Paris: ESF.

Toselli, M., P. Farneti & P. Salzarulo (1995). Infant sleep representation in the pregnant women. *Journal of Reproductive and Infant Psychology, 13,* 47–50.

Toselli, M., P. Farneti & P. Salzarulo (1998). Maternal representation and care of infant sleep. *Early Development and Parenting, 7,* 73–78.

Van Tassel, E. (1985). The relative influence of child and environmental characteristics on sleep disturbances in the first and in the second years of life. *Developmental Behavioral Pediatrics, 6,* 81–86.

Vecchierini-Blineau, M.F., B. Nogues, S. Louvet & O. Desfontaines (1994). Maturation de la motilité généralisée, spontanée au cours du sommeil, de la naissance à terme à l'âge de 6 mois. *Neurophysiologie Clinique, 24,* 141–154.

Wolf, A., & B. Lozoff (1989). Object attachment, thumbsucking and passage to sleep. *Journal of the American Academy of child and adolescent Psychiatry, 28,* 287–292.

Wolff, P. (1987). *The development of behavioural states and the expression of emotions in early infancy.* Chicago: The University Chicago Press.

Wright, P., H. Macleod & M. Cooper (1983). Waking at night: the effect of early feeding experience. *Child: care, health and developement, 9,* 309–319.

Mother–infant relationship as a modulator of night waking

Anat Scher
Faculty of Education, University of Haifa, Israel

In the course of the first year of life sleep problems, particularly settling difficulties and frequent night waking, are a cause of concern to many parents. The high prevalence of sleep problems during infancy and the associated parental concerns have been widely documented (for a review see, e.g., Messer & Richards, 1993; Salzarulo & Chevalier, 1983). Night waking is a common phenomenon throughout infancy (Moore & Ucko, 1957). Even at one year of age more than 50% of the mothers report that their infant regularly wakes up during the night (Scher, 1991). Furthermore, home-based objective sleep measures such as all-night time-lapse recordings (e.g. Anders, 1979) or actively-monitoring (e.g., Sadeh, Lavie, Scher, Tirosh, & Epstein, 1991) indicate that awakenings are even more frequent than parents perceive. In fact, brief awakenings are an integral part of sleep, occurring several times each night in infants (Hoppenbrouwers et al., 1988) and also in adults (Aserinsky and Kleitman, 1953). From a developmental perspective, a sleep-related task of infancy is often described in terms of "sleeping through the night" (e.g., Daws, 1989; Anders, Halpern, & Hua, 1992). Given that sleep architecture, as noted, involves a number of sleep segments divided by physiological awakenings (Aserinsky & Kleitman, 1953), the task is to regulate nighttime sleep–wake transitions so that from the parent's perspective the infant seems to be "sleeping through the night".

Although the achievement of uninterrupted sleep for both child and parent is a valuable challenge, parental nighttime involvement, and frequent caregiving in the course of the night, prevail throughout infancy. Since the regulation of sleep and waking states has both constitutional, (child) and contextual (social and environmental) components (e.g., Anders, 1994; Van Tassel, 1985), a complete account of the variations in sleep regulation requires examination of both child and context. The scope of the present chapter, however, is to focus on the contextual component. Maternal and demographic variables are typically incorporated in many/most studies of infants' sleep. In their pioneering study of night waking, Moore and Ucko (1957) found that neither mother's education nor age predicted night waking. But they did find a link between handling procedures, particularly deficient nursing, and night waking. Similarly, Zuckerman, Stevenson & Bailey (1987), investigating stability predictive factors and behavioural correlates of sleep problems in the first three years, found that at eight months social-economic status did not discriminate between infants with or without sleep problems, but that maternal depression and breast-feeding were associated with sleep problems. Van Tassel (1985), who investigated the relative effect of child and environmental characteristics on sleep problems in the first two years, also found that demographic background variables were not associated with night waking in the first year. By and large, this is the pattern, namely demographic variables are unrelated to sleep problems, whereas maternal well-being (e.g., Benoit et al., 1992; Zuckerman et al., 1987) and care-giving practices such as breast-feeding (e.g., Elias et al., 1986; Scher et al., 1995), or parental presence at bedtime (Adair et al., 1991), tend to be associated with infants' sleep problems.

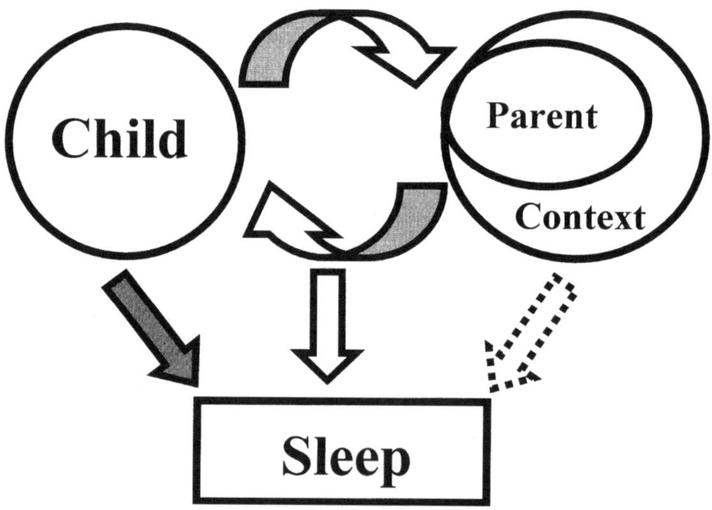

Figure 1. A transactional model of sleep regulation infancy.

Unlike the above approach, in which specific, discrete handling and bedtime routines were identified, the present standpoint is to use a broader conceptual view and examine sleep from an interpersonal perspective (see Figure 1). While the mother–child relationship has been widely conceptualized as a significant modulator of sleep (e.g., Daws, 1989; Freud, 1965; Mahler, Pine & Bergman, 1975) it has been less frequently addressed in empirical studies. The goal of the present chapter is to examine the role of the mather–child relationships as a modulator of sleep–wake regulation in the first year. The thrust of the present approach is to include psychological constructs and dimensions of mother–infant relationships, rather than background variables or specific care routines, and examine the contribution of maternal orientation, sensitivity, and attachment to the evolving sleep patterns in the first year. While some of the ideas and data outlined in this chapter have been presented before (e.g., Scher, 1991, 2001a, b, c; Scher & Blumberg, 1999), this address reviews various dimensions characterizing mather–child relationships with a view to examining their combined and unique contribution to sleep–wake variations.

A number of themes and propositions guided the selection and formalization of the concepts and measures, which are discussed here. First, from early infancy the care-giving relationship modulates the child's behavioural organization and regulatory processes (Fogel, 1993; Greenspan, 1992; Sameroff, 1989). Consequently, while sleep regulation, which relies on smooth transitions from wakefulness to sleep is primarily a biological function (Dahl, 1996), it is also modulated by psycho-social factors (Anders, 1994). Care-giving variables are considered relevant to the study of the infants' sleep, as sleep and waking patterns develop through transactions between the child's constitutional propensities and the care-giving environment (Figure 1). Second, the characteristics of mather–child sleep transactions develop within the ongoing dyadic relationships. Thus, daytime mather–child relationships are relevant for examining sleep related issues (Paret, 1983). The third proposition is that since nighttime typically involves separations from the caregiver, separation issues for both mother and child are relevant for the study of infants' sleep. Fourth, the regulating contribution of maternal care-giving variables can be examined at different levels. In the present discussion three facets or constructs are addressed: a) mother's representation of her care-giving role and of the infant's needs, b) mother–infant daytime interaction style, and c) infant–mother security of attachment. The fifth point is that as both sleep and infant–mother relationship change in the course of development, the links between the two are likely to be age-related. Thus analysis of sleep from a relational perspective should be age-specific. Finally, although objective sleep measures such as polisomnography or actigraphy are considered a choice methodology for sleep studies, questionnaires and diaries have their advantages. Given parents' involvement in putting the child to bed and in handling night waking, parental perceptions of the child's sleep characteristics and his/her nighttime needs are particularly important for understanding how sleep is regulated. Hence, the present review is based on objective and subjective sleep data.

Maternal separation anxiety

Transition to sleep and wakeful states during the course of the night are instances of separation and reunion: falling asleep each night is an instance of separation, while waking up sets the stage for a reunion (Anders, 1994). It has been argued previously that sleep-related separations are likely to be perceived as anxiety-provoking situations by both child (Mahler et al., 1975) and mother (Schaffer, 1977). Within Bowlby's attachment theory (Bowlby, 1969), such separations are expected to be accompanied by feelings of worry and anxiety, evoked as part of attachment behaviour by both mother and baby. Maternal separation anxiety has been intensively researched by Hock, who in a series of studies addressing mothers' separation concerns (e.g., Hock et al., 1983, 1989) defined maternal separation anxiety as an unpleasant emotional state, involving fear, nervousness, or guilt, associated with short-term separations from the baby. Maternal separation anxiety, according to Hock et al. (1983), is a unique dimension of motherhood which includes three facets: a) *the mother's feeling when separated from her child*; b) *her concern regarding the child's distress during separation*; c) *her belief in the adequacy of alternative care.*

The construct of maternal separation anxiety is of particular interest in the context of sleep since the degree to which the mother experiences anxiety about separation has implications for her nighttime behaviour, specifically, close proximity and immediate responsiveness to her sleepy or wakeful baby. Employing this construct, Scher (1995) found that at three months maternal separation anxiety was not related to night waking reports. By contrast, the level of separation anxiety at three months predicted night waking at nine months. *Nightwakers* at the end of infancy had mothers who presented high levels of separation anxiety in the first months. It was further found (Scher & Blumberg, 1999) that at 12 months mothers' separation anxiety induced during a brief but stressful separation in the laboratory was associated with reports of night waking. Mothers who expressed low separation anxiety reported significantly fewer awakenings than the more anxious mothers. It was further found that maternal separation anxiety was associated with settling down to sleep routines. Infants of mothers with low separation anxiety got themselves off to sleep using their own finger more often than the infants of anxious mothers. Taken together, these results support the conclusion that high maternal separation anxiety is characteristic of mothers who are involved with their child during the course of the night.

Maternal orientation: *Facilitators* vs. *Regulators*

Mothers' feelings and ideas about issues of separation from her baby and their responsiveness to his/her signals are also central to Raphael-Leff's (1986, 1991, 1993) conceptualization of parenting orientation. Drawing on clinical insights, observations, and survey data, Raphael-Leff suggested a model delineating two broad orientations of mothers towards the baby and motherhood. The *Facilitator* mother believes the baby "knows best", so the environment should be adapted to the baby; by contrast, the *Regulator* mother thinks the baby must learn to adapt to the environment. The uniqueness of these two styles is based on distinct conceptualizations of the infant's nature and needs, on differences in meaning assigned to the gestures and messages of the child, and accordingly, to different attitudes towards the maternal role and child caring strategies. According to Raphael-Leff (1991, 1993), mothers-to-be already differ in their approach to pregnancy and childbirth. Once the baby is born the basic observable difference between the two styles is that the *Facilitator* views the newborn as sociable, believes that mothering is based on intuitive "Instinct", maintains close physical/spatial contact with the baby, and fears separation. By contrast, the *Regulator* views the newborn as asocial, believes that mothering is an acquired skill, and prefers separateness (Raphael-Leff, 1991).

These orientations have identifiable implications for sleep–wake regulation as well. Specifically, the degree of mothers' involvement in regulating the infants' sleep differs: *Regulators* encourage independent settling whereas *Facilitators* are expected to be closely involved in settling at bedtime and at night. Scher (1992) measured maternal orientation at six months and found that a facilitating stance strongly predicted later night waking. At nine months, babies of *Facilitator* mothers were reported to wake up more often than babies of *Regulators*. Similarly, with one-year-old babies maternal orientation continued to be a significant predictor of the infants' sleep (Scher & Blumberg, 1999) and of attachment security (Scher, 2001a). Interestingly, mothers who fluctuated between facilitating and regulating strategies, labeled bi-polars (Scher &

Blumberg, 1992), reported more bedtime difficulties than the other mothers. Inconsistent parenting was already described by Moore and Ucko (1957) as associated with night waking continuing throughout the first year. Our findings taken together with Moore and Ucko's point to sleep-related consequences, and/or antecedents, of inconsistent parenting.

Maternal sensitivity and emotional availability

Maternal sensitivity, especially mother's ability to accurately perceive infant signals and appropriately respond to them, is one of the most frequently discussed early parenting variables. Maternal sensitivity reflects the ability to read the signs of the baby and to respond immediately in a caring way. Emotional availability within the dyad is a relational concept in which the interchanges between mother and child are seen as a key to emotional regulation (Emde, 1980). The role of emotional availability in regulating daytime behaviour has been demonstrated in a number of studies (e.g., Biringen & Robinson,1991; Robinson, Little & Biringen, 1993). Scher (2001b) examined the role of emotional availability in regulating awakenings. The actigraph recordings of emotionally available dyads were compared with the sleep of less responsively engaged dyads. It was found that while mothers' sensitivity during a daytime observation was unrelated to the child's sleep, the child's emotional availability in the play interaction was significantly related to the infants' night waking. For more involved and responsive children, a higher frequency of night waking was recorded. Note that the sleep measures in that study were based on actigraph recordings.

The finding that infants who were more involved and responsive in the daytime interaction had more fragmented sleep than infants who expressed less pleasure and eagerness in the interaction was explained in terms of the child's desire to engage his/her social companion in the course of the night as well (Scher, 2001c). Since we know that not all sleep–wake transitions result in a full awakening (e.g., Anders, 1979; Anders et al., 1992) it could well be that for the socially responsive and communicative infants brief physiological awakenings more easily turn into a quest for a social interchange. While this suggestion is theoretically interesting and could be important from a practical perspective, a number of methodological limitations of the above study should be underscored. First, the study group included only 37 dyads, so it might have been a non-representative sample. Secondly, the findings could be specific to well functioning one-year-olds, so generalizations about sleep and mather–child relationships should be avoided. A different transactional model (Sameroff, 1989), whereby disturbed mather–child relationships could be further reflected in sleep disorder (Benoit et al., 1992), should be further examined. Finally, the reported link between emotional availability and night waking may well be limited to the end of the first year. To further assess the prediction that the link between social competency and "fragile" sleep is a function of age, more studies, longitudinal and cross-sectional, are called for.

Infant–mother attachment

Attachment theory (Bowlby, 1969) is the most widely accepted view of the infant's emotional tie to the caregiver. According to the theory, infants are predisposed to form an attachment bond with their caregivers (Bowlby, 1969), and the parents likewise have a biologically based urge to care for and protect children (Bowlby, 1984). In the course of the first year, the infant directs the innate need for social interaction towards specific caregivers and becomes attached to them. By the end of the first year a "clear-cut" attachment relation to the caregiver has evolved. At this period infants show separation anxiety when proximity to the attachment figure is not maintained. Such separation, at this stage, triggers attachment related behaviours, such as, proximity seeking or crying. Infants differ in the amount of anxiety and of attachment-related behaviours demonstrated when separated, and in the comfort displayed when reunited with the attachment figure. These variations are believed to reflect the type of infant–mother attachment relationships and the degree to which the attachment figure serves as a "secure base" (Bowlby, 1988). To capture the differences between secure and insecure infant–mother attachments, Ainsworth et al. (1978) designed a laboratory procedure, called the Strange Situation, that takes the infant through a series of short episodes of separation and reunions. Based on the infants' behaviour in the Strange Situation, a classification of secure or insecure attachment is obtained. In secure relationships, infants use the parent as a secure base (Bowlby, 1988). When separated, these infants, labeled B, may or may not cry, but in either case when the parent returns they seek contact, show relief, and find comfort in the parent's presence. The insecure pattern was initially divided into two categories: the avoidant classification (A) and the resistant/ambivalent classification (C). In the avoidant pattern the infants seem unresponsive to the mother; when she leaves they are usually not distressed and during reunion they tend to avoid their mother. The resistant/ambivalent children seek contact with the mother and often fail to explore. Upon reunion they display angry behaviour and cannot easily be comforted.

From the attachment perspective, separation at bedtime, and the absent attachment figure when awakening occurs, are anxiety-provoking instances for the infant who has formed true attachment relationships with the caregiver, typically towards the end of the first year (Bowlby, 1969). At this stage, when proximity to the attachment figure is not maintained, infants signal distress and actively seek comfort. Thus, separation around sleep is likely to activate the attachment system, giving rise to attachment behaviours such as crying and proximity seeking. To date, only a few empirical studies have examined the relationship between attachment and sleep. Moore (1989) in a clinical study, reported an association between insecure attachment and sleep disturbances, and argued that the anxiously attached child feels "unsafe to sleep". Benoit et al. (1992) found an association between insecure, adult attachment classification in mothers and sleep disorders in their toddlers. Neither of these studies examined mother–infant sleep-related interactions directly. Scher (2001c) examined the sleep patterns of a group of 94 one-year-olds whose attachment security to their mothers was assessed in the Strange Situation Procedure (see Scher & Mayseles, 2000). The comparison between the sleep patterns of secure and insecure infants yielded more similarities than differences. The percentage of infants who were defined by their mothers as *nightwakers* was consistently high across the attachment groups. On the actigraph, both groups had similar levels of sleep efficiency and awakenings. Similarly, the sleep scores obtained from mothers' descriptions, and rated according to Richman's (1981) criteria for severity of sleep problems, were not a function of their infants' attachment quality. While most aspects of sleep regulation were not related to the infant's attachment classification, mother's perception of settling difficulties was linked to attachment. Bedtime was particularly difficult for the *dependently secure* infants. As pointed out (Scher, 2001c), the limited association between sleep and attachment found in a non-clinical sample does not rule out another transactional model in which disturbed mather–child relationships are further reflected in sleep disorders (Benoit et al., 1992).

Summary and conclusions

Before concluding this chapter, a word about the interrelations among the aspects of the mather–child relationship examined here is in order. From the data set which served for the present discussion, it was found that while the mothers of insecure infants tended to be more anxious about separation at 12 months, at three months the mothers of infants later to be classified as insecure did not display higher levels of separation anxiety than the secure group. Attachment security was unrelated to playtime emotional availability, possibly demonstrating that positive and negative emotional regulation involves different regulatory aspects. Finally, while mothers of secure infants were more likely to present a facilitating orientation (Scher, 2001a), the facilitator-regulator score was not correlated with separation anxiety or with emotional availability in the play interaction. Therefore it may be argued that the selected dimensions, chosen for the present discussion, tap unique, even if not independent, facets of the mather--child relationship. Consequently, the various relational constructs served to illuminate specific aspects of settling and awakening.

This chapter focused on sleep regulation, particularly settling down to sleep and nighttime awakenings, from a relational perspective. Four psychological constructs relevant to mother–infant relationship were examined as depicted in Figure 2: maternal separation anxiety (MSA), mothers' orientation to childcare (FR), emotional availability (EA) and security of attachment (ATT). In short, the following findings were highlighted: (1) Mothers' separation anxiety and their orientation towards the maternal role (i.e., facilitating or regulating), measured early in infancy predicted night waking and bedtime difficulties at the end of the first year; (2) night waking and bedtime difficulties at one year of age were partially accounted for by aspects of mother–infant relationship measured concurrently at that age. For example, interrupted sleep was

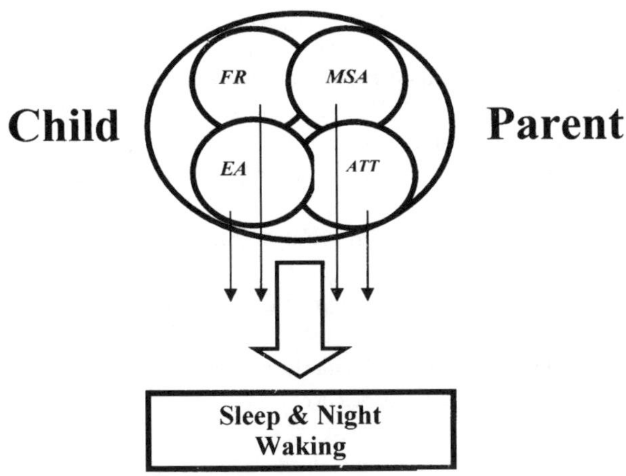

Figure 2. Relationship and dyadic variables as modulators of sleep.

characteristic of dyads in which infants were communicative and responsive when interacting with their mothers. In addition, securely, but dependently attached infants were found to be perceived by their mothers as having bedtime difficulties.

Taken together, the role of the mather–child relationship in predicting both objective sleep–wake regulation and subjective perception of sleep difficulties has been demonstrated. More research is still necessary to clarify how biology and the social-emotional contexts jointly modulate sleep–wake cycles. This task is not only theoretically important but as sleep problems are common and worrisome for parents, explaining how care-giving variables modulate sleep regulation has applied implications.

Acknowledgements

The research that served as the basis for this chapter was conducted in collaboration with a number of colleagues and graduate students who contributed in many ways. The input of Judith Harel, Peretz Lavie, Avi Sadeh, Avi Sagi, and Emanuel Tirosh is gratefully acknowledged. Thanks are extended to my former students, Tamar Amir, Orly Blumberg, Rachel Epstein, Ruth Hershkovitz and Merav Yarkoney, who combined their thesis research with the sleep project.

References

Adair, R., H. Bauchner, B. Phillipp, S. Levenson & B. Zuckerman (1991). Night waking during infancy: Role of parental presence at bedtime. *Pediatrics*, *87*, 500–504.

Ainsworth, M.D.S., M.C. Blehar, E. Waters & S. Wall (1978). *Patterns of attachment: A psychological study of strange situation*. Hillsdale, NJ: Erlbaum.

Anders, T. (1979). Night waking in infants during the first year of life. *Pediatrics*, *63*, 860–864.

Anders, T. (1994). Infant sleep, nighttime relationships and attachment. *Psychiatry*, *57*, 11–21.

Anders, T., L. Halpern & J. Hua (1992). Sleeping through the night: A developmental perspective. *Pediatrics*, *90*, 554–560.

Aserinsky, E., & N. Kleitman (1953). Regularly occurring periods of motility and concomitant phenomena during sleep. *Science*, *18*, 273–274.

Benoit, D., C. Zeanah, C. Boucher & K. Minde (1992). Sleep disorders in early childhood: Association with insecure maternal attachment. *Journal of the American Association of Child and Adolescent Psychiatry*, *31*, 86–93.

Biringen, Z., & J. Robinson (1991). Emotional availability in mather–child interactions: A reconceptualization for research. *American Journal of Orthopsychiatry, 61*, 258–272.

Bowlby, J. (1969). *Attachment and loss.* Vol. 1; *Attachment.* New York: Basic Books.

Bowlby, J. (1984). Caring for the young: Influences on development. In R. Cohen, B. Cohler, & S. Weissman (Eds), *Parenthood: A psychodynamic perspective* (269–284). New York: Guilford Press.

Bowlby, J. (1988*). A secure base: Parent-child attachment and healthy human development.* New York: Basic Books.

Dahl, R.E. (1996). The regulation of sleep and arousal: Development and psychopathology. *Development and Psychopathology, 8*, 3–27.

Daws, D. (1989). *Through the night: Helping parents and sleepless infants.* London: Free Press.

Elias, M., N. Nicholson, C. Bora & J. Johnston (1986). Sleep–wake patterns of breast-fed infants in the first two years of life. *Pediatrics, 77*, 322–329.

Emde, R.N. (1980). Emotional availability: A reciprocal reward system for infants and parents with implications for prevention of psychosocial disorders. In E. Goldson (Ed.), *Parent infant relationship* (87–115). Orlando, Fl.: Grune and Stratton.

Fogel, A. (1993). *Developing through relationships: Origins of communication, self, and culture.* New York: Harvester Wheatsheaf.

Freud, A. (1965). *Normality and pathology in childhood.* New York: International University Press.

Greenspan, S.L. (1992). *Infancy and early childhood: The practice of clinical assessment and intervention with emotional and developmental challenges.* Madison, CT: International Universities Press.

Hock, E., M. Gnezda & S. McBride (1983). *The measurement of maternal separation anxiety.* Paper presented at the biennial meeting of the Society for Research in Child Development. Detroit, US.

Hock, E., S. McBride & M. Gnezda (1989). Maternal separation anxiety: Mother–infant separation from the maternal perspective. *Child Development, 4*, 793–802.

Hoppenbrouwers, T., J. Hodgman, K. Arakawa, S. Greidel & M. Sterman (1988). Sleep and wake states in infancy: Normative studies. *Sleep, 11*, 387–401.

Mahler, M.S., F. Pine & Bergman, A. (1975). *The psychological birth of the human infant.* New York: Basic Books.

Messer, D., & M. Richards. (1993). The development of sleeping difficulties. In St. James-Roberts I., G. Harris, & D. Messer (Eds), *Infant crying feeding and sleeping.* London: Harvester-Wheatsheaf.

Moore, S.M. (1989). Disturbed attachment in children: a factor in sleep disturbance, altered dream production and immune dysfunction. *Journal of Child Psychotherapy, 15*, 99–111.

Moore, T., & L.E. Ucko (1957). Nightwaking in early infancy. *Archives of Disease in Childhood, 32*, 333–342.

Paret, I. (1983). Night waking and its relation to mather–infant interaction in the nine-month old infant. In Call, J.D., E. Galenson, & R.Z. Tyson (Eds), *Frontiers of infant psychiatry*. New York: Basic Books.

Raphael-Leff, J. (1986). Facilitators and regulators: Conscious and unconscious processes in pregnancy and early motherhood. *British Journal of Medical Psychology, 59*, 43–55.

Raphael-Leff, J. (1991). *Psychological processes of childbearing.* London: Chapman & Hall.
Raphael-Leff, J. (1993). *Pregnancy: The inside story.* London: Sheldon Press.
Richman, N. (1981). A community survey of characteristics of one-to-two olds with sleep disruptions. *Journal of the American Academy of Child Psychiatry, 20,* 281–291.
Robinson, J.L., C. Little & Z. Biringen (1993). Emotional communication in mather–toddler relationship: Evidence for early gender differences. *Merril-Palmer Quarterly, 39,* 496–517.
Sadeh, A., P. Lavie, A. Scher, E. Tirosh & R. Epstein (1991). Actigraph home-monitoring of sleep disturbed and control infants and young children: A new method for pediatric assessment of sleep–wake patterns. *Pediatrics, 87,* 494–499.
Salzarulo P., & A. Chevalier (1983). Sleep problems in children and their relationship with early disturbances of the waking-sleeping rhythms. *Sleep,* 6, 47–51.
Sameroff, A. (1989). General systems and regulation of development. In M. Gunnar & E. Thelen (Eds), *Systems and development* (219–235). Hillsdale, NJ: LEA.
Schaffer, R.S. (1977). *Mothering.* Cambridge, Mass.: Harvard University Press.
Scher, A. (1991). A longitudinal study of night waking in the first year. *Child: Care, Health and Development, 17,* 295–302.
Scher, A. (1992). Facilitators and regulators: Maternal style and separation anxiety. Paper presented at the 5th World Congress of Infant Psychiatry and Allied Disciplines. Chicago, Illinois.
Scher, A. (1995). Changes in maternal separation anxiety in the first year. Paper presented at the Meetings of the Society for Research in Child Development. Indianapolis.
Scher, A. (2001a). Facilitators and regulators: maternal orientation as an antecedent of attachment security. *Journal of Infant and Reproductive Psychology, 19,* 325–333.
Scher, A. (2001b). Mother–child interaction and sleep regulation in one-year olds. *Infant Mental Health Journal, 22,* 515–528.
Scher, A. (2001c). Attachment and sleep regulation: a study of night waking among one-year olds. *Developmental Psychobiology, 38,* 274–285.
Scher, A., & O. Blumberg (1992). Facilitators and regulators: Cross-cultural and methodological considerations. *British Journal of Medical Psychology, 65,* 327–331.
Scher, A., & O. Blumberg (1999). Nightwaking among 1-year-olds: A study of maternal separation anxiety. *Child: Health, Care and Development, 25,* 323–334.
Scher, A., E. Tirosh, M. Jaffe, L. Rubin, A. Sadeh & P. Lavie (1995). Sleep patterns of infants and yound children in Israel. *International Journal of Behavioral Development, 18,* 701–711.
Scher, A., & M. Mayseles (2000). Mothers of anxious-ambivalent infants: Maternal characteristics and child-care context. *Child Development, 71,* 1629–1639.
Van Tassel, E.B. (1985). The relative influence of child and environmental characteristics on sleep disturbances in the first and second years of life. *Developmental and Behavioral Paediatrics,* 6, 81–86.
Zuckerman, B., J. Stevenson & V. Bailey (1987). Sleep problems in early childhood: Continuities, predictive factors, and behavioral correlates. *Pediatrics, 80,* 664–671.

Sleep fragmentation and awakening during development

Insights from actigraphic studies

Avi Sadeh
Department of Psychology, Tel Aviv University, Israel

This chapter introduces actigraphy (ambulatory activity monitoring) and the data on sleep fragmentation and night waking during development obtained by using of actigraphy. The ability to objectively record sleep in infants and children for extended periods in their natural sleep environment with a cost-effective method led to improved access to the answers to developmental and clinical questions related to sleep fragmentation and night-wakings. The data suggest that night-wakings are more prevalent in the course of development than previously thought. Actigraphy documents fragmented sleep in many non-referred and children not suspected to have sleep problems. The implications of this sleep fragmentation phenomenon are still unclear and more research is needed to identify the sources of undetected sleep fragmentation as well as the implications of this phenomenon.

Night waking during development

Most of the studies on night waking phenomena in childhood have been based on parental reports (Adair, Bauchner, Philipp, Levenson, & Zuckerman, 1991; Bernal, 1973; Klackenberg, 1982; Ottaviano, Giannotti, Cortesi, Bruni, & Ottaviano, 1996; Owens, Spirito, McGuinn, & Nobile, 2000; Pollock, 1994; Scher et al., 1995; Thunstrom, 1999; Weissbluth, Davis, & Poncher, 1984; Wooding, Boyd, & Geddis, 1990). These reports varied between global assessments on questionnaires or more specific and detailed responses on daily sleep logs.

Overall it has been recognized that night waking problems are among the most prevalent parental complaints in early childhood. Various surveys suggest that between 20 and 30 percent of all children suffer from sleep problems associated with night-wakings (Mindell, 1993; Mindell, Owens, & Carskadon, 1999; Richman, 1987; Sadeh & Anders, 1993). Furthermore, studies have linked night-waking problems with more difficult temperament and behavior problems (Carey, 1974; Kaplan, McNicol, Conte, & Moghadam, 1987; Keener, Zeanah, & Anders, 1988; Sadeh, Lavie, & Scher, 1994), medical problems (Dahl, Bernhiselbroadbent, Scanlonholdford, Sampson, & Lupo, 1995; Kahn, Mozin, Rebuffat, Sottiaux, & Muller, 1989; Reuveni, Chapnick, Tal, & Tarasiuk, 1999) and interaction with parents or parental characteristics (Adair et al., 1991; Paret, 1983; Scher & Blumberg, 1999; Thunstrom, 1999; Weissbluth et al., 1984; Wooding et al., 1990).

Notwithstanding the significant knowledge obtained from many studies on night-wakings based on parental reports, it is important to emphasize the limitations of these studies. Studies using both objective and subjective measures, suggested that parents are not always aware of night-waking phenomena and that some of the individual differences may be related to the question of whether the child signals to his or her parents upon awakening or is able to resume sleep without help (Anders, Halpern, & Hua, 1992; Gaylor, Goodlin-Jones, & Anders, 2001; Keener et al., 1988; Sadeh, 1994, 1996a; Sadeh, Lavie, Scher, Tirosh, & Epstein, 1991).

Why actigraphy?

Activity monitoring has been used in research for many years to assess motility patterns associated with diverse physiological phenomena and medical conditions (Tryon, 1991). Interestingly, one of the earlier studies on developmental processes in sleep used a mechanical device to monitor crib movements for documenting sleep patterns in infants (Kleitman & Engelmann, 1953). Modern technology has led to the miniaturizing of the devices required to collect activity data and modern actigraphs are wristwatch-like devices that can collect motility data for extended periods (e.g., one week or longer). Collected data is stored in the device's internal memory and downloaded to a computer for display and analysis. Computerized sleep-wake algorithms for providing sleep measures (i.e., sleep onset time, sleep duration, night-wakings) have been developed and validated for different age groups.

Over the last two decades the use of actigraphy in sleep research and sleep medicine has been established (Sadeh, Hauri, Kripke, & Lavie, 1995), and has gained professional recognition leading to the development of Standards of Practice by the American Sleep Disorders Associations (American-Sleep-Disorders-Association, 1995).

Specific research efforts have been invested in testing the use of actigraphs with infants and children and developing scoring algorithms validated against established methods such as polysomnography (Sadeh, Alster, Urbach, & Lavie, 1989; Sadeh et al., 1991; Sadeh, Sharkey, & Carskadon, 1994) and direct obser-

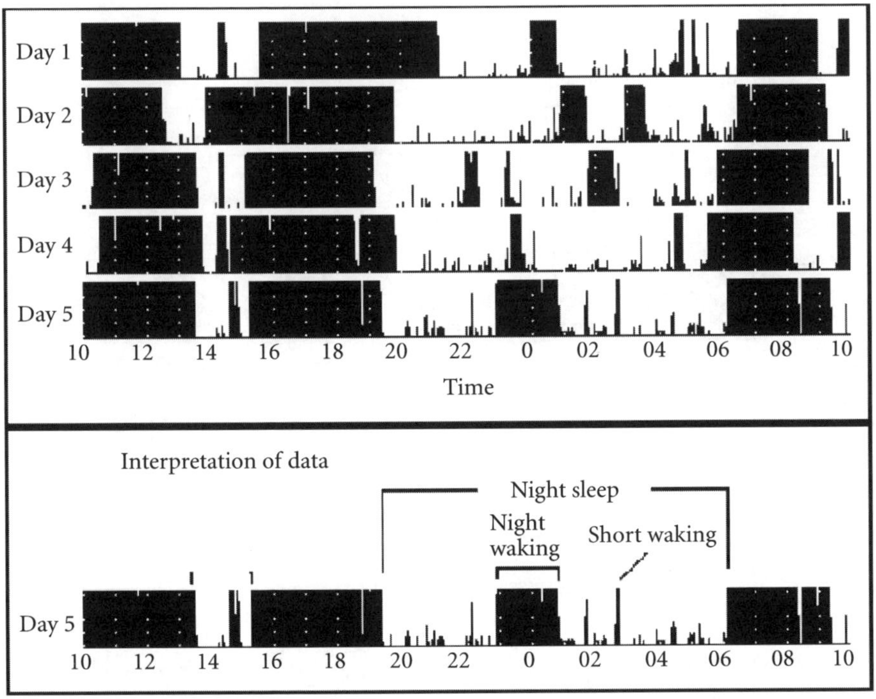

Figure 1. A sample record of a one year-old baby's sleep-wake patterns over the course of five consecutive twenty-four hour periods. The detailed explanation in the lower frame represents the last night of the diagram. The baby's activity level each and every minute is recorded. The "black" areas are those of great activity, usually identified as wakefulness. The quiet areas with low levels of activity are usually identified as quiet or active sleep.
(From Sadeh, A. (2001). "Sleeping Like a Baby: A Sensitive and Sensible Approach to Solving Your Child's Sleep Problems", Connecticut: Yale University Press. Reprinted with permission.)

vations and breathing monitoring (Sadeh et al., 1995). Overall these studies have indicated that actigraphy can be used for distinguishing between sleep and wake minutes with an accuracy level of above 85% in comparison to the previously established methods.

Actigraphic studies on night-wakings: Developmental trends

To date, there are a number of relatively large-scale actigraphic studies documenting sleep in non-clinical samples of infants and children (Sadeh, Dark, &

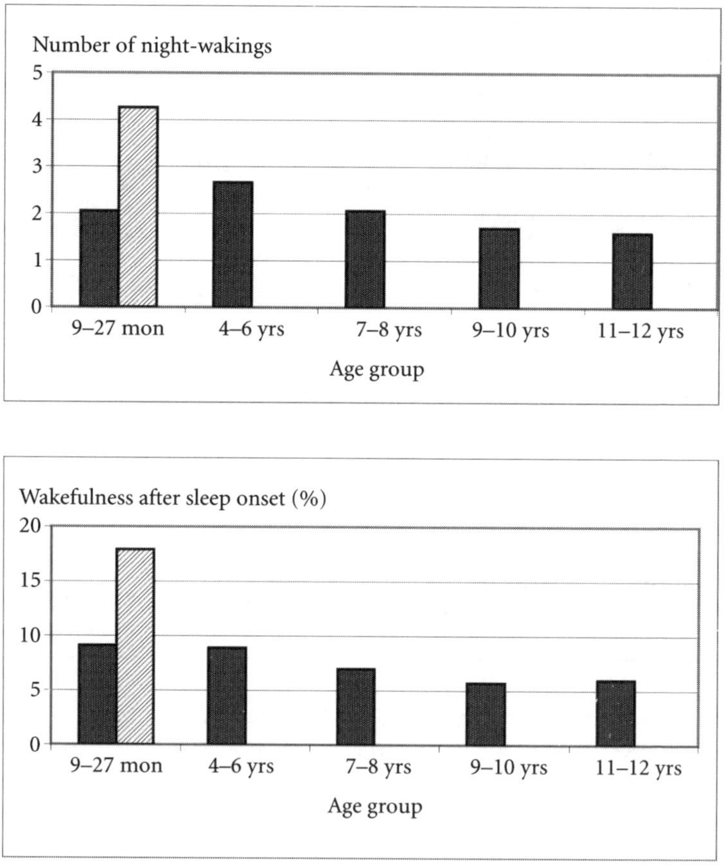

Figure 2. Number of night-wakings and percentage of wakefulness after sleep onset in 3 different studies across development. The younger age group consists of a clinical sample of sleep disturbed infants and a control non-sleep-disturbed infants.

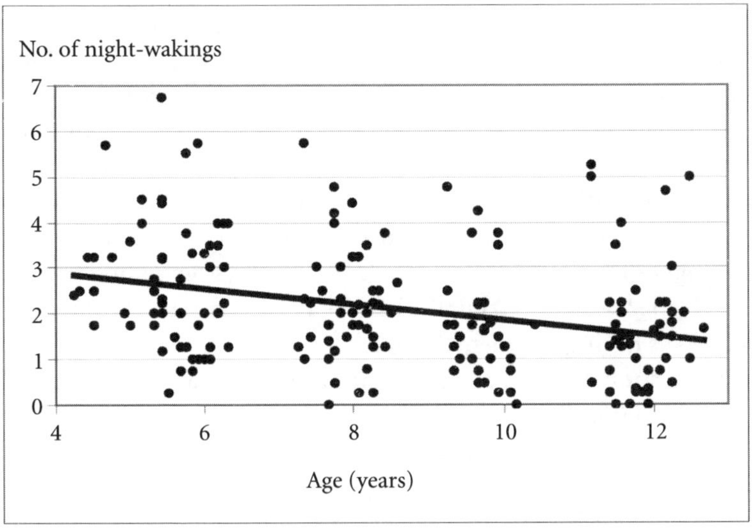

Figure 3. Distribution of night-wakings across development: Scatter plot of average number of night-wakings for each individual child.

Vohr, 1996; Sadeh et al., 1991; Sadeh, Raviv, & Gruber, 2000; Tikotzky & Sadeh, in press). Although not all of these studies were originally designed to focus on night-waking, relevant data are available for infants and toddlers (Sadeh et al., 1991), for 4–6 year old children (Tikotzky & Sadeh, 2001), and for school age children (Sadeh et al., 2000). Figure 2 summarizes the results of these studies with regard to night-waking phenomena.

In the first study, Sadeh et al., (1991) compared actigraphic sleep measures in 63 referred sleep-disturbed infants and young children (aged 9 to 27 months) with 34 control non-disturbed infants. The sleep measures were averaged across the nights of monitoring. A night-waking was defined as any actigraphically identified awakening lasting 5 minutes or longer. Sleep-disturbed infants woke-up (4.26 ±1.33) more than twice as much as the infants from the non-referred control group (2.05 ±1.17). Furthermore, the sleep-disturbed infants spent much more time in wakefulness after sleep onset (17.87% of total sleep time) in comparison to their controls (9.06%). It is important to note that although this study documents night-wakings in early childhood, both groups were selected for "poor" and "non-poor" sleep and thus it makes sense to conclude that the results of a normative sample would have been somewhere between the extremes of these groups.

In the second study, sleep patterns of 140 school age children were assessed for 4–5 nights using actigraphy. These children were sampled from 3 different age groups (2nd grade, 4 grade and 6th grade) with no sleep-related selection criteria and therefore they could be considered as a more representative sample. The findings indicate that night-wakings are quite prevalent during the school age period although a tendency toward improvement from earlier ages is noted. "Poor sleep" was defined using two criteria: 1) three night-wakings or more per night on average; 2) more than 10% of the sleep period was spent in wakefulness after sleep onset. On the basis of these criteria 18% of the children were defined as having fragmented sleep.

The third study focused on kindergarten children (aged 4–6 years) (Tikotzky & Sadeh, 2001). Fifty-nine children were monitored with actigraphy for 4–5 consecutive nights. Night-wakings were found to be very prevalent in this age group with an average of 2.66 wakings per night. Using the same criteria as above, 41% of the children were characterized as having fragmented sleep.

Overall, our actigraphic studies indicate that a trend toward sleep consolidation and a reduction in night-wakings exists across childhood. This trend has been reported for various age ranges in laboratory studies using EEG (Coble, Kupfer, Taska, & Kane, 1984; Ficca, Fagioli, Giganti, & Salzarulo, 1999), time-lapse video (Anders, 1979; Anders & Keener, 1985), and questionnaires (Klackenberg, 1982; Ottaviano et al., 1996).

Gender differences vis-à-vis night-wakings were not found in any of the actigraphic studies in the children described above. Gender differences were found on other measures reflecting that girls are more likely to sleep longer than boys in the school age period (Sadeh et al., 2000).

Finally, from a different developmental angle, the relationships between the development of sleep and melatonin secretion patterns have been studied in 6–8 month old infants (Sadeh, 1997). Fragmented sleep (i.e., increased number of night-wakings and lower sleep percent) was associated with inappropriate melatonin secretion patterns. Similar relationships between sleep fragmentation and melatonin secretion patterns were found in a clinical sample of blind children (Tzischinsky, Skene, Epstein, & Lavie, 1991).

Distribution of wakings across the night

To assess the distribution of awakenings across the night I reanalyzed the data from our two recent studies (Sadeh et al., 2000; Tikotzky & Sadeh, 2001). The percentage of time spent in wakefulness after sleep onset was calculated for

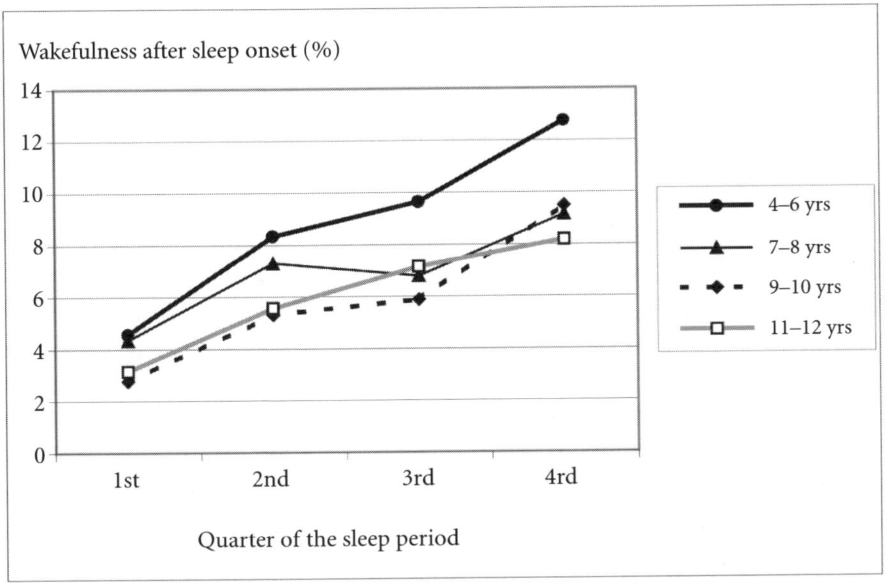

Figure 4. Distribution of wakefulness across the night in different age groups: Average percentage of wakefulness in each quarter of the night.

each quarter of the sleep period in each of the age groups. MANOVA revealed significant Quarter effect ($F = 64$; $p < .0001$). As demonstrated in Figure 4, wakefulness increases gradually throughout the night in all age groups. This tendency is in accord with the well-established trend that occurs from deep sleep stages that are concentrated in the first section of the night to the more shallow sleep stages and REM episodes during the later sections of the night (Carskadon, Keenan, & Dement, 1987).

Actigraphic studies on night-wakings: Clinical and methodological issues

Subjective versus objective findings

A number of actigraphic studies reflected the limited knowledge of parents on night-waking phenomena. It has been repeatedly documented that parents are not aware of many of their children's night-wakings (Sadeh, 1994, 1996a; Sadeh et al., 1991; Tikotzky & Sadeh, 2001). It has been demonstrated that the process of completing daily logs for an extended period during treatment follow-up is exhausting and may lead to parents reporting less and less night-wakings due to attrition, which may lead to a false impression of treatment success (Sadeh, 1994).

Night-wakings in clinical settings

The question of what is the real difference between referred sleep-disturbed children and non-referred controls in terms of night-waking has been partially answered. Sleep-referred infants do wake up more often and spend more time in wakefulness during the night, and in addition, they require more parental help to settle back to sleep (Sadeh et al., 1991). A similar question was raised with regard to what actually happens with night-wakings during behavioral intervention for sleep-disturbed infants. Most studies indicate that according to parental reports, most infants improve their sleep quite rapidly in response to behavioral intervention (Mindell, 1999; Owens, France, & Wiggs, 1999; Sadeh & Anders, 1993). However, it was not clear whether these infants actually learn to sleep through the night without waking up or just learned to resume sleep on their own without signaling their parents, and therefore their parents reported improved sleep. The ability to monitor sleep for extended treatment follow-up assessment with actigraphy yielded information suggesting that both processes do occur (Sadeh, 1994). In an actigraphic assessment of behavioral intervention with 50 sleep-disturbed infants, a decrease in the number of night-wakings from an average of 4.4 during the baseline period to 3.2 during the treatment follow-up period (2–3 weeks) was documented. However, the parents reported a much larger decrease in the number of night-wakings, suggesting that the infants also learned to soothe themselves back to sleep after waking up in the middle of night.

Night wakings and developmental psychopathology

Fragmented sleep has been often associated with stress, illness and psychopathology in children (Dahl, 1996; Moore, 1989; Sadeh, 1996b; Sadeh & Gruber, 1998). A growing number of studies have indeed documented such relationships using actigraphy (Franck et al., 1999; Glod, Teicher, Hartman, & Harakal, 1997; Pillar et al., 2000; Sadeh et al., 2000). However, some studies failed to detect significant relationships between sleep fragmentation and psychopathology (Gruber, Sadeh, & Raviv, 2000; Hering, Epstein, Elroy, Iancu, & Zelnik, 1999).

Sleep fragmentation is a major component of many sleep disorders (Philip, Stoohs, & Guilleminault, 1994). Studies of experimental sleep fragmentation have suggested that it leads to an increase in less-restorative sleep and a relative decrease in deeper and more restorative sleep stages (Philip et al., 1994; Roehrs, Merlotti, Petrucelli, Stepanski, & Roth, 1994; Wesensten, Balkin, & Belenky, 1999). These alterations in sleep structure may lead to detrimental effects on subsequent alertness and performance. In a recent study, fragmented sleep (multiple and/or prolonged night wakings documented by actigraphy) has been associated with poor neurobehavioural functioning on computerized tests in school-age children (Sadeh, Gruber & Raviv, in press).

Conclusions and future research questions

Actigraphy provides a cost-effective, non-intrusive way to assess sleep under regular sleep circumstances during development. Actigraphic studies have yielded important information on sleep fragmentation across development that has validated and extended the knowledge obtained by other assessment methods.

The major findings include the following points:

- Sleep consolidation progresses with maturation and a moderate trend of decrease in the number and length of night-wakings has been demonstrated.
- Night-wakings continue to be prevalent phenomena during development and most children do wake up during the night.
- Parental knowledge on night-waking phenomena is very limited and depends on the child's needs for parental help for resuming sleep.
- Sleep-disturbed infants tend to wake-up more than non-disturbed infants and require more help to resume sleep.
- Following behavioral intervention for sleep-disturbed infants, the number and the length of their night-wakings decrease and the infants require fewer interventions to resume their sleep.
- Night wakings are associated with other psychosocial and medical phenomena such as stress, psychopathology and impaired neurobehavioural functioning.

There are many research topics that await further exploration and deeper understanding. There is a need to fill the gaps in the normative data collected so far for various age groups, particularly in the early years and the adolescent period. Future research should address the following issues:

- What are the underlying causes for the prevalent night-wakings in children beyond the early process of consolidation of "sleeping through the night"? Are these night-wakings caused by environmental, medical or psychological factors or by an independent biologically driven "internal clock"?
- What is the level of continuity in night-waking phenomena across development? Are some individuals prone to night-wakings and continue to wake more often throughout their lives?
- What are the behavioural correlates and consequences of night-wakings in children?
- Is there any method to improve sleep in children with fragmented sleep without detected underlying cause?

Actigraphy provides an opportunity for large-scale studies with longitudinal designs that can identify and map the night-waking phenomenon in population-based samples and for intervention follow-up studies. EEG studies and complementary methods would enable zooming in on smaller clinical samples and exploring the underlying mechanisms of this prevalent phenomenon of night-wakings.

References

Adair, R., Bauchner, H., Philipp, B., Levenson, S., & Zuckerman, B. (1991). Night waking during infancy: role of parental presence at bedtime. *Pediatrics, 87*(4), 500–504.

American Sleep Disorders Association. (1995). Practice parameters for the use of actigraphy in the clinical assessment of sleep disorders. *Sleep, 18*(4), 285–287.

Anders, T.F. (1979). Night-waking in infants during the first year of life. *Pediatrics, 63*(6), 860–864.

Anders, T.F., Halpern, L.F., & Hua, J. (1992). Sleeping through the night: a developmental perspective. *Pediatrics, 90*(4), 554–560.

Anders, T.F., & Keener, M. (1985). Developmental course of nighttime sleep-wake patterns in full-term and premature infants during the first year of life. I. *Sleep, 8*(3), 173–192.

Bernal, J.F. (1973). Night waking in infants during the first 14 months. *Developmental Medicine and Child Neurology, 15*(6), 760–769.

Carey, W.B. (1974). Night waking and temperament in infancy. *Journal De Pediatria, 84*(5), 756–758.

Carskadon, M.A., Keenan, S., & Dement, W.C. (1987). Nighttime sleep and daytime sleep tendency in preadolescents. In C. Guilleminault (Ed.), *Sleep and its disorders in children* (43–52). New-York: Raven Press.

Coble, P.A., Kupfer, D.J., Taska, L.S., & Kane, J. (1984). EEG sleep of normal healthy children. Part I: Findings using standard measurement methods. *Sleep, 7*(4), 289–303.

Dahl, R.E. (1996). The regulation of sleep and arousal: Development and psychopathology. *Development and Psychopathology, 8*(1), 3–27.

Dahl, R.E., Bernhiselbroadbent, J., Scanlonholdford, S., Sampson, H.A., & Lupo, M. (1995). Sleep Disturbances in Children with Atopic-Dermatitis. *Archives of Pediatrics & Adolescent Medicine, 149*(8), 856–860.

Ficca, G., Fagioli, I., Giganti, F., & Salzarulo, P. (1999). Spontaneous awakenings from sleep in the first year of life. *Early Human Development, 55*(3), 219–228.

Franck, L.S., Johnson, L.M., Lee, K., Hepner, C., Lambert, L., Passeri, M., Manio, E., Dorenbaum, A., & Wara, D. (1999). Sleep disturbances in children with human immunodeficiency virus infection. *Pediatrics, 104*(5), J1–J5.

Gaylor, E.E., Goodlin-Jones, B.L., & Anders, T.F. (2001). Classification of young children's sleep problems: A pilot study. *Journal of the American Academy of Child and Adolescent Psychiatry, 40*(1), 61–67.

Glod, C.A., Teicher, M.H., Hartman, C.R., & Harakal, T. (1997). Increased nocturnal activity and impaired sleep maintenance in abused children. *Journal of the American Academy of Child and Adolescent Psychiatry, 36*(9), 1236–1243.

Gruber, R., Sadeh, A., & Raviv, A. (2000). Instability of sleep patterns in children with attention – deficit/hyperactivity disorder. *Journal of the American Academy of Child and Adolescent Psychiatry, 39*(4), 495–501.

Hering, E., Epstein, R., Elroy, S., Iancu, D.R., & Zelnik, N. (1999). Sleep patterns in autistic children. *Journal of Autism and Developmental Disorders, 29*(2), 143–147.

Kahn, A., Mozin, M.J., Rebuffat, E., Sottiaux, M., & Muller, M.F. (1989). Milk intolerance in children with persistent sleeplessness: a prospective double-blind crossover evaluation. *Pediatrics, 84*(4), 595–603.

Kaplan, B.J., McNicol, J., Conte, R.A., & Moghadam, H.K. (1987). Sleep disturbance in preschool-aged hyperactive and nonhyperactive children. *Pediatrics, 80*(6), 839–844.

Keener, M.A., Zeanah, C.H., & Anders, T.F. (1988). Infant temperament, sleep organization, and nighttime parental interventions. *Pediatrics, 81*(6), 762–771.

Klackenberg, G. (1982). Sleep behaviour studied longitudinally. Data from 4–16 years on duration, night-awakening and bed-sharing. *Acta Paediatrica Scandinavica, 71*(3), 501–506.

Kleitman, N., & Engelmann, T.G. (1953). Sleep characteristics of infants. *Journal of Applied Physiology, 6*, 269–282.

Mindell, J.A. (1993). Sleep disorders in children. *Health Psychology, 12*(2), 151–162.

Mindell, J.A. (1999). Empirically supported treatments in pediatric psychology: bedtime refusal and night wakings in young children. *Journal of Pediatric Psychology, 24*(6), 465–481.

Mindell, J.A., Owens, J.A., & Carskadon, M.A. (1999). Developmental features of sleep. *Child and Adolescent Psychiatric Clinics of North America, 8*(4), 695–725.

Moore, M.S. (1989). Disturbed attachment in children: A factor in sleep disturbance, altered dream production and immune dysfunction: I. Not safe to sleep: Chronic sleep disturbance in anxious attachment. *Journal of Child Psychotherapy, 15*(1), 99–111.

Ottaviano, S., Giannotti, F., Cortesi, F., Bruni, O., & Ottaviano, C. (1996). Sleep characteristics in healthy children from birth to 6 years of age in the urban area of Rome. *Sleep, 19*(1), 1–3.

Owens, J.A., Spirito, A., McGuinn, M., & Nobile, C. (2000). Sleep habits and sleep disturbance in elementary school-aged children. *Journal of Developmental and Behavioral Pediatrics, 21*(1), 27–36.

Owens, J.L., France, K.G., & Wiggs, L. (1999). Behavioural and cognitive-behavioural interventions for sleep disorders in infants and children: A review. *Sleep Medicine Reviews, 3*(4), 281–302.

Paret, I. (1983). Night waking and its relation to mother-infant interaction in nine-month-old infants. In J. Call & E. Galenson & R. Tyson (Eds), *Frontiers of infant psychiatry* (171–177). New York: Basic Books.

Philip, P., Stoohs, R., & Guilleminault, C. (1994). Sleep fragmentation in normals: A model for sleepiness associated with upper airway resistance syndrome. *Sleep, 17*(3), 242–247.

Pillar, G., Shahar, E., Peled, N., Ravid, S., Lavie, P., & Etzioni, A. (2000). Melatonin improves sleep-wake patterns in psychomotor retarded children. *Pediatric Neurology, 23*(3), 225–228.

Pollock, J.I. (1994). Night-waking at five years of age: predictors and prognosis. *Journal of Child Psychology and Psychiatry, 35*(4), 699–708.

Reuveni, H., Chapnick, G., Tal, A., & Tarasiuk, A. (1999). Sleep fragmentation in children with atopic dermatitis. *Archives of pediatrics and adolescent medicine, 153*(3), 249–253.

Richman, N. (1987). Surveys of sleep disorders in child in a general population. In C. Guilleminault (Ed.), *Sleep and its disorders in children* (115–127). New-York: Raven Press.

Roehrs, T., Merlotti, L., Petrucelli, N., Stepanski, E., & Roth, T. (1994). Experimental sleep fragmentation. *Sleep, 17*(5), 438–443.

Sadeh, A. (1994). Assessment of intervention for infant night waking: parental reports and activity-based home monitoring. *Journal of Consulting and Clinical Psychology, 62*(1), 63–68.

Sadeh, A. (1996a). Evaluating night wakings in sleep-disturbed infants: a methodological study of parental reports and actigraphy. *Sleep, 19*(10), 757–762.

Sadeh, A. (1996b). Stress, Trauma, and Sleep in Children. *Child and Adolescent Psychiatric Clinics of North America, 5*(3), 685–700.

Sadeh, A. (1997). Sleep and melatonin in infants: A preliminary study. *Sleep, 20*(3), 185–191.

Sadeh, A., Gruber, R. & Raviv, A. (in press). Sleep, neurobehavioral functioning and behavior problems in school-age children. *Child Development.*

Sadeh, A., Acebo, C., Seifer, R., Aytur, S., & et al. (1995). Activity-based assessment of sleep-wake patterns during the 1st year of life. *Infant Behavior and Development, 18*(3), 329–337.

Sadeh, A., Alster, J., Urbach, D., & Lavie, P. (1989). Actigraphically based automatic bedtime sleep-wake scoring: Validity and clinical applications. *Jounal of Ambulatory Monitoring, 2*(3), 209–216.

Sadeh, A., & Anders, T.F. (1993). Infant sleep problems: Origins, assessment, interventions. *Infant Mental Health Journal, 14*(1), 17–34.

Sadeh, A., Dark, I., & Vohr, B.R. (1996). Newborns' sleep-wake patterns: The role of maternal, delivery and infant factors. *Early Human Development, 44*(2), 113–126.

Sadeh, A., & Gruber, R. (1998). Sleep Disorders. In T. Ollendick (Ed.), *Comprehensive clinical psychology* (Vol. 5., pp. 629–653). Oxford, England UK: Pergamon/Elsevier Science.

Sadeh, A., Hauri, P.J., Kripke, D.F., & Lavie, P. (1995). The role of actigraphy in the evaluation of sleep disorders. *Sleep, 18*(4), 288–302.

Sadeh, A., Lavie, P., & Scher, A. (1994). Maternal perceptions of temperament of sleep-disturbed toddlers. *Early education and development, 5*, 311–322.

Sadeh, A., Lavie, P., Scher, A., Tirosh, E., & Epstein, R. (1991). Actigraphic home-monitoring sleep-disturbed and control infants and young children: a new method for pediatric assessment of sleep-wake patterns. *Pediatrics, 87*(4), 494–499.

Sadeh, A., McGuire, J.P., Sachs, H., Seifer, R., Tremblay, A., Civita, R., & Hayden, R.M. (1995). Sleep and psychological characteristics of children on a psychiatric inpatient unit. *Journal of the American Academy of Child and Adolescent Psychiatry, 34*(6), 813–819.

Sadeh, A., Raviv, A., & Gruber, R. (2000). Sleep patterns and sleep disruptions in school-age children. *Developmental Psychology, 36*(3), 291–301.

Sadeh, A., Sharkey, K.M., & Carskadon, M.A. (1994). Activity-based sleep-wake identification: an empirical test of methodological issues. *Sleep, 17*(3), 201–207.

Scher, A., & Blumberg, O. (1999). Night waking among 1-year olds: a study of maternal separation anxiety. *Child: Care, Health and Development, 25*(5), 323–334.

Scher, A., Tirosh, E., Jaffe, M., Rubin, L., Sadeh, A., & Lavie, P. (1995). Sleep patterns of infants and young children in Israel. *International Journal of Behavioral Development, 18*(4), 701–711.

Thunstrom, M. (1999). Severe sleep problems among infants in a normal population in Sweden: prevalence, severity and correlates. *Acta Paediatrica, 88*(12), 1356–1363.

Tikotzky, L., & Sadeh, A. (2001). Sleep patterns and sleep disruptions in kindergarten children. *Journal of Clinical Child Psychology, 30*, 579–589.

Tryon, W.W. (1991). *Activity measurement in psychology and medicine.* New York: Plenum Press.

Tzischinsky, O., Skene, D., Epstein, R., & Lavie, P. (1991). Circadian rhythms in 6-sulphatoxymelatonin and nocturnal sleep in blind children. *Chronobiology International, 8*(3), 168–175.

Weissbluth, M., Davis, A.T., & Poncher, J. (1984). Night waking in 4- to 8-month-old infants. *Journal of Pediatrics, 104*(3), 477–480.

Wesensten, N.J., Balkin, T.J., & Belenky, G. (1999). Does sleep fragmentation impact recuperation? A review and reanalysis. *Journal of Sleep Research, 8*(4), 237–245.

Wooding, A.R., Boyd, J., & Geddis, D.C. (1990). Sleep patterns of New Zealand infants during the first 12 months of life. *Journal of Paediatrics and Child Health, 26*(2), 85–88.

Arousals and awakenings in infancy

Evaluation for clinical context

Marie-Françoise Vecchierini and Yvonne Navelet
Hôpital Bichat, INSERM and Centre Hospitalier de Bicêtre, Paris

Introduction

Arousals and awakenings, during sleep, in infants and children, are still controversial subjects ought to a lack of pediatric definitions.

Arousals and awakenings can occur spontaneously or be provoked by external stimuli. Spontaneous arousals are either "non-stimulus related", appearing for unknown causes or "stimulus related", that is related to a suspected ethiology, as a respiratory, cardiac, digestive event. Provoked (or exogenous) arousals can follow a change in the sleep environment (noise, light, and so on).

The spontaneous non-stimulus related (or endogenous) awakenings occur as a part of the regular physiological process of the sleep-wake rhythm; they undergo a maturational evolution leading to a reduction of the number and length of nocturnal wakefulness episodes. Arousals and awakenings are also secondary to a suspected cause, most often a respiratory event, such as obstructive or central apnea, or hypopnea or increased inspiratory effort. In such case, they are important physiological defense mechanisms against potentially dangerous situations.

The interest in arousals and awakenings during sleep in infants has been growing up; the field of the chronobiogical research for the sleep-wake organisation has been more and more studied. The lack of arousal after a dangerous event was considered to put the infants at risk for life-threatening events and eventually for sudden infant death syndrome. It was reported in the literature that near-miss infants had less spontaneous awakenings (Navelet et al., 1984; Vecchierini-Blineau et al., 1988; Kahn et al., 1992) and less body movements

(Coons & Guilleminault, 1985; Vecchierini-Blineau et al., 1988) during sleep than control infants.

This chapter, after some rapid definitions and methodological considerations, will mainly review 1) spontaneous non-stimulus related arousals and awakenings which, when too numerous, may lead to "insomnia" and 2) respiratory related arousals in infants. Some other clinical circumstances such as parasomnias by arousal disorders or periodic leg movements known to be associated with arousals will be mentioned.

Definitions

Arousals and awakenings can be defined by behavioural and polysomnographic criteria.

During awakenings, the infant may be quiet or restless, eyes open, usually grimacing or moving and sometimes crying.

On the polysomnographic recording, an awakening is usually scored when changes in EEG frequency, presence of eye movements, increase in muscle tone, modifications in cardio-respiratory rates and often artifacts, remain stable for at least 1 or 2 minutes (Ficca et al., 1999; Vecchierini-Blineau et al., 2001).

Arousals are more difficult to assess. Behavioural criteria were first studied; they were mainly based on motor events: body movements according to their intensity and their length (twitches, startles, partial or global movements) and sighs or augmented breaths. The trouble is that each author defines his own behaviour arousal criteria, and criteria change from one study to an other one.

Polygraphic arousals have been defined in adults on transient EEG and EMG changes (ASDA, 1992). Authors studying arousals in infants and children have either used adults'criteria or modified some ASDA criteria and considered arousals as soon as they lasted one second (Mograss et al., 1994; Mc Namara, 1996). Finally others have emphasized that adult criteria were not appropriate for neonates and infants (Curzi-Dascalova et al., 2000) for at least two reasons: spontaneous important EEG and EMG pattern variations occur during sleep and the time between a stimulus and the arousal is not taken into account making difficult the evaluation of such a relationship. Consequently, in Kahn et al. meeting of the Pediatric wake up club it was proposed to score arousal in infants on the association of changes in at least three recorded signals: EEG frequency shift for at least one second or increase in EMG amplitude (chin or limb muscles), or occurrence of a body movement, or change in heart rate or changes in respiratory rate or breathing amplitude. These modifications could be evaluated in comparison with a pre-arousal period, preceding the arousal by at least 10 seconds (Curzi-Dascalova et al., 2000).

These methodological proposals taking in account EEG, motor and autonomic nervous system activation, have not yet been validated. It would be important to establish a consensus to score arousals in infants improving the comparison of results from different studies.

Technical issues

Difficulties in scoring arousals involve technical issues which will be detailed in another chapter of this book. We wanted just to emphasize some points.

Behavioural observation of the infant implies that a well-trained nurse notices every external event and change of the infant; a video recording may allow a more precise analysis of movements and posture changes.

Polygraphic recording of an arousal requires EEG recording with at least 4 electrodes (system 10–20 – Guidelines two, 1994) with a frontal lead. Quantitative EEG analysis may complete visual analysis. EMG of the chin muscle is always recorded but EMG of some limb muscles such as tibialis muscle and of respiratory muscles are useful in some clinical contexts. Body movements are always recorded by actimeters, piezo-electric quartz transducers or by the charge sensitive mattress; increase in EMG channels and artefacts on other leads help in detecting some movements. Electrocardiogram and respiratory parameters will be carefully recorded according to previous recommendations (American Thoracic Society, 1996; Davidson-Ward & Marcus, 1996). It is noticeable that respiratory inductive plethysmography allows a quantitative evaluation of respiratory effort. Guilleminault et al. (1996) recommended oesophageal pressure recording though being an invasive method. Nasal pressure using a nasal canula is still under evaluation in infants. Blood gas is appreciated, at least by SaO_2 value, recorded by pulse oxymetry; pulse wave form changes allow to distinguish true desaturations from movement artifacts. End tidal partial pressure in CO_2 is usually recorded.

Factors that influence arousals during sleep

As already mentioned, spontaneous arousals occur without apparent external stimulation and great care must be taken to exclude any stimulation from the environment or from the sleeper. Some factors are known to modify the arousal threshold in infants and must be investigated and controlled when studying arousals in clinical context.

Prenatal exposure to drug abuse must be considered because marijuana exposure has been shown (Dahl et al., 1995) to disturb sleep until 3 years age. Ward et al. (1992) reported delayed arousal response to hypoxia and hypercapnia in infants of substance – abusing mothers. *Prenatal nicotine exposure* would be a major and independent risk for SIDS in infants (Kahn et al., 1997). Franco et al. (1999) have shown that arousal threshold (tested by auditory stimuli) was higher in infants born from smoking mothers.

In infants, the use of *sedative drugs* such as phenothiazines decrease spontaneous arousals (Kahn & Blum, 1982).

Room and infant temperature must be verified though the effect of air temperature on sleep architecture, body movements and respiratory pauses were only tested in the newborn (Bach et al., 1994). Respiratory tract infections would decrease arousal responses to different stimuli in infants (Pickens et al., 1989) and in young animals (Lindgren et al., 1996; Toth & Chandhory, 1998).

The use of a pacifier, breast-feeding and bedsharing are conditions known to increase spontaneous arousals (see text later). *Prone* compared to supine sleep position has deleterious effects, decreasing the number and duration of spontaneous awakenings during sleep, in infants, (Kahn et al. 1993) with an increase in the auditory arousal threshold (Franco et al. 1998). Moreover, an altered autonomic function was described in these prone sleeping infants (Franco et al. 1996; Galland et al. 1998). Jeffery et al. (1999) found a decrease in airway protective reflexes, after pharyngeal infusion of water in healthy newborn in prone sleep position, during active sleep, without a compensatory increase in arousal. Finally, Galland et al. (2000) described in prone sleeping infants, poorer ventilatory responses to mild asphyxia during active sleep.

Arousal threshold was shown to be *sleep state dependent*, being lower in active than in quiet sleep, but arousability in quiet sleep increased with the length of time that the infant had been asleep (Read et al., 1998). Finally, *sleep deprivation*, in healthy three months old infants, has been studied by Thomas et al. (1996) showing no effect on spontaneous awakenings, on spontaneous movement arousals or on provoked arousals.

Maturational processes

Different technical processes were used to study spontaneous awakenings in infants as video somnography (Anders & Keener, 1985) interviews (Eaton-Evans & Dugdale, 1988) actigraphy (Sadeh, 1991). Night sleep polygraphic recordings as well as longer duration polygraphic recordings were performed in several studies.

Wakefulness is a constitutive part of a normal sleep episode and its distribution through the nycthemere depends on a regular chronobiological evolution. In normal babies between 4 and 30 weeks of age, Navelet et al. (1982) described a diminution of the intrasleep wakefulness from 32.8% to 13.4% during the night. For Samson-Dollfus et al. (1988), the total waking time represented 10%–20% of all night polygraphic sleep recordings in six months old babies. Navelet et al. (1982) evidenced a decreased number of awakening episodes ≥ 5 minutes with an increase in their mean duration and a change in the distribution of nocturnal intervening wakefulness whose first episode latency increases. In the second semester of life, night wakings may increase again (Eaton – Evans & Dugdale 1988, Anders & Keener 1985).

In infants from 1 to 54 weeks, Ficca et al. (1999) identified awakenings by means of a combination of electrophysiological and behavioural signals already described in previous publications of their group. Awakenings were scored if followed by a period of wakefulness lasting at least 2 minutes.

When studying 24 hours sleep-wake patterns polygraphically recorded in hospitalised infants, Schulz et al. (1985) established that infants awoke preferentially out of REM-sleep, and less often out of NREM-sleep. They hypothesised that brain activity during REM-sleep, facilitates the transition from sleep to wakefulness, especially in the youngest infant. In Louis et al. longitudinal study (1997), 24-h home polygraphic recordings in normal infants showed an increase in waking time during the diurnal part of the nycthemere with a decrease in number and duration of nocturnal awakenings and body movements. Ficca et al. (1999) in infants 1 to 7 weeks old evidenced a bimodal distribution of the awakenings through the night with two main peaks of awakenings. Awakenings out of NREM sleep were followed by longer periods of wakefulness than those out of REM sleep. Over the same period, sleep onset changes from REM to NREM sleep.

Clinical implications

Numerous epidemiological and clinical studies (Ferber 1985; Sheldon et al. 1992) have featured the main traits of sleep disorders in infants and toddlers, pointing out the role of both internal and external synchronizers (Thirion & Challamel, 1995; Mc Graw et al., 1999). The emergence and consolidation of a stable sleep wake pattern in the first months of life depends on several factors, the maturation of CNS structures playing a major role in the modulation of this phenomenon. From birth to late infancy the care-giving, parent-child interaction and the early social influences will converge to help the changes from an unstable ultradian sleep-wake rhythm to a progressive more mature 24 h circadian cycle. The circadian process involves not only the wake and sleep rhythm, but also the main physiological functions: temperature, cortisol and melatonin secretion (Mc Graw et al. 1999), as well as respiration and heart rates.

In a clinical context, insomnia in small children is the most often unsolved problem. For Anders & Keener (1985), Mc Kenna et al. (1993), sleep problems have become the most frequent complaint of parents during well-baby visits. For Navelet (1996) insomnia in less than 5 years old children represents 51.4% of sleep troubles referred to a consultation of pediatric sleep disorders. Insomnia as a lack of sleep is rare between 2 and 15 years of age for Salzarulo & Chevalier (1983) who described night wakings being more frequent in the youngest age. In the same study, other sleep problems as falling asleep disturbances occured more often in older children having had previous disorders of the sleep-wake rhythm in the first year of life.

For Chambry et al. (2000), half of the children suffered previous medical problems (digestive, respiratory, allergic, etc.). More often than chronic medical problems or illness requiring hospitalization (Tirosh et al., 1993) the environmental factors as well as the maturational factors are determinant to trigger insomnia in infants. The parental practices with their different cultural aspects will interfere with the ontogenetic process. Parents capability to help the baby to settle and selfsooth alone at bedtime, and by the way to develop a self-capacity to go back to sleep alone when awaken during the night, depends on personal parents' psychological and social involvement. Infant-parents interactions and relationship will determine behavioural strategies in the way the parents will manage interventions at bedtime and during the night. Using a pacifier (Franco et al., 2000) as well as breastfeeding (Eaton-Evans & Dugdale, 1988) and bedsharing (Mc Kenna et al., 1993; Mc Kenna & Mosko, 1994), when prolonged or when associated, may facilitate repeated night awakenings and postpone weaning to a later age. For Mosko et al. (1997) bedsharing induces a high degree of close proximity between mother and child, increases environmental CO_2 from maternal respiration stimulating infant respiration, and maximises the sensory impact of the mother on the infant. Finally the feeding schedule controlled by hunger (Mc Graw et al., 1999) does not influence the occurrence of awakenings and the stabilization of the sleep-wake rhythm (Salzarulo et al., 2000).

Parents' ideas on babies sleep and education are culturally determined and influence behaviour at bedtime and during the night (Lozoff, 1995). In most epidemiological studies, among all age groups, a statistical link was pointed out between the mother's depression and the child's sleep trouble (Ferber, 1995; Stoleru et al., 1997). It may be essential to know the parents' story, their personal attitude and reactions to understand the child's trouble (De Leersnyder, 1998). For illustration, in a group of 120 children less than 5 years old, a different parental attitude was described (Chambry et al., 2000) when either isolated and repeated nocturnal awakenings associated with bedtime difficulties occured. In isolated awakenings, parents were very anxious, mother suffering and feeling guilty from the nocturnal separation from the child, sleep representing a potential danger. Fathers were unable to reassure their wives in spite of a very strong parents-child attachement. In awakenings associated with bedtime difficulties, the family dynamic seemed different, the mother feeling lonely to assume the educational and parental responsabilities without close maternal model. She was often depressed and unable to give a self security feeling to the child. The motherhood failure led the child to an excited state and prevented him from falling asleep. These findings are close to constatations of Bruni et al. (2000) in poor sleepers preschool children with a high rate of behavioural problems presenting night wakings without bedtime problems and bedtime resistance without sleepwaking.

Arousals after respiratory events in infants

Central apneas are common events in infants. Obstructive apneas are rare in healthy infants (<2/H of sleep) and their number decreases from birth to 3–4 months of age.

When numerous, obstructive sleep apneas or upper airway obstruction episodes realise an obstructive sleep apnea syndrome (OSAS) usually secondary to adeno-tensillar hypertrophy but also observed in cranio-facial dysostosis with or without hindbrain herniation, in neuro-muscular diseases, in some genetic syndromes such as the Down syndrome (Levanon et al., 1999). Obesity is always a worsening factor. The link between gastro-oesophageal reflux and apneas is more controversial. Kahn et al. (1991) found that proximal acid oesophageal reflux increased the number of behavioural arousals. Thach (1997) showed that regurgition can cause an hyperactive laryngeal chemoreflex and episodic prolonged apneas in infants. On the opposite, Page & Jeffery (1998) in full term neonates showed that pharyngeal fluid stimulation did not induce apnea but swallowing. This airway defense response occurred more frequently in active sleep.

Effect of sleep apnea on sleep pattern

Whatever the cause, sleep apnea or upper airway obstruction was described to modify sleep patterns in infants, but not in children (Suen et al., 1995; Mc Grath et al., 1992). Mc Namara & Sullivan (1996) described in infants less REM sleep because of many arousals due to apneas, which shortened REM sleep episodes. The authors hypothesised that sleep fragmentation might result in a cumulative effect on the severity of sleep apnea and alter arousal responsiveness.

Behavioural arousal

Behavioural criteria used to define arousal are different from a study to another as already mentioned. Thoppil and al. (1991) proposed a classification based on video-image with definitive criteria (cry or eye opening > 5 sec), major criteria (sustained movement of the head, neck, trunck or both upper or lower limbs) and minor criteria (eye opening < 5 sec, frown, grimaces, smiles...) within 5 sec of apneas termination; twitches or movement just after the apnea called miniarousals. An arousal was scored on the presence of one definitive, or three major or two major plus three minor criteria. Spontaneous arousal rate was significantly higher in apneic periods but only 42% of obstructive apneas was terminated by an arousal response. The occurrence of arousals is significantly higher in long (>15sec) versus short apneas, in obstructive versus central apneas, in severe (important hypoxemia) versus mild apneas and in apneas with versus without bradycardia.

Taking into account twitches and movements during or at the end of apneas called miniarousals, Hoppenbrouwers et al. (1993) found that motor events were seen after 46, 54 and 86% of apnea episodes respectively at one, three and six months of age. Considering only miniarousals after apneas their percentage declines with age, 30% at 1 month, 9% at 3 months and 0% at 6 months of age. The number of miniarousals after apneas was not different in active sleep (AS) from quiet sleep (QS) and in the later part of the night from the earlier part. These two studies found a lack of arousal after a great number of apneic episodes suggesting that behavioural arousal is not essential for the termination of apnea in infants.

Behavioural and EEG arousals

Polygraphic criteria (with EEG and body movements recording) were used in more recent studies.

Mograss et al. (1994) classified the arousals as respiratory, "technician-induced" or spontaneous. Respiratory movement arousals, as numerous in AS as in QS, occurred at the termination of nearly all the obstructive events, re-establishing airway potency. Goh et al. (2000) showed that the arousal apnea indices increased from the beginning to the end of the REM periods across the night; such a change was not present during quiet sleep. Spontaneous arousals were frequent in NREM sleep in the same children.

Mc Namara et al. (1996) using the same criteria as Mograss et al. (1994) for scoring arousals found also a majority of obstructive apneas in active sleep but 61% of the respiratory events were not terminated with an arousal. Arousals occurred more frequently after obstructive than after central apneas. They concluded that arousal was not an important mechanism in the termination of sleep apnea in infants and children.

The same group (Thach & Lijowska, 1996; Lijowska et al., 1997; Wulbrand et al., 1998) described a consistent arousal sequence in infants after a tactile stimulus but also after an hypoxic-hypercapnic respiratory stimulus. End tidal CO_2 reached 40–50 Torr and SaO_2 did not fall usually below 94%. This stimulus provoked the appareance of four stereotyped successive behaviours: an augmented breath, a startle (usually a rapid neck extension) then a body movement and asymmetrical limb movements called thrashing by the authors. At the end of the sequence, the infant either resumed sleep or progressed to a full awakening. So, spontaneous and respiratory related sighs and startles could be considered as part of an arousal. Moreover, these phenomena have been found to be associated with an EEG interspindle interval prolongation, itself positively correlated with the intensity of occlusion and of the evoked startle. This EEG spindle suppression had a physiological meaning of brain-stem arousal. These arousal responses usually succeeded in clearing the airway. Such arousal sequences could occur spontaneously and periodically. The authors hypothesised that the airway defensive responses consist of an increase in the frequency and complexity of an endogeneously regulated sequence of arousal behaviour. Considering augmented breath, partial and global movement as a part of the arousal response, Vecchierini-Blineau et al. (2001) studied such parameters and EEG modifications after isolated, short apneas in infants suspected of upper airway problems. Isolated, non repetitive apneas were only considered to avoid habituation and a depressed arousal response (Mc Namara et al., 1999; Mc Namara & Sullivan, 1999). Only 22% of apneas, mainly obstructive, were followed by a motor event, either an augmented breath (7.9%) or a body movement (14.1%) and only 1.6% of apneas were terminated by an awakening. So short apneas (< 12 sec) were rarely accompanied by a motor event, nevertheless these respiratory related events were more frequent than spontaneous events. These percentages are similar to those published by Don et al. (2000) who found 29% of obstructive and mixed apnea terminated by an arousal. In Vecchierini et al. (2001), EEG frequency calculated by a semi-automatically analysis was found to increase after 60% of apnea, followed or not by a motor event, whatever the sleep state and apnea type. This EEG frequency increase was greater than spontaneous EEG frequency variation in the same sleep state and could be consistent with cortical arousal. A decrease in EEG amplitude, quantified by power spectrum evaluation, was described during active sleep by Schramm et al. (2000), being interpretated as an arousal reaction.

Finally, Don et al. (2000) showed that during obstructive events, successive respiratory efforts increased in amplitude with a full arousal after 17% of apneas (23% obstructive against 7.3% central apnea). They defined a respiratory arousal as a large change in at least two independent channels (EMGs or respiratory effort channels) without EEG disturbance.

Cardio-respiratory arousal

Wulbrand and al. (1995) described a “cardio-respiratory arousal”, in infants, terminating apneas without a change in sleep phase. This arousal was characterized by (1) a phasic simultaneous increase in submental and diaphragmatic muscles EMG, (2) correlated with the extent of tcp O_2 decline in REM sleep and (3) associated with bradycardia which ceased at the end of apnea. No change in EEG activity was found.

Muscle activation: Co-activation of submental and diaphragmatic muscles was found at the end of 64% and 79% of REM and NREM sleep apnea. Praud et al. (1988) had previously described such a mechanism at the temination of apneas in children. In infants, this coactivation of submental and diaphragmatic muscles occurred in parallel with a “gasp”. Auto rescusciting gasp in relation to apnea was already described in infants. This gasp was a combination of short expiration and deep inspiration apparently triggered by the decline of tcp O_2 in REM sleep allowing the recovery of mixed and obstructive apnea. This observation emphasized the importance of simultaneous both submental and diaphragmatic EMG activation. This co-contraction required a well developed integration of afferent and efferent neuronal pathways. As this co-contraction occurred in relationship with the decrease in tcp O_2, Wulbrand et al. (1995) pointed out the role of peripheral and central chemoreceptors in the apnea termination mechanism. Nevertheless, such a relationship between genio-glossus muscle activation and decrease in tcp O_2 was not found in children. So not only reflexes from chemical stimuli but also reflexes from mechanoreceptors in upper airways might play a role in the apnea termination (review in Berry & Gleeson 1997).

Changes in heart rate: a decrease in heart rate after apnea was described by several authors. Heart rate deceleration was greater after long apnea (Carbone et al., 1999) was more frequent in QS (Haddad et al., 1984) but greater in AS than in QS, (Vecchierini-Blineau, 2001). When apnea was followed by a gasp (Wulbrand et al., 1995) bradycardia ceased rapidly at the end of apnea. Moreover, when apnea provoked a body movement or miniarousal, heart rate deceleration was replaced by a heart rate acceleration (Hoppenbrouwers et al., 1993; Vecchierini-Blineau et al., 2001). This potentially protective response was less present in siblings and was less active at the age of highest risk for SIDS (Hoppenbrouwers et al., 1993).

Comparing heart rate power spectral analysis before and after obstructive apnea, in REM sleep, Franco et al. (1999) found that in normal infants but not in the future SIDS infants, low frequency to high frequency power ratio decreased after obstructive, long apnea. In their experimental procedure, Wulbrand et al. (1998) observed that heart rate first increased during 3.5 ± 0.9 sec then decreased and reached its minimum after 9.4 ± 0.8 sec. Startle intensity correlated with the percentage of heart rate increase and decrease.

Katz-Salomon and Milerad (1998) described also a significant decrease in heart rate, in infants with severe apnea compared to healthy infants in case of provoked hypercapnia by inhaled CO_2.

Mechanisms of heart rate change after apnea are unclear. Schechtman et al. (1998) suggested that repetitive apneas may impair sympathetic mechanisms and consequently elicit repeated vagal excitation creating an impairement in the balance between sympathetic and vagal activity. An increase in vagal tonus facilited the occurrence of bradycardia.

Interestingly, apneas ended by a body movement with or without an EEG frequency shift were not followed by a decrease but rather by an increase in heart rate. Sympathetic drive contingent on somatic activity may override the usual deceleration. After obstructive and central apneas, bradycardia but also hypoxia are noticed.

What is the role of hypoxia or/and hypercapnia in respiratory related arousals?

The longer are the apneas, the more important and rapid is the decrease in heart rate, SaO_2 or tcP O_2. As the length of the apneic interval increased, the interval between the onset of apnea and an associated drop in heart rate and in SaO_2 also increased. If apnea heart rate and SaO_2 drops are closely associated events, SaO_2 decrease cannot be assessed by heart rate drop.

There is no relationship between bradycardia and hypoxia (Carbone et al., 1999). Moreover, no constant relation was found between hypoxia and arousal, in healthy as well as in near- miss infants. Infants with severe apneas have a higher mean Pa O_2 level at which arousal occurred compared to normal infants. More apneic infants than healthy infants failed to arouse to hypoxic challenge (Newman et al. 1986). Some studies submitted normal and apneic infant to mild hypoxia in 6 weeks infants (Milerad et al., 1989) or to an increasing asphyxia measured by Fi CO_2 value, in healthy infants, at birth then at 3 and 6 months of age (Campbell et al., 1998). Infants responded to hypoxia or hypercapnia during sleep, by an increase in ventilation, sometimes by periodic breathing and by an arousal. Arousal in healthy infants were more frequent in REM sleep whatever the age, and in newborn than at 6 months of age. This decrease in arousal threshold to chemical stimuli, with age, was confirmed by some studies but not by others (see Campbell et al., 1998). In infants with severe apneas, the baseline tcP O_2 value was significantly lower than in control infants. This low baseline value was not related to the occurrence of arousal during the hypoxic challenge.

The arousal frequency was similar in apneic and control infants. No relationship was found between arousal and the mean rate of tcP O_2 decrease or the ventilatory slope. No threshold levels of tcP O_2 or tcP CO_2 for arousals were found. So, tcP O_2 and tcP CO_2 values realise a weak feed-back control of breathing. These results do not support the hypothesis of a deficient hypoxic response in infants with apneic events. In older healthy and OSAS children, Marcus et al. (1998) demonstrated that hypoxemia was a poor stimulus to arouse. On the opposite, hypercapnia or hypoxic – hypercapnia were potent stimuli to arouse. Children with OSAS have a slightly blunted arousal response to hypercapnia.

Other clinical contexts

In older children, up to school age, some sleep disorders in relation with awakenings may appear due to physiological changes in infants sleep. In infants NREM sleep has a tendency to appear in alternate cycles through the night with a higher amount of slow wave sleep in the first cycle (Bes et al., 1991). Cycles are more numerous and of shorter duration than in older children and in adults (Bes et al., 1991; Louis et al., 1997). In some infants up to two years of age, there is still an ability to have REM sleep onsets in the middle of the night (Louis, 1998). In 5 to 11 years old children Leygonie & Garma (1973) described a partial REM episode with persistence of slow wave EEG pattern, most often at the end of the first NREM state. Such a pattern was more rarely observed in the second cycle and not later in the night.

In parasomnias associated with NREM sleep, there is a continuum of manifestations in arousal disorders with a hierarchical model from partial arousal: confusional arousal or sleep drunkeness, night terrors, somnambulism (Ferber 1985; Sheldon et al., 1992). They occur from slow wave sleep in the first third of the night with unusual motor behaviour. In night terrors autonomic manifestations are very intense, related to dysfunction in sleep state transitions and partial arousals from NREM stages 3 and 4 sleep (Sheldon et al., 1992; Rosen et al., 1995). Partial arousals most often occur at the transition from NREM sleep to the next sleep cycle; therefore, the child appears "caught" in a dissociated state between deep NREM sleep and full arousal (Rosen et al., 1995).

The first night terrors, the partial arousals with drunkeness may occur several times during the night at fairly fixed hours in the same child. During EEG sleep recordings (Rosen et al., 1995), observed a combination of alpha, theta and delta frequencies, as described by Schenck et al. (1998), in adults with night terrors and sleepwalking after each behavioural and nonbehavioural slow wave sleep (SWS) arousal.

Night terrors are often described by the parents as nightmares. Both are impressive and frightful to the observer, since the child seems to endure an intense pain with cries, confusion and agitation. Theorically these two kinds of events are easy to differenciate. They do not occur at the same time in the night, the clinical manifestations are different. After the nightmare, the child recovers a full consciousness and is able to tell the story of his bad dream. The occurrence of parasomnias was reported to be positively associated with anxiety and significant family life-events. In a large controlled study, from 3 to 13 years of age, night terrors were more frequent in 3–10 years children than at older ages, associated to high anxiety levels but not to significant sociodemographic variables (Laberge et al., 2000).

Hyperactivity disorders were more often described in older children and adolescents (Dugas, 2000), in association with sleep troubles and movements / arousals manifestations (Mograss et al., 1994), as restless leg syndrome (Walters et al., 1996) and periodic leg syndrome (Picchietti & Walters, 1999).

Conclusion

Behavioural or/and electrophysiological awakenings are easier to recognize than arousals. Awakenings are frequent and decrease during infancy following a physiological maturational process. When too numerous, in some pathological or psycho-social circumstances, they may require parents assistance. If persistent, they lead to insomnia. In some older infants, awakenings, clear-out behavioural or EEG arousals are observed as parasomnia manifestations, when SWS amount is very high in the first two sleep cycles of the night. After respiratory events, awakenings are very rare, arousals are more frequent (more numerous than if a random association had occurred) especially after obstructive and long apnea whatever the sleep state. Arousals have a broad range of transient behavioural and electrophysiological manifestations: augmented breath, startles, partial or global body movements, spindle suppressions or shifts in EEG frequency as well as EEG amplitude modifications. Heart rate change and inspiratory effort level are important parts of the arousal response. Nevertheless, minimal behavioural and electrophysiological events significant of an arousal process, in infancy, have still to be defined.

References

American Sleep Disorders Association (ASDA) and Sleep Reasearch Society report (1992). EEG arousals: scoring rules and examples. The Atlas Task Force. *Sleep, 15,* 173–184.

American Thoracic Society (1996). Standards and indications for cardiopulmonary sleep studies in children. *American Journal of Respiratory and Critical Care Medicine, 153,* 866–878.

Anders, Thomas F. & Maria Keener (1985). Developmental course of nighttime sleep-wake patterns in full term and premature infants during the first year of life. I. *Sleep, 8,* 173–192.

Bach, Véronique, Belkacem Bouferrache, Odile Kremp, Yves Maingourd & Jean-Pierre Libert (1994). Regulation of sleep and body temperature in response to exposure to cool and warm environments in neonates. *Pediatrics, 93*(5), 789–796.

Berry, Richard B., & Kevin Gleeson (1997). Respiratory arousal from sleep: mechanisms and significance. *Sleep, 20*(8), 654–675.

Bes, Frederick, Harmut Schulz, Yvonne Navelet & Piero Salzarulo (1991). The distribution of slow-wave sleep accross the night: a comparison for infants, children and adults. *Sleep, 14,* 5–12.

Bruni, Oliviero, F. Lo Reto, S. Miano & S. Ottaviano (2000). Clinical Neurophysiology at the beginning of the 21st century (Supplement to Clinical Neurophysiology, vol 53). In Ambler, Z., S. Nevsimalova, Z. Kadanka, P.M. Rossini, (Eds), *Daytime behavioural correlates of awakenings and bedtime resistance in preschool children* (pp. 358–361). Amsterdam: Elsevier.

Campbell, A.J, D.P.G Bolton, B.J Taylor & R.M.Sayers (1998). Responses to an increasing asphyxia in infants: effects of age and sleep state. *Respiratory Physiology, 112,* 51–58.

Carbone, Tracy, Luis C. Marrero, Johanna Weiss, Mark Hiatt & Thomas Hegyi (1999). Heart rate and oxygen saturation correlates of infants apnea. *Journal of Perinatology, 19*(1) 44–47.

Chambry, Jean, Yvonne Navelet & Pierre Ferrari (2000). Insomnia in children. *Journal of Sleep Research, 9,* suppl. 1, 34.

Coons, Susan & Christian Guilleminault (1985). Motility and arousal in near miss sudden infant death syndrome. *Journal of Pediatrics, 107,* 728–732.

Curzi-Dascalova, Lilia, Juliette Bloch, Marie-Françoise Vecchierini, Antoine Bedu & Patricia Vignolo (2000). Physiological Parameters Evaluation following apnea in healthy premature infants. *Biology of the Neonate, 77,* 203–211.

Dahl, Ronald E., Mark S. Scher, Douglas E. Williamson, Nadine Robles & Nancy Day (1995). A longitudinal study of prenatal marijuana use. Effects on sleep and arousal at age three years. *Archives of Pediatric and Adolescent Medicine, 149,* 145–150.

Davidson-Ward, Susan & Carole L. Marcus (1996). Obstructive sleep apnea in infants and young children. *Journal of Clinical Neurophysiology, 13,* 3, 198–207.

De Leersnyder, Hélène(1998). *L'enfant et son sommeil.* Paris: Editions Robert Laffont, SA.

Don, Garrick W., Turkka Kirjavainen, Catherine Broome, Chris Seton & Karen A. Waters (2000). Site and mechanics of spontaneous, sleep-associated obstructive apnea in infants. *Journal of Applied Physiology, 89,* 2453–2462.

Dugas, Michel (2000). Hyperactivité, hyperkinésie et troubles déficitaires de l'attention. In D. Houzel, M. Emmanuelli, F. Moggio (Eds), *Dictionnaire de Psychopathologie de l'enfant et de l'adolescent.* (pp. 326–329). Paris: P.U.F.

Eaton-Evans, J., & A.E. Dugdale (1988). Sleep patterns of infants in the first year of life. *Archives of Disease in Childhood, 63,* 647–649.

Ferber, Richard (1985). *Solve your child's sleep problems.* New York: Simon and Schuster.

Ferber, Richard (1995). Sleeplessness in children. In Ferber, R., M. Kryger (Eds), *Principles and pratice of sleep medicine in the child* (pp. 79–89). Philadelphia: W.B. Saunders Co.

Ficca, Gianluca, Igino Fagioli, Fiorenza Giganti & Piero Salzarulo (1999). Spontaneous awakenings from sleep across the first year of life. *Early Human Development, 55,* 219–228.

Franco, Patricia, José Groswasser, Martine Sottiaux, Ema Broodfield & André Kahn (1996). Decreased cardiac responses to auditory stimulation during prone sleep. *Pediatrics, 97*, 2, 174–178.

Franco, Patricia, Anne Pardou, Sergio Hassid, Paul Lurquin, José Groswasser & André Kahn (1998). Auditory arousal thresholds are higher when infants sleep in the prone position. *Journal of Pediatrics, 132*, 240–243.

Franco, Patricia, José Grosswasser, Sergio Hassid, Jean-Pierre Lanquart, Sonia Scaillet & André Kahn (1999). Prenatal exposure to cigarette smoking is associated with a decrease in arousal in infants. *Journal of Pediatrics, 135*, 34–38.

Franco, Patricia, Henri Szliwoski, Michelle Dramaise and André Kahn (1999). Decreased autonomic responses to obstructive sleep events in future victims of sudden infant death syndrome. *Pediatric Research, 46*, 33–39.

Franco, Patricia, J. Scaillet, V. Wermenbol, F. Valente, José Groswasser & André Kahn (2000). The influence of a pacifier on infant's arousal from sleep. *Journal of Pediatrics, 136*(6), 775–779.

Galland, Barbara C., G. Reeves, B.J. Taylor & D.P.G. Bolton (1998). Sleep position, autonomic fonction, and arousal. *Archives of Disease in Childhood Fetal Neonatal Ed., 78*, F189–F194.

Galland, Barbara C., D.P.G. Bolton, B.J. Taylor, R.M. Sayers & S.M. Williams (2000). Ventilatory sensitivity to mild asphyxia: prone versus supine sleep position. *Archives of Disease in Childhood, 83*, 423–428.

Goh, Daniel, Patricia Galster & Carole L. Marcus (2000). Sleep architecture and respiratory disturbances in children with obstructive sleep apnea. *American Journal of Respiratory and Critical Care Medicine, 162*, 682–686.

Guideline Two: Minimal technical standards for pediatric electroencephalography (1994). *Journal of Clinical Neurophysiology, 11*, 6–9.

Guilleminault, Christian, Rafael Pelayo, Damien Leger, Alex Clerk & Robert C.Z. Bociam (1996). Recognition of sleep-disordered breathing in children. *Pediatrics, 98*, 871–882.

Haddad, G.G., A.R. Bazzy, S.L. Chang & R.B. Mellins (1984). Heart rate pattern during respiratory pauses in normal infants during sleep. *Journal of Developmental Physiology, 6*, 329–337.

Hoppenbrouwers, Toke, Joan E. Hodgman & Luis Cabal (1993). Obstructive apnea, associated patterns of movement, heart rate and oxygenation in infants at low and increased risk for SIDS. *Pediatric Pulmonology, 15*, 1–12.

Jeffery, Heather E., J.H.E. Megevand & A. Page (1999). Why the prone position is a risk factor for sudden infant death syndrome. *Pediatrics, 104*, 263–269.

Kahn, André & Denise Blum (1982). Phenothiazines and sudden infant death syndrome. *Pediatrics, 70*, 75–78.

Kahn, André, Elizabeth Rebuffat, Martin Sottiaux, D. Dufour, S. Cadranel & F. Reiterer (1991). Arousals induced by proximal oesophageal reflux in infants. *Sleep, 14*(1), 39–42.

Kahn, André, José Groswasser, Elizabeth Rebuffat, Martin Sottiaux, Denise Blum, M. Foerster, Patricia Franco, A. Bochner, M. Alexander & A. Bachy (1992). Sleep and cardiorespiratory characteristics of infants victims of sudden death: a prospective case-control study. *Sleep, 15*, 287–292.

Kahn, André, José Groswasser, Martin Sottiaux, Elizabeth Rebuffat, Patricia Franco & Philippe Dramaix (1993). Prone or supine body position and sleep characteristics in infants. *Pediatrics, 91*(6), 1112–1115.

Kahn, André, Patricia Franco, Sonia Scaillet, José Groswasser & Bernard Dan (1997). Development of cardio-pulmonary integration and the role of arousability from sleep. *Current Opinions in Pulmonary Medicine, 3*, 440–444.

Katz-Salomon, Miriam, & Joseph Milerad (1998). The divergent ventilatory and heart rate response to moderate hypercapnia in infants with apnea of infancy. *Archives of Disease in Childhood, 79*, 231–236.

Laberge, Luc, Richard E. Tremblay, Franck Vitaro & Jacques Montplaisir (2000) Development of parasomnias from childhood to early adolescence. *Pediatrics, 106*, 67–74.

Levanon, Asaf, Ariel Tarasiuk & Asher Tal (1999). Sleep characteristics in children with Down syndrome. *Journal of Pediatrics, 134*, 755–760.

Leygonie, Françoise, & Lucile Garma (1973). Sleep 73. In W.P. Koella and P. Levin (Eds), *First cycle of sleep in normal children* (pp. 372–373). Basel: S. Karger.

Lijowska, Anna, Nevada Reed, Barbara Mertins Chiodini & Bradley T.Thach (1997). Sequential arousal and airway defensive behaviour of infants in asphyxial sleep environments. *Journal of Applied Physiology, 83*(1), 219–228.

Lindgren, C., J. Lin, B.S. Grahan, M.E. Gray, R.A. Parker & H.W. Sundell (1996). Respiratory syncytial virus infection enhances the response to laryngeal chemo-stimulation and inhibits arousal from sleep in young lambs. *Acta Paediatrica, 85*, 789–797.

Louis, Jacqueline (1998). Maturation du sommeil pendant les deux premières années de vie: aspects quantitatif, structurel et circadien. *Neurophysiologie Clinique, 28*, 477–491.

Louis, Jacqueline, Christine Cannard, Hélène Bastuji & Marie-José Challamel (1997). Sleep ontogenesis revisited: a longitudinal 24-Hour home polygraphic study on 15 normal infants during the first two years of life. *Sleep, 20*, 323–333.

Lozoff, Betsy (1995). Principles and Practices of sleep medicine in the child. In R. Ferber, M. Kryger (Eds), *Culture and family: influences on childhood sleep practices and problems* (69–73). Philadelphia: W.B. Saunders Co.

Mc Grath, S.A., J.L. Carroll, S.A. Mc Colley, Carole L. Marcus, P. Pyzik & G.M. Loughlin (1992). Normal sleep structure found in children with obstructive sleep apnea. *American Review of Respiratory Disorders, 145*, A 176.

Mc Graw, Kate, Robert Hoffmann, Chris Harker & John Herman (1999). The development of circadian rythms in human infant. *Sleep, 22*, 303–310.

Mc Kenna, James J., Evelyn B. Thoman, Thomas F. Anders, Abraham Sadeh, Vicki L. Schechtman & Steven F. Glotzbach (1993). Infant-parent co-sleeping in an evolutionary perspective: implications for understanding infant sleep development and the sudden infant death syndrome. *Sleep, 16*, 263–282.

Mac Kenna, James J., & Sarah S. Mosko (1994). Sleep and arousal, synchrony and independence, among mothers and infants sleeping apart and together (same bed): an experiment in evolutionary medicine. *Acta Paediatrica*, Suppl. 397, 94–102.

McNamara, Frances, & Colin E.Sullivan (1996). Sleep disordered breathing and its effects on sleep in infants. *Sleep, 19*(1), 4–12.

McNamara, Frances, Faiq G. Issa & Colin E. Sullivan (1996). Arousal pattern following central and obstructive breathing abnormalities in infants and children. *Journal of Applied Physiology, 81*(6), 2651–2657.

McNamara, Frances, & Colin E. Sullivan (1999). Effects of nasal CPAP therapy on respiratory and spontaneous arousals in infants with OSAS. *Journal of Applied Physiology, 87*(3), 889–893.

McNamara, Frances, Henning Wulbrand H. & Bradley T. Thach (1999). Habituation of the infant arousal response. *Sleep, 22*(3), 320–326.

Marcus, Carole L., Janita Lutz, John L. Carroll & Owen Bamford (1998). Arousal and ventilatory responses during sleep apnea. *Journal of Applied Physiology, 84*(6), 1926–1936.

Milerad, J., T. Hertzberg, G. Wennergren & Hugo Lagercrantz (1989). Respiratory and arousal responses to hypoxia in apnoeic infants reinvestigated. *European Journal of Pediatrics, 148*, 565–570.

Mograss, M.A., F.M. Ducharme & Robert T. Brouillette (1994). Movement/arousals. Description, classification, and relationship to sleep apnea in children. *American Journal of Respiratory and Critical Care Medicine, 150*, 1690–1696.

Mosko, Sarah, Chritopher, Richard, James Mc Kenna, S. Drummond & D. Mukai (1997). Maternal proximity and infant CO_2 environment during bedsharing and possible implications for SIDS research. *American Journal of Physical Anthropology*, 103, 315–328.

Navelet, Yvonne, Odile Benoit & Ginette Bouard (1982). Nocturnal sleep organization during the first months of life. *Electroencephalography and Clinical Neurophysiology, 54*, 71–78.

Navelet, Yvonne, Christine Payan, Alain Guilhaume & Odile Benoit (1984). Nocturnal sleep organization in infants "at risk" for Sudden Infant Death Syndrome. *Pediatric Research, 18*(7), 654–657.

Navelet, Yvonne (1996). Insomnia in the child and adolescent. *Sleep, 19*, S23–S28.

Newman, N.M., J.A. Trinder, K.A. Phillips, K. Jordan & J. Cruickshank (1989). Arousal deficit: mechanism of the sudden infant death syndrome. *Australian Pediatric Journal, 25*, 196–201.

Page, Megan, & Heather E. Jeffery (1998). Airway protection in sleeping infants in response to pharyngeal fluid stimulation in the supine position. *Pediatric Research, 44*, 691–698.

Picchietti, Daniel L. & Arthur S. Walters. Moderate to severe periodic limb movement disorder in childhood and adolescence. *Sleep, 22*, 297–300.

Pickens, D.L., G.L. Schefft, G.A. Storch & Bradley T. Thach (1989). Characterization of prolonged apneic episodes associated with respiratory syncitial viral infection. *Pediatric Pulmonology, 6*, 195–201.

Praud, Jean-Paul, Anne-Marie D'Allest, Marie-France Delaperche, Serge Bobin & Claude Gaultier (1988). Diaphragmatic and genioglossus electromyographic activity at the onset and at the end of obstructive apnea in children with obstructive sleep apnea syndrome. *Pediatric Research, 23*, 1–4.

Read, Paul A., Rosemary S.C. Horne, Susan M. Cranage, Adrian M. Walker, David W. Walker & Michael Adamson (1998). Dynamic changes in arousal threshold during sleep in the human infant. *Pediatric Research, 43*, 697–703.

Rosen, Gerald, Mark W. Mahowald & Richard Ferber (1995). Principles and practices of sleep medicine in the child. In R. Ferber, M. Kryger, (Eds), *Sleep walking, confusional arousals and sleep terrors in the child* (pp. 99–106). Philadelphia: W.B. Saunders Co.

Sadeh, Avi, Peretz Lavie, Anat Scher, Emanuel Tirosh & Rachel Epstein (1991). Actigraphic home-monitoring sleep-disturbed and control infants and young children: a new method for pediatric assessment of sleep-wake patterns. *Pediatrics, 87*, 494–499.

Salzarulo, Piero, & A. Chevalier (1983). Sleep problems in children and their relationship with early disturbances of the wakingsleeping rhythms. *Sleep, 6*, 46–51.

Salzarulo, Piero, Fiorenza Giganti, Gianluca Ficca, Igino Fagioli & Monica Toselli (2000). Gates to awakening in early development. *Clinical Neurophysiology, 53*, S352–S354.

Samson-Dollfus, Dominique, Gérard Delapierre, Béatrice Nogues & Isabelle Bertoldi (1988). Sleep organization in children at risk for sudden infant death syndrome. *Sleep, 11*, 277–285.

Schechtman, Vicki L., Judith A. Henslee & Ronald M. Harper (1998). Developmental patterns of heart rate and variability in infants with persistent apnea of infancy. *Early Human Development, 50*, 251–262.

Schenck, Carlos H., Juan A. Pareja, Andrea L. Patterson & Mark E. Mahowald (1998). Analysis of polysomnographic events surrounding 252 slow-wave sleep arousals in thirty-eight adults with injurious sleep walking and sleep terrors. *Journal of Clinical Neurophysiology, 15*, 159–166.

Schramm, D., B. Scheidt, A. Hübler, J. Frenzel, K. Holthausen & O. Breidbach (2000). Spectral analysis of electroencephalogram during sleep-related apneas in preterm and term born infant in the first weeks of life. *Clinical Neurophysiology, 111*, 1788–1791.

Schulz, Harmut, Roberto Massetani, Igino Fagioli & Piero Salzarulo (1985). Spontaneous awakening from sleep in infants. *Electroencephalography and Clinical Neurophysiology, 61*, 267–271.

Sheldon, Stephen H., Jean-Paul Spire & Howard B. Levy (Eds) (1992). *Pediatric sleep medicine*. Philadelphia: W.B. Saunders Co.

Stoleru, Serge, Editha D. Nottelmann, Barbara Belmont & D. Ronsaville (1997). Sleep problems in children of affectively ill mothers. *Journal of Child Psychology and Psychiatry, 38*, 831–841.

Suen, J.S., J.E. Arnold & L.J. Brooks (1995). Adenotonsillectomy for treatment of obstructive sleep apnea in children. *Archives of Otolaryngology-Head and Neck Surgery, 121*, 525–530.

Thach, Bradley T. (1997). Reflux associated apnea in infants: evidence for a laryngeal chemoreflexe. *American Journal of Medicine, 103*, 5A, 120S–124S.

Thach, Bradley T., & Anna Lijowska (1996). Arousals in infants. *Sleep, 19*(10), S271–S273.

Thirion, Marie, & Marie-Josèphe Challamel (1995). *Le sommeil, le rêve et l'enfant*. Paris: Albin Michel.

Thomas, D.A., K. Poole, E.K. Mc Ardle, P.C. Goodenough, J. Thompson, C.S. Beardsmore & H. Simpson (1996). The effect of sleep deprivation on sleep states, breathing events, peripheral chemoresponsiveness and arousal propensity in healthy 3 month old infants. *European Respiratory Journal, 9*, 932–938.

Thoppil, C.K., M.A. Belan, C.P. Cowen & O.P. Mathew (1991). Behavioural arousal in newborn infants and its association with termination of apnea. *Journal of Applied Physiology, 70*(6), 2479–2484.

Tirosh, Emanuel, Anat Scher, Avi Sadeh, M. Jaffe, A. Rubin & Peretz Lavie (1993). The effects of illness on sleep behaviour in infants. *European Journal of Pediatrics, 152*, 15–17.

Toth, Linda A., & Mohamed A. Chaudhary (1997). Developmental alterations in auditory arousal from sleep in healthy and virus infected cats. *Sleep, 21*(2), 143–152.

Vecchierini-Blineau, Marie-Françoise, Beatrice Nogues & Jacques Colin (1988), Sleep 86. In Koella, W.P., F. Obal, H. Schultz and P. Visser (Eds), *Awake periods during sleep in infants: a comparison between control and near-miss infants* (pp. 435–437). Stuttgart, New-York: Gustav Fischer Verlag.

Vecchierini-Blineau, Marie-Françoise, Beatrice Nogues & Sylvain Louvet (1988). Sleep 86. In Koella, W.P., F. Obal, H Schultz and P. Visser (Eds), *Gross body movements during sleep in controls, sudden infant death siblings and near-miss infants* (pp. 432–434). Stuttgart, New-York: Gustav Fischer Verlag.

Vecchierini-Blineau, Marie-Françoise, Lilia Curzi-Dascalova, Ha Trang-Pham, Juliette Bloch & Claude Gaultier (2001). Patterns of EEG frequency, motor activity, heart rate and oxygenation following isolated short apneas in infants. *Pediatric Research, 49*(2), 1–9.

Walters, A.S., K Hickey, J. Maltzman, T. Verrico, D. Joseph, W. Hening, V. Wilson & S. Chokroverty (1996). A questionnaire study of 138 patients with restless legs syndrome: the "night-walkers survey". *Neurology, 46*, 92–95.

Ward, Susan L., D.B. Bautista, M.S. Woo, M. Chang, S. Scheutz, L. Wachsman, S. Sehgal & X.Bean (1992). Responses to hypoxia and hypercapnia in infants of substance-abusing mothers. *Journal of Pediatrics, 121*, 704–709.

Wulbrand, Henning, Georges Von Zezschwitz & Karl H. P. Bentele (1995). Submental and diaphragmatic muscles activity during and at resolution of mixed and obstructive apneas and cardiorespiratory arousal in preterm infants. *Pediatric Research, 38*, 298–305.

Wulbrand, Henning, Frances McNamara & Bradley T. Thach (1998). Suppression of sigma spindle electroencephalographic activity as a measure of transient arousal after spontaneous and occlusion evoked sighs and startles. *Pediatric Research, 44*, 767–773.

Wulbrand, Henning, Frances McNamara & Bradley T. Thach (1998). Indicators of arousal activity in the infant's ascending reticular system: sighs, startles, EEG spindle suppression and heart rate changes. 16th conference on apnea of infancy. *Pediatric Pulmonology, 24*, 453.

Arousal responses to hypercapnia and hypoxia in infants and children

Claude Gaultier
Service de Physiologie, Hôpital Robert Debré, Université Paris

Arousal from sleep is considered an important protective response to life-threatening stimuli such as hypoxia and hypercapnia (Phillipson & Sullivan, 1978). It has been suggested that failure to arouse in response to hypoxia and/or hypercapnia may put infants at risk for sudden infant death syndrome (SIDS) (McCulloch et al., 1982; Hunt, 1981). This chapter reviews data on arousal responses to hypoxia and/or hypercapnia in infants and children who are healthy or have respiratory disorders.

Mechanisms of arousal to chemical stimuli

Mechanisms of arousal from sleep in response to respiratory stimuli, i.e., hypoxia, hypercapnia, or both (asphyxia), remain incompletely understood. The arousal system may be stimulated directly or indirectly via either the chemoreceptors or the respiratory mechanoreceptors (Bowes et al., 1981; Berry et al., 1997). A role for peripheral chemoreceptors in the arousal response to isocapnic hypoxia has been shown in dogs studied before and after carotid body denervation (Bowes et al., 1981). The arterial oxygen saturation associated with arousal from both non-rapid-eye-movement (NREM) and rapid-eye-movement (REM) sleep decreased after carotid body denervation, suggesting a simple model of hypoxic arousal in which the peripheral chemoreceptors send impulses directly to areas of the brain responsible for arousal, such as the reticular activating system, causing cortical activation. However, another study in chemodenervated cats suggested a possible direct effect of hypoxia independent from peripheral chemoreceptor output (Neubauer et al., 1981). Similarly, increasing the arterial partial pressure of CO_2 may cause arousal by directly stimulating specific brain areas (such as the locus coeruleus and the midline raphe) (Pineda & Aghajanian, 1997; Bernard et al., 1996). A role for peripheral chemoreceptors in arousal from hypercapnia is plausible, since a decreased frequency of arousal responses to hypercapnia has been reported in lambs with carotid denervation (Fewell et al., 1989).

Other studies indicate that respiratory mechanoreceptors can contribute to arousal in response to chemical stimuli because they send impulses to the reticular activating system when they detect an increase in ventilatory efforts (Yasuma et al., 1991; Berry & Gleeson, 1997). Gleeson et al. showed that arousal in human adults in response to hypoxia, hypercapnia, and increased resistive load occurred at similar levels of ventilatory effort, as measured by peak esophageal pressure (Gleeson et al., 1990). These findings have been interpreted as suggesting that afferents from respiratory mechanoreceptors may play a prominent role in arousal mechanisms to chemical stimuli (Berry & Gleeson, 1997). If this is indeed the case, then a ventilatory response, i.e., increased respiratory efforts, may be required for arousal to occur. However, a recent study showed that respiratory mechanoreceptor input was not required for arousal to hypercapnia (Ayas et al., 2000). Humans with neurologically complete proximal spinal cord section abolishing changes in respiratory mechanoreceptor input showed arousal in response to hypercapnia. CO_2 may act on arousal centres directly or via projections from chemoreceptors in these patients. Therefore, further studies are needed to determine the relative contributions of potential mechanisms of arousal to chemical stimuli in adult humans or animals.

Because most studies of arousal responses to chemical stimuli have been performed in adults, the postnatal development of this response is poorly understood. In particular, it is unclear whether the main triggers of this response are the same throughout development. We recently reported a study on the arousal response to hypoxia in newborn mice aged 3 hours (H3), 12 hours, and 48 hours, respectively (Dauger et al., 2001). These ages corresponded to the periods before, during, and after peripheral chemoreceptor resetting, which in mice, occurs at approximately 12 hours of age (Dauger et al., 2001). Behaviour during arousal was a characteristic pattern of motor responses, including extension of the head, neck, and forepaws. This arousal response was present at all the ages studied, including H3, when the hyperpneic response to hypoxia was minimal. Furthermore, at all three ages, arousal occurred after the peak of the ventilatory response to hypoxia, i.e., during the hypoxic ventilatory decline. These data indicate that neither the afferents from chemoreceptors nor those from ventilatory muscles are critical triggers of the arousal response to hypoxia in newborn mice.

Criteria for arousal response to chemical stimuli

The term "arousal from sleep" denotes the change from a state of sleep to a state of wakefulness (Phillipson & Sullivan, 1978). The Atlas Task Force of the American Sleep Disorders Association has developed a set of criteria, including electroencephalogram (EEG) and electromyogram (EMG) criteria, for scoring arousal in NREM and REM sleep in human adults (American Sleep Disorders Association, 1992). However, these cortical EEG criteria currently used to define EEG arousal in adults may overlook the potential importance of subcortical arousal (Pitson & Stradling, 1998). Furthermore, criteria for EEG arousal in infants and children are not agreed on (McNamara et al., 1996; Mograss et al., 1994). Studies of hypoxic or hypercapnic arousal responses in infants and children have used a variety of criteria for defining arousal. However, most used behavioural criteria, defining arousal in infants as awakening with eye opening and crying (Dunne et al., 1992; Davidson-Ward et al., 1986; Van der Hal et al., 1986; Gingras et al., 1994; Milerad et al., 1989; Lewis & Bosque, 1995; Davidson-Ward et al., 1992; Garg et al., 1988). One recent study found that the arousal sequence to a hypercapnic stimulus in infants (Lijowska et al., 1997) consisted of a spinal withdrawal reflex followed by an augmented breath, then a startle, and finally EEG arousal. Thus, arousal involved progression of central nervous system activation from the spinal to the cortical level. This arousal sequence first described after a respiratory (hypercapnic) stimulus (Lijowska et al., 1997) has been found also after a non-respiratory (tactile) stimulus in infants (McNamara et al., 1999).

Measurement conditions of arousal responses to chemical stimuli

Conditions for measuring arousal responses to chemical stimuli have not been standardized. Because they vary across studies, results are difficult to compare.

1. Most studies were performed during day-time naps in infants. It is not known whether arousal responses during daytime naps differ from those during nighttime sleep.

2. Although a plastic hood was used to administer the gas mixture in most studies, some authors used a face mask (Ariagno et al., 1980; Praud et al., 1991; Marcus et al., 1998), a device that may contribute to arousal.
3. In one study, some of the infants with apnoea, but none of the healthy infants, received 30 mg/kg of chloral hydrate to facilitate sleep (Van der Hal et al., 1986). Because sedatives have been shown to depress arousal in animals, their use is not recommmended before testing arousal responses to any kind of stimulus.
4. Sleep state has been shown to influence arousal responses to chemical stimuli in newborn and adult animals (Fewell & Baker, 1987; Phillipson et al., 1978). Most of the studies in human infants were done during quiet (NREM) sleep, as defined by behavioural criteria.
5. The testing protocol varied among studies: some studies analysed arousal responses at the end of a hypoxic or hypercapnic ventilatory response test (Praud et al., 1991; Campbell et al., 1998), whereas others used a test specifically designed to evaluate arousal responses.
6. The method of hypoxic or hypercapnic challenge also differed across studies. Nevertheless, with the exception of the earliest work, available studies fall into two categories. In the first category (method 1, Tables 1–4), the hypoxic or hypercapnic challenge lasted no more than 3 minutes. During the hypoxic challenge, the inspired fraction of O_2 (FIO_2) was 11%, leading to a fall in arterial partial pressure of O_2 to 45- to 40-mmHg. During the hypercapnic challenge, the inspired CO_2 fraction was 10%, producing a rise in end-tidal partial pressure of CO_2 ($P_{ET}CO_2$) up to 60 to 65 mmHg. The hypoxic or hypercapnic challenges were stopped immediately upon arousal or at the end of the 3 minutes. In the second category (method 2, Tables 1–4), $P_{ET}CO_2$ was increased stepwise or F_IO_2 decreased stepwise over 10 to 15 minutes. The levels of hypoxemia or hypercapnia were similar to those with method 1. The hypoxic or hypercapnic challenge was stopped at arousal or at the end of the challenge. Method 2 is more accurate for determining hypoxic or hypercapnic arousal thresholds (Ayas et al., 2000).
7. The composition of the gas mixture was hyperoxic for all hypercapnic challenges, except in one study (Marcus et al., 1998). During hypoxic challenges, no effort was made to maintain isocapnia and, consequently, hypocapnia occurred.
8. The number of trials varied among studies. Data were expressed either using the total number of trials with arousal in the study group or the percentage of subjects with arousal to one or more trials. Tables 1–4 in this chapter indicate the percentages of subjects with arousal.

Table 1. Arousal to hypercapnia in healthy infants and children in NREM sleep

nb	PNA	method	%A	$P_{ET}CO_2$ at A mmHg	Reference
18	4.6±1.7 d	2	100	50.9	Dunne et al., 1992
17	45±6.2 d	2	100	52.8	Dunne et al., 1992
16	87±7.9 d	2	100	53.0	Dunne et al., 1992
22	7.3±0.7 wk	2	100	*48.4 ±1.4	McCulloch et al., 1982
29	8.7±1.3 wk	2	100	48.3 ±5.4	Lewis & Bosque 1995
6	8.4±3.2 mo	1	100	51.6 ±2.6	Davidson-Ward et al., 1986
9	6.8±1.1 mo	1	100	51.6 ±2	Van der Hal et al., 1986
7	4.4±1.1 yr	1	100	51	Campbell et al., 1998
10 +	9.2±2 yr	1	100	58 ±2	Marcus et al., 1998
9 +	14.2±2.6 yr	1	100	46 ±1.7	Brady et al., 1985

Note: nb: number of subjects; PNA: postnatal age; d: day; wk: week; mo: month; yr: year; method 1: rapid increase in $P_{ET}CO_2$ (maximum 3 minutes); method 2: slow increase in $P_{ET}CO_2$; during 12 minutes. %A: percentage of subjects who aroused. A: arousal; $P_{ET}CO_2$: end-tidal partial pressure in CO_2; * mean +SD; + electroencephalographic signals recorded.

Table 2. Arousal to hypercapnia in infants and children with respiratory disorders in NREM sleep

Disorder	nb	PNA	meth-od	%A	$P_{ET}CO_2$ at A mmHg	Reference
Apnea of infancy	56	6.8 ±1.1 mo	1	100	54.7 ±1.3	Van der Hal et al., 1986
Near-Miss SIDS	9	9.3 ±1.4 wk	2	91	54.9 ±2.3*	McCulloch et al., 1982
SIDS sibling	19	4.4 ±1.5 d	2	100	53.4	
	15	44 ±6.2 d	2	100	53.6	Dunne et al., 1992
	20	86 ±7.9 d	2	100	53.7	
Prenatal cigarette smoke exposure	11	10.4 ±2.8 wk	2	100	50.3 ±4.5	Lewis & Bosque, 1995
Myelomeningocele	5	15.2 ±4.8 mo	1	60	61.0 ±3.3*	Davidson-Ward et al., 1986
OSAS	15 +	8 ±2 yr	1	100	60.0 ±5*	Marcus et al., 1998
CCHS	8	5.8 ±1.2 yr	1	88	53	Marcus et al., 1991
PWS	10 +	17.7 ±2.5 yr	1	100	53 ±1*	Livingston et al., 1995

Note: SIDS: sudden infant death syndrome; OSAS: obstructive sleep apnea syndrome; CCHS: congenital central hypoventilation syndrome; PWS: Prader Willi syndrome; for other abbreviations see legend of Table 1; * significantly different from $P_{ET}CO_2$ at A in controls (see $P_{ET}CO_2$ values in Table 1).

Table 3. Arousal to hypoxia in healthy infants, children and adults in NREM sleep

nb	PNA	method	%A	Reference
10	2.7 d	1	100	Gingras et al., 1994
18	4.6 ±1.7 d	2		
17	45 ±6.2 d	2	67 °	Dunne et al., 1992
16	87 ±7.9 d	2		
18	1.5 d - 14 wk	2	33	Milerad et al., 1989
22	7.3 ±0.7 wk	2	70	McCulloch et al., 1982
34	8.7 ±1.3 wk	2	85	Lewis & Bosque, 1995
18	12.1 ±1.7 wk	1	44	Davidson-Ward et al., 1989
9	6.8 ±1.1 mo	1	100	Van der Hal et al., 1986
6	8.4 ±3.2 mo	1	89	Davidson-Ward et al., 1986
10 +	9 ±2 yr	1	26	Marcus et al., 1998
11 +	28 ±5.4 yr	1	64	Arens et al., 1996

Method 1: rapid fall in inspired fraction of O_2 from 21 to 11% (maximum: 3 minutes; method 2: exposure to an inspired fraction of O_2 equal to 15% during 15 minutes or to 17%, 15% and 13% during 5 minutes; °: mean percentage for the three groups; for other abbreviations and symbols see legend of Table 1.

Table 4. Arousal to hypoxia in infants, children and adults with respiratory disorders in NREM sleep

Disorder	nb	PNA	method	%A	Reference
Prenatal cocaine exposure	15	4.1 ±1.7 d	1	60*	Gingras et al., 1994
ALTE	21	5.5 ±2.2 wk			
			2	32 °	Milerad et al., 1989
	15	16.2 ±4.7 wk			
ALTE	32	42 – 112 d	2	22*	Dunne et al., 1992
Near-Miss SIDS	11	9.3 ±1.4 wk	2	9*	McCulloch et al., 1982
SIDS Sibling	54	4 – 103 d	2	40*	Dunne et al., 1992
Prenatal cigarette smoke exposure	13	10.7 ±2.8 wk	1	46*	Lewis & Bosque, 1995
BPD	12	48 ±1.3 wk	1	92	Garg et al., 1988
Apnea of infancy	50	8.4 ±3.2 mo	1	38*	Van der Hal et al., 1986
Myelomeningocele	5	15.2 ±4.8 mo	1	29*	Davidson-Ward et al., 1986
OSAS	15 +	8 ±2 yr	1	21	Marcus et al., 1998
PWS	13 +	23 ±3.7 yr	1	8*	Arens et al., 1996

ALTE: apparent-life-threatening event; BPD: bronchopulmonary dysplasia; * significantly different from the percentage in controls (see references in Table 3); o: mean percentage for the two groups; for other abbreviations and symbols see legend of Table 1.

Arousal response to hypercapnia

The arousal response to hypercapnia was studied during NREM sleep in most studies of infants and children, whether healthy or suffering from respiratory disorders. Three studies, two in infants (Ariagno et al., 1980; Praud et al., 1991) and one in children (Marcus et al., 1998), investigated arousal responses to hypercapnia during both NREM and REM sleep. A hypercapnic gas mixture was delivered through a plastic hood in all the studies but three, in which a face mask was used (Prand et al., 1991; Ariagno et al., 1980; Marcus et al., 1998). Methods 1 and 2 (as described above) were used to set the duration of the challenge, except in two studies (Ariagno et al., 1980; Praud et al., 1991).

Data in healthy infants and children

Hypercapnia is a potent arousal stimulus during NREM sleep. Table 1 shows data from healthy infants and children. All subjects in all age groups from the early neonatal period to adolescence aroused to hypercapnia. Mean $P_{ET}CO_2$ at arousal, a measurement of the arousal threshold, was between 46 mmHg and 51.6 mmHg in all age groups but one, a group of prepubertal children with a mean $P_{ET}CO_2$ at arousal of 58 mm Hg (Marcus et al., 1998). Interestingly, in this group, time to arousal was longer in slow-wave sleep than in stage-2 NREM sleep (36±12s and 78±39s respectively, $p< 0.05$).

Three studies looked at arousal responses during NREM and REM sleep. Ariagno et al. found no differences in arousal occurrence between these two sleep states in a small group of infants (Ariagno et al., 1980). In a study in which the occurrence of arousal was recorded at the end of a rebreathing test performed to quantify the ventilatory response to hypercapnia, Praud et al. found that arousal was significantly less common during REM than NREM sleep (Praud et al., 1991). Finally, in a group of prepubertal children, Marcus et al. found similar hypercapnic arousal thresholds during NREM and REM sleep (Marcus et al., 1998).

Data in infants, children, and young adults with respiratory disorders

Hypercapnic arousal responses have been tested in infants with apnoea of infancy (McCulloch et al., 1982), in near-miss SIDS infants (McCulloch et al., 1982; Hunt, 1981; Brady & McCann, 1985), in siblings of SIDS infants (Dunne et al., 1982), in infants whose mothers smoked during pregnancy (Lewis & Bosque, 1995), in infants and young children with myelomeningocele

(Davidson-Ward et al., 1986), in children with obstructive apnoea syndrome (OSAS) (Marcus et al., 1998) or congenital hypoventilation syndrome (CCHS) (Marcus et al., 1991), and in adolescents and young adults with Prader-Willi syndrome (PWS) (Livingston et al., 1995). Data from these studies, but two (Hunt, 1981; Brady & McCann, 1985) are reported in Table 2.

All tested patients with apnoea of infancy (although some were sedated) (McCulloch et al., 1982) and all infants with an SIDS sibling (Dunne et al., 1992) aroused to hypercapnia at a similar $P_{ET}CO_2$ as the controls (Table 1). One of the tested near-miss infants failed to arouse to hypercapnia, and $P_{ET}CO_2$ at arousal in the other near-miss infants was significantly higher than in the controls (Table 1). Five infants with myelomeningocele and Arnold-Chiari malformation who had central hypoventilation and/or apnoea were tested (Davidson-Ward et al., 1986). Two of the five infants failed to arouse to hypercapnia. Because they had hypoventilation at baseline, the three remaining infants had significantly higher $P_{ET}CO_2$ levels at arousal than the controls (Table 1).

In a group of eight children with CCHS, Marcus et al. studied arousal during sleep while normal ventilation was maintained using a home ventilator (Marcus et al., 1991). Although hypercapnia caused arousal in seven of these eight children, the $P_{ET}CO_2$ change needed to produce arousal (21±3 mmHg) was larger than in the controls (12±2 mmHg) because the baseline $P_{ET}CO_2$ was lower (32±3 mmHg vs. 39±1 mmHg, respectively, $p < 0.05$). CCHS is known to be associated with absence of ventilatory responses to chemical stimuli (Gozal, 1998). This implies that arousal to hypercapnia in CCHS patients results from a direct effect of CO_2 on the central nervous system areas involved in arousal. Nevertheless, it remains unclear why these mechanically ventilated CCHS patients exhibited an arousal response to induced hypercapnia during sleep, whereas in other studies CCHS patients had no arousals during spontaneous breathing despite severe hypercapnia and hypoxia (Gaultier et al., 1997).

A group of 15 prepubertal children with OSAS was tested during nighttime sleep. All 15 children aroused to hypercapnia during NREM and REM sleep, but at higher $P_{ET}CO_2$ levels than the controls (Marcus et al., 1998). Furthermore, arousal thresholds to hypercapnia were highest in the patients with the highest apnoea index values ($p < 0.05$) (Marcus et al., 1998). Interestingly, after treatment of the OSAS, $P_{ET}CO_2$ at arousal decreased to the range seen in control children (Table 1) (Marcus et al., 1998).

Adolescents with PWS showed arousal to hypercapnia, but at higher $P_{ET}CO_2$ levels than controls (Livingston et al., 1995), a finding that has been attributed to the deficient peripheral chemoreceptor function reported in PWS patients (Gozal et al., 1994).

In summary, given that 100% of healthy infants and children show arousal to a hypercapnic challenge involving slow or rapid $P_{ET}CO_2$ elevation to 60 mmHg, the absence of arousal to hypercapnia can be considered abnormal. Although the numbers of tested patients were small, the brainstem lesions associated with myelomeningocele and Arnold-Chiari malformation seem to increase the risk of failure to arouse to hypercapnia. The usefulness of determining the hypercapnic arousal threshold has been shown in patients with PWS (Livingston et al., 1995), as well as in patients with OSAS (Marcus et al., 1998) before and after specific treatment.

Arousal response to hypoxia

Again, the arousal response to hypoxia was investigated during NREM sleep in most studies in infants and children who were healthy or had respiratory disorders. Two studies, one in infants (Ariagno et al., 1980) and one in children (Marcus et al., 1998), evaluated hypoxic arousal responses during both NREM and REM sleep. A hypoxic mixture was delivered through a plastic hood in all the studies but one (Marcus et al., 1998). In none of the studies was isocapnia maintained during the hypoxic challenge. Methods 1 or 2 (as described above) were used to set the duration of the hypoxic challenge, except in one study (Ariagno et al., 1980), which is not included in Table 3.

Data in healthy infants and children

As shown in Table 3, hypoxia is a less potent arousal stimulus than hypercapnia. In all the studies but two (Van der Hal et al., 1986; Gingras et al., 1994), some healthy subjects failed to arouse to hypoxia. Two studies conducted during the first days of life showed that 67% and 100% of the newborns aroused to hypoxia (Dunne et al., 1992; Gingras et al., 1994). Two early studies suggest that the arousal response may weaken transiently from two to four months of age, which is the period of peak SIDS occurrence (Milerad et al., 1989; Davidson-Ward et al., 1992). Davidson-Ward et al. (1992) tested 18 infants aged 4 to 28 weeks and found that infants younger than nine weeks were more likely to arouse to hypoxia than older infants, although the difference was not statistically significant. Milerad et al. (1989) reported that healthy infants younger than 10 weeks of age were more likely to arouse than older infants, but their report does not specify the level of statistical significance. In contrast to these two early studies, a recent study found no difference across percentages of infants with arousal in three groups tested one week, six weeks, and 13 weeks after birth (Dunne et al., 1992). Hypoxic arousal occurred on average in 67% of the infants in the three groups. Therefore, to date, there are no statistically significant data supporting a weakening of the arousal response to hypoxia during the period of peak SIDS occurrence. Furthermore, Table 3 shows that the percentage of infants with arousal in the seven- to 12-week age range varied widely among studies, from 44% (Davidson-Ward et al., 1992) to 85% (Lewis & Bosque, 1995). The lower percentage was obtained using method 1 (Davidson-Ward et al., 1992) and the two higher percentages using method 2 for the hypoxic challenge (McCulloch et al., 1982; Lewis & Bosque, 1995). Thus, a stepwise decrease in arterial partial pressure of O_2 may be a more potent arousal stimulus than a rapid decrease. Two studies in older infants with a mean age of 6.8 and 8.4 months respectively found hypoxic arousal in 89% and 100% of the infants, respectively (Davidson-Ward et al., 1986; Van der Hal, 1986).

In a group of 15 pubertal children, only 26% of the subjects aroused to hypoxia (Marcus et al., 1998), as compared to 64% of a group of young adults (Arens et al., 1996).

Data in infants, children, and young adults with respiratory disorders

Hypoxic arousal responses during NREM sleep have been tested in newborns exposed prenatally to cocaine (Gingras et al., 1994) and in infants born to mothers who smoked during pregnancy (Lewis & Bosque, 1995); in infants with apparently life-threatening events (ALTEs) (Dunne et al., 1992; Milerad et al., 1989), near-miss SIDS (McCulloch et al., 1982), or in SIDS sibling (Dunne et al., 1992), in infants with apnoea of infancy (Van der Hal et al., 1986), myelomeningocele (Davidson-Ward et al., 1986), or bronchopulmonary dysplasia (Garg et al., 1988); in children with OSAS (Marcus et al., 1998); and in young adults with PWS (Arens et al., 1996) (Table 4).

Gingras et al. found that only 60% of neonates exposed prenatally to cocaine aroused to hypoxia versus 100% of unexposed neonates (see Table 3) (Gingras et al., 1994), suggesting that prenatal exposure to cocaine may be a risk factor for failed hypoxic arousal. However, the percentage of newborns with prenatal cocaine exposure who aroused to hypoxia (60%) was close to the percentage of unexposed newborns who aroused to hypoxia in another study (Dunne et al., 1992) (Tables 3 and 4).

Lewis & Bosque (1995) studied infants born to mothers who smoked during pregnancy. Mean age of the infants at the time of the study was 10.7±2.8 weeks. Forty-six percent aroused to hypoxia as compared to 70% of the control infants. This finding indicating that prenatal exposure to nicotine may predispose to deficient hypoxic arousal is in keeping with a study in lambs (Hafstrom et al., 2000). However, again, the percentage of infants with arousal to hypoxia in this population exposed prenatally to nicotine (46%) was close to the percentage found in unexposed infants of similar age range in another study (44%) (Davidson-Ward et al., 1992) (Table 3 and 4).

Hypoxic arousal responses have been studied in two groups of infants with ALTEs (Dunne et al., 1992; Milerad et al., 1989). In both studies, the percentage of infants who aroused to hypoxia was significantly lower than in the ALTE than the control group. In a group of near-miss SIDS infants, only 9% aroused to hypoxia (McCulloch et al., 1982). Similarly, a significantly smaller percentage of siblings of SIDS patients aroused to hypoxia, as compared to a control group (Dunne et al., 1992). Thus, some patients with ALTE, near-miss SIDS, or a sibling with SIDS seem to have deficient arousal to hypoxia. However, the predictive value of absence of hypoxic arousal is not high enough to enable detection of individual infants at risk for SIDS.

Arousal to hypoxia has been tested in five infants with myelomeningocele and Arnold-Chiari malformation who had hypoventilation and/or apnoea (Davidson-Ward et al., 1986). Only two aroused to hypoxia, suggesting that brainstem lesions may impair hypoxic as well as hypercapnic arousal responses (Davidson-Ward et al., 1986).

Garg et al. examined hypoxic arousal responses in 12 infants with bronchopulmonary dysplasia (BPD) at 41.4±1.3 weeks postconceptional age (Garg et al., 1988). Eleven (92%) aroused to hypoxia. However, all these infants required vigorous stimulation and supplemental oxygen after the arousal response, eight experienced prolonged apnoea with bradycardia, and four required brief ventilatory assistance to restore normal breathing. Thus, these BPD infants were unable to protect themselves from the hypoxic challenge. This may be ascribable, at least in part, to the blunted peripheral chemoreceptor response previously reported in infants with BPD (Katz-Salomon et al., 1995).

In a large group of older infants (mean age, 8.4±3.2 months) with apnoea of infancy (Van der Hal et al., 1986), hypoxic arousal occurred in only 38% of the patients, as compared to 100% in the controls. However, 40% of the patients were sedated to facilitate sleep, and this may have depressed the hypoxic arousal response in some cases.

Marcus et al. examined hypoxic arousal responses in a group of children with OSAS (Marcus et al., 1998). The percentage of children who aroused to hypoxia was not significantly different in the OSAS group and in the control group (21% and 26%, respectively); neither was any significant within-group difference found between NREM and REM sleep.

In a study of young adults with PWS, all but one patient failed to arouse to hypoxia (Arens et al., 1996). Furthermore, during hypoxia, heart rate increased by only 9±2% in the PWS group as compared to 22±4% in the control group ($p < 0.005$). These findings suggest that abnormal arousal and heart rate responses to hypoxia may be common in PWS patients. Failure of hypoxic arousal mechanisms may be related to absent peripheral chemoreceptor function in PWS patients (Gozal et al., 1994).

In summary, not all healthy subjects from the early neonatal period to adulthood aroused to hypoxia. Therefore, the absence of hypoxic arousal in an individual subject cannot be considered abnormal per se. Furthermore, more data is needed so that we can determine proportions of normal subjects with hypoxic arousal from infancy to adulthood, as has been done for the arousal response to auditory stimuli (Busby et al., 1994). Nevertheless, comparisons of proportions of healthy or ill infants and children with arousal responses suggest that some respiratory disorders and some prenatal environmental factors may predispose to deficient hypoxic arousal.

Arousal responses to asphyxia

Asphyxia (hypoxia and hypercapnia) occurs spontaneously at the end of obstructive events during sleep, whereas isolated hypercapnia probably does not occur naturally. Three recent studies, two in infants and one in children, examined arousal responses to induced asphyxia (Marcus et al., 1998; Campbell et al., 1998; Galland et al., 2000).

Campbell et al. examined the arousal response to mild asphyxia during NREM and REM sleep in 29 infants during the neonatal period and at three and six months of age (Campbell et al., 1998). Most of the infants were tested longitudinally. A gas delivery hood was used to slowly change inspired gas to a maximum stimulus of 5% CO_2 and 13% O_2 in nitrogen. Duration of the test was up to 5 min. Arousal occurred more frequently in REM than in NREM sleep ($p < 0.005$) and in the neonatal period than at six months ($p < 0.005$). Galland et al. used a similar challenge in infants during the neonatal period and at three months of age (Galland et al., 2000). In contrast to Campbell et al. (1998), they found that arousal to asphyxia was more likely to occur at three months than in the neonatal period ($p < 0.01$). However, in agreement with Campbell et al., they found that arousal was more common during REM than NREM sleep ($p < 0.001$) (Campbell et al., 1998; Galland et al., 2000). Furthermore, they found that placing the infants prone as opposed to supine significantly increased the likelihood of arousal ($p < 0.04$).

Marcus et al. studied the arousal response to asphyxia in prepubertal children with and without OSAS (Marcus et al., 1998). Nitrogen and CO_2 were delivered until pulse oximeter saturation fell to 75% and $P_{ET}CO_2$ reached 65 mmHg for a maximum of three minutes. In the control children, arousals occurred faster and at a lower $P_{ET}CO_2$ than with hypercapnia alone (53±5 mmHg and 58±2 mmHg, respectively, $p < 0.005$). Children with OSAS showed a similar trend, which did not reach statistical significance. Therefore, as expected, the arousal threshold was lower for hypercapnia combined with hypoxia than for hypercapnia alone. No difference was observed between NREM and REM sleep.

Factors depressing the arousal responses to chemical stimuli

Several factors have been shown to depress arousal responses to chemical stimuli in humans or animals. As noted above, prenatal exposure to cocaine (Gingras et al., 1994) and to nicotine or other components of tobacco (Lewis & Bosque, 1995) may lead to a deficient hypoxic arousal response after birth. Sedatives, such as promethazine and diazepam, have been shown to depress arousal responses to airflow obstruction in sleeping lambs, leading to severe hypoxia (Jakubowska et al., 1996). Therefore, arousal responses should be tested during natural sleep. Sleep deprivation has been reported to depress arousal responses in adult humans with OSAS (Guilleminault, 1980) and in adult dogs (Phillipson et al., 1980). However, brief sleep deprivation had only a slight effect on arousal in lambs (Fewell, 1987). Furthermore, a short period of evening sleep deprivation in 3-month-old infants did not induce detectable alterations in spontaneous arousals or in arousals produced by auditory stimuli (Thomas et al., 1996). Sleeping in the prone position as compared to the supine position has been shown to decrease the number of spontaneous arousals in infants (Kahn et al., 1993) and of arousals produced by auditory stimuli (Franco et al., 1996). However, as noted above, Galland et al. reported that arousal to asphyxia was more common in infants sleeping prone than supine (Galland et al., 2000).

Repetition of a stimulus, such as airflow obstruction, has been shown to depress arousal responses in lambs (Harding et al., 1997). Repetitive mild hypoxia rapidly depressed arousal during REM but not NREM sleep in lambs (Johnston et al., 1998). These findings suggest that hypoxic arousal mechanisms may be particularly vulnerable to failure during REM sleep. No similar studies have been performed in infants. However, it has recently been shown that habituation of the infant arousal response to tactile stimuli occurred more rapidly during REM than NREM sleep (McNamara et al., 1999). Although habituation may be appropriate if the stimulus is harmless, it may be deleterious, or even life-threatening, if the stimulus is hypoxia and/or hypercapnia, particularly during REM sleep, which is the predominant sleep state in young infants.

Interactions between ventilatory and arousal responses to chemical stimuli

If respiratory mechanoreceptors play a major role in arousal responses to chemical stimuli, then arousal responses should be depressed in subjects without ventilatory responses. In contrast, if chemical stimuli act on arousal areas, either directly or indirectly via the chemoreceptors, then arousal responses would be expected to occur in the absence of ventilatory responses. Data in human patients have varied across disorders. In two disorders, PWS and myelomeningocele, both arousal responses to chemical stimuli and ventilatory responses were depressed (Davidson-Ward et al., 1986; Gozal et al., 1994; Livingston, et al., 1995; Swaminatan et al., 1989). In contrast, arousal to hypercapnia has been shown in a group patients with CCHS (Marcus et al., 1991), a condition in which lack of a ventilatory response to hypercapnia is a major characteristic (Gozal, 1998). Thus, arousal to hypercapnia may occur in the absence of a hypercapnic ventilatory response. Further investigations in patients should explore both ventilatory and arousal responses to chemical stimuli in order to improve our understanding of the interactions between ventilatory and arousal responses to chemical stimuli at various developmental stages and during various sleep stages.

In summary

Available data on arousal responses to chemical stimuli suggest the following considerations and recommendations for further clinical research investigations in infants and children:

- neither the mechanisms underlying arousal responses to chemical stimuli nor the impact of developmental processes on arousal responses is fully understood;
- criteria for arousal in infants and children need to be standardized;
- arousal responses to induced hypoxic, hypercapnic, or asphyxic challenges should be tested using standardized methods;
- care should be taken to avoid potential confounding by factors reported to depress arousal responses;
- multicenter studies using standardized methods should be performed in healthy infants and children to determine whether responses to hypoxia and/or asphyxia vary with the developmental stage;
- investigations in patients should include evaluations of both the ventilatory and the arousal responses to chemical stimuli, including not only respiratory variables but also variables reflecting sympathetic activation;
- arousal responses to chemical stimuli should be studied in both NREM and REM sleep.

References

American Sleep Disorders Association (1992). EEG arousals: scoring rules and examples: a preliminary report from the sleep disorders atlas task force of the American Sleep Disorders Association. *Sleep, 15*: 174–184.

Arens, Raanan, David Gozal, Brian C. Burrell, Sandra L. Bailey, Daisy B. Bautista, Thomas G. Keens & Sally L. Davidson-Ward (1996). Arousal and cardiorespiratory responses to hypoxia in Prader-Willi syndrome. *American Journal of Respiratory and Critical Care Medicine, 153*: 283–287.

Ariagno, Ronald, Lynn Nagel & Christian Guilleminault (1980). Waking and ventilatory responses during sleep in infants near-miss for sudden infant death syndrome. *Sleep, 3*: 351–359.

Ayas, Najib T., Robert Brown & Steven A. Shea (2000). Hypercapnia can induce arousal from sleep in the absence of altered respiratory mechanoreception. *American Journal of Respiration and Critical Care Medicine, 162*: 1001–1008.

Bernard, D.G., A. Li & Eugene E. Nattie (1996). Evidence for central chemoreception in the middle raphe. *Journal of Applied Physiolology, 80*: 108–115.

Berry, Richard B., & Kevin Gleeson (1997). Respiratory arousal from sleep: mechanisms and significance. *Sleep, 20*: 654–675.

Bowes, G., E.R. Towsend, Louise F. Kozar, S.M. Bromley & Eliot A. Phillipson (1981). Effect of carotid body denervation on arousal response to hypoxia in sleeping dogs. *Journal of Applied Physiology, 51*: 40–45.

Brady, June P., & Ellen M. McCann (1985). Control of ventilation in subsequent siblings of victims of sudden infant death syndrome. *Journal of Pediatrics, 106*: 212–217.

Busby, Keith A., Lise Mercier & R.T. Pivik (1994). Ontogenetic variations in auditory arousal threshold during sleep. *Psychophysiology, 31*: 182–188.

Campbell, A.J., D.P.G. Bolton, B.J. Taylor & R.M. Sayer (1998). Responses to an increasing asphyxia in infants: effects of age and sleep state. *Respiratory Physiology, 112*: 51–58.

Dauger, Stéphane, Sophie Aisenfisz, Estelle Durand, Sylvain Renolleau, Guy Vardon, Claude Gaultier & Jorge Gallego (2001). Arousal response to hypoxia in newborn mice. *Respiratory Physiology, 128*: 235–240.

Davidson-Ward, Sally L., Bruce G. Nickerson, Andre Van der Hal, Antonio M. Rodriguez, Robert A. Jacobs, and Thomas G. Keens (1986). Absent hypoxic and hypercapneic arousal responses in children with myelomeningocele and apnea. *Pediatrics, 78*: 44–50.

Davidson-Ward, Sally L., Daisy B. Bautista & Thomas G. Keens (1992). Hypoxic arousal responses in normal infants. *Pediatrics, 89*: 860–864.

Dunne, K.P., G.P. Fox, M. O' Regan & T.G. Matthews (1992). Arousal responses in babies at risk of sudden infant death syndrome at different postnatal ages. *Irish Medicine Journal, 85*: 19–22.

Fewell, James E. (1987). The effect of short-term sleep fragmentation produced by intense auditory stimuli on the arousal response to upper airway obstruction in lambs. *Journal of Developmental Physiology, 9*: 409–417.

Fewell, James E., & Susan B. Baker (1987). Arousal from sleep during rapidly developing hypoxemia in lambs. *Pediatric Research, 22*: 471–477.

Fewell, James E., Colleen S. Kondo, Victor Dascalu & Sonya Filyk (1989). Influence of carotid denervation on the arousal and cardiopulmonary response to rapidly developing hypoxemia in lambs. *Pediatric Research, 25*: 473–477.

Franco, Patricia, Jose Groswasser, Martine Sottiaux, Ema Broadfield & André Kahn (1996). Decreased cardiac responses to auditory stimulation during prone sleep. *Pediatrics, 97*: 174–178.

Galland, B.C., D.P.G. Bolton, B.J. Taylor, R.M. Sayers & S.M. Williams (2000). Ventilatory sensitivity to mild asphyxia: prone versus supine sleep position. *Archives of Disease in Childhood, 83*: 423–428.

Garg, Meena, Sharon I. Kurzner, Daisy B. Bautista & Thomas G. Keens (1988). Hypoxic arousal responses in infants with bronchopulmonary dysplasia. *Pediatrics, 82*: 59–63.

Gaultier, Claude, Ha Trang-Pham, Jean-Paul Praud & Jorge Gallego (1997). Cardiorespiratory control during sleep in the congenital central hypoventilation syndrome. *Pediatric Pulmonology, 23*: 140–142.

Gingras, Jeannine L., Andre Muelenaer, Linda B. Dalley & Karen J. O'Donnell (1994). Prenatal cocaine exposure alters postnatal hypoxic arousal responses and hypercarbic ventilatory responses but not pneumocardiograms in prenatally cocaine-exposed term infants. *Pediatric Pulmonology, 18*: 13–20.

Gleeson, Kevin, Clifford W. Zwillich & David P. White (1990). The influence of increasing ventilatory effort on arousal from sleep. *American Revew of Respiratory Disorders, 142*: 295–300.

Gozal, David (1998). Congenital central hypoventilation syndrome: an update. *Pediatric Pulmonology, 26*: 273–282.

Gozal, David, Raanan Arens, Kenneth J. Omlin, Sally L. Davidson-Ward & Thomas G. Keens (1994). Absent peripheral chemosensitivity in Prader-Willi syndrome. *Journal of Applied Physiology, 77*: 2231–2236.

Guilleminault, Christian (1980). Sleep apnea syndromes: impact of sleep and sleep states. *Sleep, 3*: 227–234.

Hafstrom, Ola, Joseph Millerad, Natarajan Asokan, Stanley D. Poole & Hakan W. Sundell (2000). Nicotine delays arousal during hypoxemia in lambs. *Pediatric Research, 47*: 646–652.

Harding, Richard, Alexandra E. Jakubowska & Graeme J. McCrabb (1997). Arousal and cardiorespiratory responses to airflow obstruction in sleeping lambs: effects of sleep state, age, and repeated obstruction. *Sleep, 20*: 693--701.

Hunt, Carl E. (1981). Abnormal, hypercarbic and hypoxic sleep arousal responses in near-miss SIDS infants. *Pediatric Research, 15*: 1462–1464.

Jakubowska, Alexandra E., Graeme J. McCrabb and Richard Harding (1996). Influence of sedation on arousal and cardiorespiratory responses to airflow obstruction in sleeping lambs. *Pediatric Research, 40*: 564–570.

Johnston, Renea V., Daniel A. Grant, Malcolm H. Wilkinson & Adrian M. Walker (1998). Repetitive hypoxia rapidly depresses arousal from active sleep in newborn lambs. *Journal of Physiology, 2*: 651–659.

Kahn, André, José Grosswasser, Martine Sottiaux, Patricia Franco & M. Drantals (1993). Prone and supine body position and sleep characteristics in infants. *Pediatrics, 91*: 112–115.

Katz-Salamon, Myriam, B. Jonsson & Hugo Lagercrantz (1995). Blunted peripheral chemoreceptor response to hypoxia in a group of infants with bronchopulmonary dysplasia. *Pediatric Pulmonology, 20*: 101–106.

Lewis, Kathleen W., & Elena M. Bosque (1995). Deficient hypoxia awakening response in infants of smoking mothers: possible relationship to sudden infant death syndrome. *Journal of Pediatrics, 127*: 691–699.

Lijowska, Anna S., N. Reed, B.A. Mertins-Chiodini & Bradley T. Thach (1997). Sequential arousal and airway defensive behavior of infants in asphyxic sleep environments. *Journal of Applied Physiolology, 83*: 219–228.

Livingston, Floyd R., Raanan Arens, Sandra L. Bailey, Thomas G. Keens & Sally L. Davidson-Ward (1995). Hypercapnic Arousal responses in Prader-Willi syndrome. *Chest, 108*: 1627–1631.

Marcus, Carole L., Daisy B. Bautista, Amma Amihyia, Sally L. Davidson-Ward and Thomas G. Keens (1991). Hypercapneic arousal responses in children with congenital central hypoventilation syndrome. *Pediatrics, 88*: 993–998.

Marcus, Carole L., Janita Lutz, John L. Carroll & Owen Bamford (1998). Arousal and ventilatory responses during sleep in children with obstructive sleep apnea. *Journal of Applied Physiolology, 84*: 1926–1936.

McCulloch, Kristine, Robert T. Brouillette, Anthony J. Guzetta & Carl E. Hunt (1982). Arousal responses in near-miss sudden infant death syndrome and in normal infants. *Journal of Pediatrics, 101*: 911–917.

McNamara, Frances., Faiq G. Issa & Colin E. Sullivan (1996). Arousal pattern following central and obstructive breathing abnormalities in infants and children. *Journal of Applied Physiolology, 81*: 2651–2657.

McNamara, Frances, Henning Wulbrand & Bradley T. Thach (1999). Habituation of the infant arousal response. *Sleep, 22*: 320–326.

Milerad, J., T. Hertzberg, G. Wennergen & Hugo Lagercrantz (1989). Respiratory and arousal responses to hypoxia in apnoeic infants reinvestigated. *European Journal of Pediatrics, 148*: 565–570.

Mograss, M.A., F.M. Ducharme & Robert T. Brouillette (1994). Movement/Arousals, Description, classification, and relationship to sleep apnea in children. *American Journal of Respiratory and Critical Care Medicine, 150*: 1690–1696.

Neubauer, Judith A., Teodoro V. Santiago & Norman H. Edelman (1981). Hypoxic arousal in intact and carotid chemodenervated sleeping cats. *Journal of Applied Physiology, 51*: 1294–1299.

Phillipson, Eliot A., & Colin E. Sullivan (1978). Arousal: the forgotten response to respiratory stimuli. *American Revew of Respiratory Disorders, 118*: 807–808.

Phillipson, Eliot A., Colin E. Sullivan, David J.C Read, E. Murphy & Louise F. Kozar (1978). Ventilatory and waking responses to hypoxia in sleeping dogs. *Journal of Applied Physiolology, 44*: 512–520.

Phillipson, Eliot A., G. Bowes, Colin E. Sullivan & G.M. Woolf (1980). The influence of sleep fragmentation on arousal and ventilatory responses to respiratory stimuli. *Sleep, 3*: 281–288.

Pineda, J., & G.A. Aghajanian (1997). Carbon dioxide regulates the tonic activity of locus coeruleus neurons by modulating a proton and polyamine sensitive inward rectifier potassium current. *Neuroscience, 77*: 723–743.

Pitson, D.J., & John R. Stradling (1998). Autonomic markers of arousal during sleep in patients undergoing investigation for obstructive sleep apnoea, their relationship to EEG arousals, respiratory events and subjective sleepiness. *Journal of Sleep Research, 7*: 53–59.

Praud, Jean-Paul, Laurent Egreteau, Malik Benlabed, Lilia Curzi-Dascalova, Hélène Nedelcoux & Claude Gaultier (1991). Abdominal muscle activity during CO2 rebreathing in sleeping neonates. *Journal of Applied Physiolology, 70*: 1344–1350.

Swaminatan, Soumya, James Y. Paton, Sally L. Davidson-Ward, Robert A. Jacobs, Charles W. Sargent & Thomas G. Keens (1989). Abnormal control of ventilation in adolescents with myelodysplasia. *Journal of Pediatrics, 115*: 898–903.

Thomas, D.A., K. Poole, E.K. Mc Ardle, P.C. Goodenough, J. Thompson, Caroline S. Beardsmore & H. Simpson (1996). The effect of sleep deprivation on sleep states, breathing events, peripheral chemoresponsiveness and arousal propensity in healthy 3 month old infants. *European Respiratory Journal, 9*: 932–938.

Van der Hal, Andre L., Antonio M. Rodriguez, Charles W. Sargent, Arnold C.G. Platzker & Thomas G. Keens (1986). Hypoxic and hypercapneic arousal responses and prediction of subsequent apnea in apnea of infancy. *Pediatrics, 75*: 848–854.

Yasuma, Fumihiko, Louise F. Kozar, R. John Kilmoff, Bradley T. Douglas & Eliot A Philippson (1991). Interaction of chemical and mechanical respiratory stimuli in the arousal response to hypoxia in sleeping dogs. *American Revew of Respiratory Disorders*, *143*: 1274–1277.

The scoring of arousals in infants

A report on the ongoing work of the pediatric "Wake-up Club"

J. Groswasser, Patricia Franco, T. Simon, Sonia Scaillet, Filomena Valente, Alain De Broca, and A. Kahn

Pediatric Sleep Unit, Erasmus Hospital / Pediatric Sleep Unit, University Children's Hospital / Department of Biostatistics, School of Public Health, Free University of Brussels/CHU d'Amiens, Hôpital Nord

1. Introduction

Infants' arousability from sleep has direct implications in various clinical conditions. An excessive propensity to arouse is found in infants suffering from insomnia and sleep disruptions (Guilleminault & Souquet, 1979). An insufficient propensity to arouse could lower the chance to survive in infants exposed to noxious conditions during sleep, possibly increasing the risk for infant death sudden. However, there is yet no uniform definition of arousals in infants, leading to severe methodological limitations when comparing the research reports from various sleep laboratories. In the young infant, the well-known spontaneous variability in respiration, body movements and heart rate significantly complicate the evaluation of arousals. It was felt that a consensus on the scoring of arousals in infants was needed. When methodological issues are resolved, researchers on arousal characteristics in infants will be able to share information in various clinical contexts.

Scientific debate within the Wake Up Club, an international scientific work force for the definition of arousals from sleep in infants, concerns a number of controversial points such as:

1. The definition of "arousal" and its classification.

2. The major variables needed for the scoring of arousal reactions in infants.
3. The common protocol for sleep-wake recordings, necessary to collect comparable data from all laboratories.

The present paper reports on the first experimental findings, adopting temptative criteria for the scoring of arousals in infants, with regard to spontaneous arousals and arousals induced by noise challenges. Hopefully, these data will turn out to be crucial for validation of the consensus criteria, when eventually they will have been produced by the Wake Up Club task force.

2. The analysis of spontaneously occurring arousals in infants

Patients and methods

All data were collected from healthy infants born at term.

Recordings of spontaneously occurring arousals were obtained from various sleep sessions recorded in various sleep research laboratories (Table 1).

All infants slept in their usual position, without restraint. Recording started around 21.00 h. The infants were observed continuously during recording. They were fed on demand. Their behaviour and any nursing intervention were charted. The following variables were recorded simultaneously: 2 scalp electroencephalograms with central and occipital leads (C4/02 and C3/01); 2 electrooculograms, electrocardiogram. Thoracic and abdominal respiratory movements were detected by piezo electric belts and airflow with a thermistor taped under both nostrils and over the upper lip. Gross body movements were detected using an actigram placed on one arm and/or on artefacts on the oxygen saturometer placed on the opposite lower limb.

Table 1.

Nr arousals	53
Nr infants	9
Gender M/F	4/5
Gestational age (weeks)	40 (36–40)*
Age (months)	5 (1–11)*
Body position	supine: 37
	prone: 1
	unknown: 15 (in 1 infant)

* median (range) values.

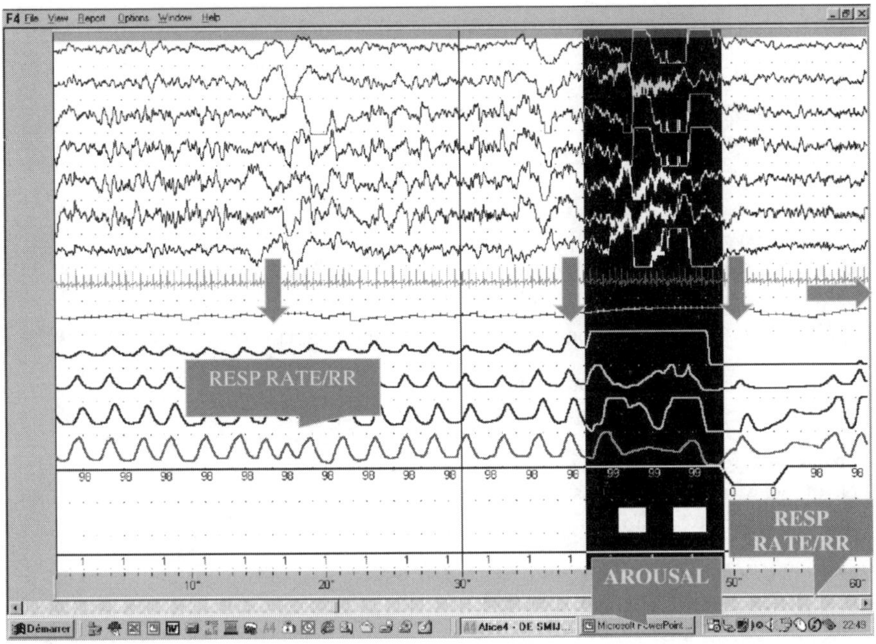

Figure 1. Spontaneous non-system related arousal.

For the calculation of changes in EEG, ECG and respiration characteristics, a 20-second reference period was used preceding either the arousal or the event that provoked the arousal (i.e. central apnea, obstructive apnea). This period was compared with the period of the arousal and the 20-second period directly following the termination of the arousal. To avoid the smoothing effect of the duration of the period on the calculation of heart rate, the changes in heart rate were evaluated on RR intervals.

Following the methodology defined by the previous consensus meetings of the Pediatric Wake Up Club, an "ad hoc" canvas was used for data collection (Table 2).

Arousals were classified as "system related" if preceded by a respiratory event visible on the recording, and "non system related" if no event could be seen on the recording during the period directly preceding the arousal. Figure 1 shows a "non system related" arousal.

Figure 2 represents an arousal that occurred following a mixed apnea.

Statistical analysis was performed with the SPSS software. For comparison between periods, Wilcoxon Rank test was performed; Mann Whitney was per-

Table 2.

N° of recording in the series
INITIALS OF PATIENT
BIRTH-WEIGHT
GESTATIONAL AGE
LEGAL AGE
GENDER
LOCATION OF STUDY (home, laboratory, intensive care unit, ward...)
REASON FOR WHICH POLYSOMNOGRAPHY WAS PERFORMED:
exclude NEUROLOGICAL & CARDIAC PATHOLOGY
smoking, illicit drugs, alcohol, medication... During pregnancy

currently taken or taken before by patient
describe. The purpose is to know if patient is sleep-deprived

breast milk, formula...
N° of recording in your series of recording
time of extract used room temperature

according to age group: <6 months QS/AS/IS/WAKE
time the patient has been in this sleep stage
NO, CA, OA, MA, bradycardia... if external, describe + sequence. Chose recording in 30-seconds free of any other event periods of the event
DELAY BETWEEN THE START OF THE EVENT AND THE START OF THE AROUSAL
DELAY BETWEEN THE END OF THE EVENT AND THE START OF THE AROUSAL
DESCRIBE: open, move ...
DESCRIBE any modification. THE PREFERRED MONTAGE IS FRONTO-CENTRAL BIPOLAR & CENTRO-OCCIPITAL REFERENTIAL
DESCRIBE any modification and location of EMG
N° of recording in the series
MODIFICATION OF HEART RATE CALCULATED BEAT TO BEAT
DESCRIBE ANY MODIFICATION OF AMPLITUDE OR FREQUENCY, POSITION OF CAPTORS, TYPE OF CAPTORS
DESCRIBE ANY MODIFICATION AND TECHNIQUE USED TO MEASURE (SaO_2, $TcPO_2$)
DESCRIBE ANY MODIFICATION AND TECHNIQUE USED TO MEASURE (end tidal, $TcPCO_2$)
any change in oesophageal pH
DESCRIBE TECHNIQUE USED TO MEASURE MOBILITY and TYPE OF MOVEMENT (limbs, face, whole body...)
DESCRIBE TECHNIQUE USED and BEHAVIOUR OF PATIENT
DESCRIBE TECHNIQUE USED and ANY NOISE (cry, snoring...)
ANY MODIFICATION OF SLEEP STAGE FOLLOWING THE AROUSAL
THE DURATION OF THE AROUSAL DESCRIBED
N° of recording in the series

HOW WOULD YOU CLASSIFY THE AROUSAL?

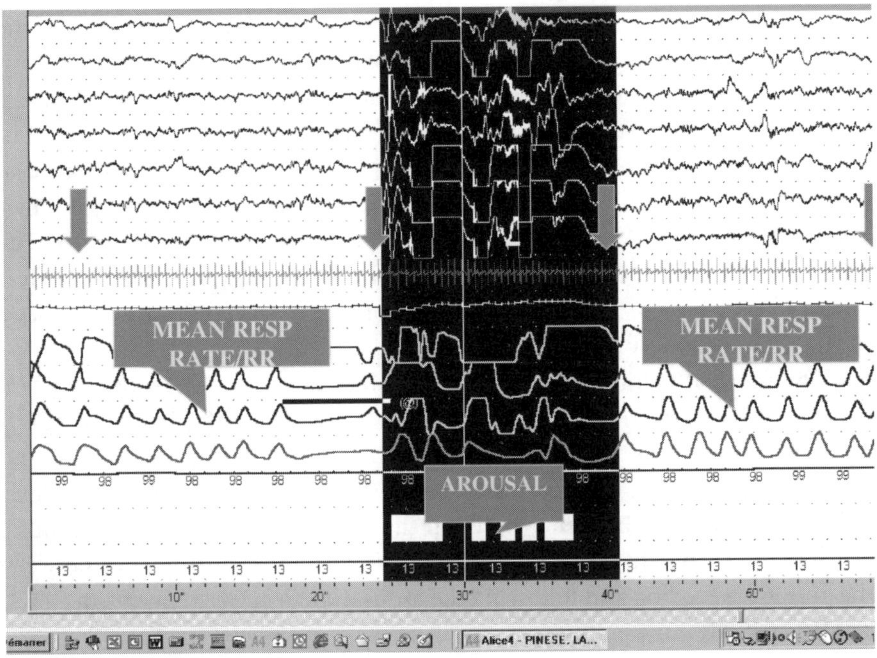

Figure 2. System-related (mixed apnea) spontaneous behavioural arousal.

formed when comparing arousals in different sleep stage or system and non system related arousals.

Main findings

Of all arousals, 36 occurred in active sleep, 16 in quiet sleep and 1 in indeterminate sleep. The median duration of the sleep stage preceding the arousal was 20 minutes (range 3 to 39 minutes). Of the 36 arousals, 9 accompanied sleep stage changes.

Of the 53 arousals, 30 were not preceded by any visible event, while 23 were preceded by an event: a central apnea in 7 cases (2 with bradycardia); an obstructive apnea in 7 cases (4 with bradycardia); a mixed apnea in 5 cases (1 with bradycardia) and 4 by movements.

The median duration of the arousals was 13.5 seconds (range from 4 to 70 seconds). For the arousals preceded by an event, the median delay from the start of the event to the start of the arousal was 5 seconds (range from 0 to

15.5 seconds), and the mean delay from the end of the event to the start of the arousal was 0 sec (range from 0 sec to 10 seconds).

The respiratory rate during the 20 seconds preceding the arousal or the event which preceded the arousal, was 31 breaths per minute (range from 21 to 62bpm). It increased to 35 bpm (range from 16 to 60 bpm) during the arousal (calculated on 13 arousals). The respiratory rate during the 20 seconds following the arousal was 28 breaths per minute (range from 17 to 51 bpm). The difference in respiratory rate between the period preceding and the period following was –3 breaths per minute (range from +9 to –14 bpm) or –9% (range from +36 to –49%) ($p = 0.003$).

The mean RR during the 20 seconds preceding the arousal or the event which preceded the arousal, was 500 msec. (range from 390 to 600 msec). It decreased to 450 msec (range from 340 to 595 msec) during the arousal and increased to 530 msec (range from 375 to 670 msec) during the period following the arousal. The difference between the period preceding and the arousal was –13.6% (range from –31 to +17%) ($p < 0.001$). The difference between the periods preceding and following the arousal was +4.8% (range from –11 to +31%) ($p < 0.001$).

The longest RR interval during the arousal was 650 msec. (range from 445 to 985 msec); compared to the mean RR interval in the period preceding the arousal, it showed an increase of +32% (range from –3 to +51%) ($p < 0.001$). The shortest RR interval during the arousal was 410 msec (range from 300 to 510 mesec); compared to the mean RR interval in the period preceding the arousal, it was decreased by –24% (range from –43 to +6%) ($p < 0.001$).

Eye movements or artefacts were detected in 39 arousals, no eye movement was noticed in 11 arousals, while in 3 cases, the absence or presence of eye movements could not be determined.

On the electroencephalogram, movement artefacts were present in 28 cases, an absence of change was noted in 7. An increased amplitude was found in 8 arousals while a decreased amplitude could be seen in 5. An increased frequency could be seen in 7 arousals while a decrease in frequency with appearance of delta waves was noted in 3 cases. In one case rhythmic delta waves were seen.

Movements were detected in all arousals: 41 by the actigraph, 18 on the pulse oxymeter and 7 by the nurse. A change in respiration, either in frequency or in amplitude, occurred in 45 of the 53 arousals. A change in the RR intervals occurred in all arousals. From the 53 arousals, 32 were accompanied by changes in 5 criteria, 14 in 4 criteria, 3 in 3 criteria and 4 in 2 criteria.

Table 3.

Referring to the arousals:	Non system	Obstructive events	P
Respiratory rate before (breaths/min.)	37 (22–62)	30 (21–62)	0.05
Mean RR before (msec.)	470 (390–510)	510 (390–600)	0.01
Mean RR after (msec.)	490 (375–465)	540 (430–625)	0.03

Obstructive events represent the sum of obstructive and mixed apneas.

Table 4.

	Central apneas	Obstructive apneas	P
Mean RR before (msec.)	500 (485–575)	470 (390–515)	0.02
Mean RR after (msec.)	540 (520–665)	485 (375–565)	0.01

The arousals preceded by an obstructive event were compared with the non system related arousals (Table 3).

Likewise, arousals preceded by a central apnea were compared with those preceded by an obstructive apnea (Table 4).

Arousals occurring in quiet or active sleep differed only by their duration: in quiet sleep, they lasted 11 seconds (range from 4 to 32 sec), while in active sleep, their duration was 14 seconds (range from 4 to 70 sec) ($p=0.05$).

2.1 Comments

Movements and changes in RR intervals were seen in all examples of arousals. These characteristics could be related to the selection of complete spontaneous arousals. Changes in respiration were found in 45 of 53 arousals, and changes in EEG occurred in 18. No change was seen in only 7 (13%) arousals. In 28 cases, movement artefacts prevented the analysis. Eye movements or EOG artefacts were found in 42 (79%) arousals. For the majority of arousals, changes were found in the physiological parameters chosen, and arousals were associated with changes in at least two of the five parameters studied.

Due to the selection of the recordings, no conclusion can be drawn regarding the occurrence of arousals without movement. Further studies should be undertaken to confirm this characteristics.

Conclusions

Our study showed that the quantitative characteristics of spontaneously occurring arousals depend on the circumstances of the arousal. Arousals were shorter in active sleep. Respiratory rate before and RR interval before and after the arousal were different in system and non system arousals. RR intervals were different in arousals associated with central or obstructive apnea.

3. The analysis of induced arousals in infants

Patients and methods

Eleven infants were selected successively from a larger group of infants recruited for a research program on sleep-related behaviour. The infants were eligible for the study if they met the following criteria: they were born at term, from non-smoking parents, with no family history of SIDS. At the time of recording the infants were about 11 weeks old, they were healthy and usually slept supine. The major characteristics of the infants included in the analysis are shown in Table 5.

The recording procedures were similar to those reported in II.B, but in the present study, the data was collected on computerized polygraph recorders (Morpheus System, Medatec, Belgium).

To study auditory arousal thresholds, white noise of increasing intensity was presented for 3 seconds via a loudspeaker (SCR Electronics, Paris, France) to either ear, at a distance of 3 cm (Franco et al., 1996). The sound level was increased by 10 dB, ranging from 50 dB (A) to 100 dB (A). The time between each presentation was 1 minute. The auditory signal was identified on the sleep recording. Infants were tested during type 2 Non Rapid Eye Movement sleep (NREM) sleep and Rapid Eye Movement (REM) sleep. Infants were tested after their first sleep cycle, after a minimum of 5 minutes in the sleep stage.

Table 5.

Number of infants	11
Gender (M/F)	4/7
Gestational age (weeks)	40 (37–41)
Age at sleep study (weeks)	9 (8–12)
Birth weight (g)	3300 (2690–4160)

Note: The figures represent median and range values.

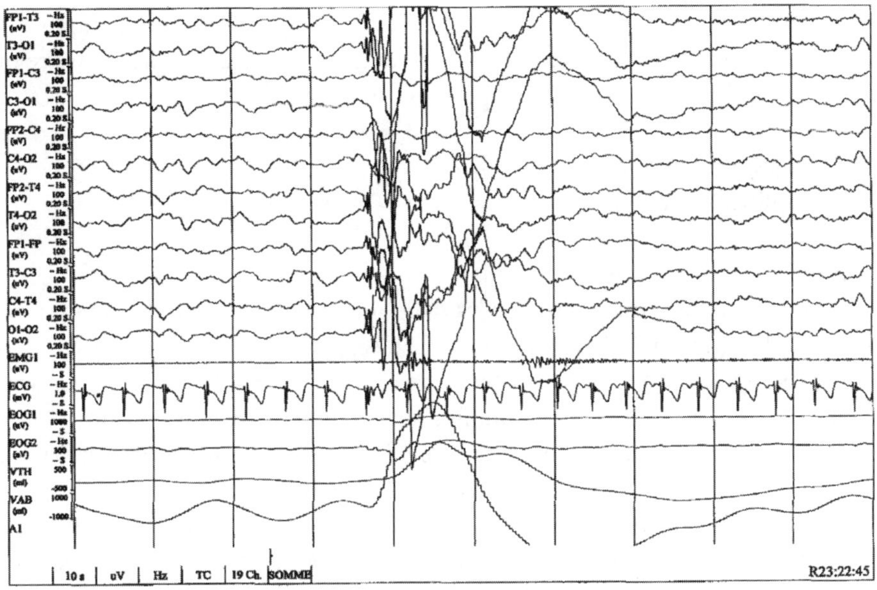

Figure 3. Global arousal in REM sleep inducing simultaneously changes in EEG, EMG, heart rate and breathing amplitude.

Every thirty-second periods of the recordings were divided into NREM sleep, REM sleep, indeterminate sleep, or wakefulness. Sleep efficiency was defined as the time spent sleeping divided by the total recording time, multiplied by 100. Scoring was done visually by two independent scorers to ensure reliability. Inter-rater agreement was 95%. Scoring discrepancies were discussed and codes thus agreed upon were used in the data analysis.

An arousal was scored if within 10 seconds after the start of an auditory stimulation, abrupt changes in polysomnographic parameters occurred. These parameters were compared with those recorded during the 20 seconds preceding the auditory challenge. These polygraphic changes were quantitatively analysed. The reaction values were divided by the basal values (ratio after/before). The parameter change's frequency was evaluated for all the infants (frequency of changes).

The polysomnographic changes included:

– Changes in EEG

The EEG montage was referentiated with ear reference (F3-A1, C3-A1, T3-A1, O1-A1). We analysed the frequency of EEG by autoregressive spectral frequency analysis and by visual analysis (EEG sampling at 200 Hz), the amplitude of EEG by computer analysis with a resolution of +/- 0.25 μV, the presence of artifacts, and for NREM sleep the presence of spindles.

– *Changes in EOG*
The amplitude of EOG (same resolution as that of EEG).

– *Changes in breathing*
Thoracic and abdominal amplitudes were measured by computer analysis as the breathing frequency. The presence of sleep apneas was noticed. Sleep apneas were scored only if they lasted 3 seconds or more. A central apnea was scored when flat tracings were obtained simultaneously from the strain gauges and the thermistors. Sighs isolated or followed by central or mixed apnea were defined by a twofold increase in breathing amplitude. Periodic breathing was defined by at least 3 central apneas separated by less than 20 seconds of breathing movements. An obstructive apnea was scored when continuous deflections were obtained from the strain gauges, while a flat tracing was recorded from the thermistors. Mixed apneas were defined as a central apnea directly followed by an obstructive episode and were scored together with the obstructive apneas.

– *Changes in EMG amplitude*
EMG amplitudes were evaluated by computer analysis.

– *Changes in heart rate and oxygen saturation*
Median values for oxygen saturation, heart rate were calculated on 20 seconds preceding the stimulation. A drop or a rise in heart rate (HR) referred to changes from basal values (%). Overall HR variability was defined as the standard deviation of the RR values.

Statistical analysis was performed with the use of Wilcoxon's matched paired test with a level of significance of <0.05.

Main findings

The major sleep characteristics of the infants included in the analysis are shown in Table 6.

Table 6. Major sleep characteristics of the infants studied (As absolute, median and range values)

Total recording time (min)	585 (520–600)
Total sleep time (min)	412 (381–495)
Sleep efficiency (%)	73 (67–85)
NREM sleep (%)	40.15 (28.9–47.5)
REM sleep (%)	31.65 (25.4–39.6)
Movement (%)	5.55 (2.6–11.7)
Awake (%)	22.6 (6.4–25.4)
Central apneas	
N°/ hour of sleep	1.94 (0.46–6.98)
Duration (sec)	6.15 (4.2–7.9)
Periodic breathing (%)	0.2 (0–16.3)
Obstructive apneas	
N°/hour of sleep	0.55 (0–1.26)
Duration (sec)	5.9 (3.4–8.2)
Heart rate (Bpm)	
NREM sleep	122 (111–158.5)
REM sleep	122.5 (115–153)
Heart rate variation (Bpm)	
NREM sleep	2.91 (1.5–6.81)
REM sleep	4.44 (2.14–8.98)
Breathing rate (Breath/min)	
NREM sleep	30 (22–49)
REM sleep	33 (18–52)
Saturation in oxygen	98 (93–99)

Auditory arousals during REM sleep

There were 2 challenges in REM sleep per infant. At 50 dB (A), 14 of 22 challenges induced an immediate global arousal (64%). The median delay of arousal was 0 sec (range 0 to 10 sec), and the mean duration was 15.5 sec (range 6 to 60 sec). The median hour of auditory stimulations was 1:54 AM (range 23:17 PM to 3:33 AM). In 12 of 14 cases, there was no change in sleep stage following the arousal response and in two cases, the infants awoke.

The global arousals (Fig. 3) were simultaneously associated with changes in (Table 7).

1. *EEG*

- Decreases in frequency (mainly on the occipital leads) of about 50%.
- Increases in amplitude (mainly on the temporal leads) ($\geq 2 \times$ of basal values).
- Appearances of EEG waves superior to 8 Hz in at less one lead (100%).

Table 7. Quantitative data of global reaction during REM sleep

REM sleep	Before	After	Frequency of changes %	Ratio after/ before(×)	P
EEG Frequency (Hz)					
Spectral					
Decrease all leads	4.60 (1.2–12.1)	1.10 (0.5–8.3)	93	0.27 (0.09–2.13)	<.001
Decrease O1 lead			**100**	**0.28 (0.10–0.74)**	.001
Increase all leads	4.60 (1.2–12.1)	9.20 (1–20.9)	62.5	1.98 (0.21–13.75)	<.001
Visual	5 (2.5–9)	2 (0.5–6)	89	0.42 (0.07–1.5)	<.001
EEG Amplitude (μV) All leads	54 (18.3–87.3)	262 (55–609)	94.6	(0.57–19.7)	<.001
Increase T3 lead			**100**	**6.29 (2.66–19.70)**	.001
EOG Amplitude (μV)	11 (2–71)	256 (7–256)	**100**	**15.24 (1.40–125.5)**	<.001
EMG Amplitude (μV)	0 (0–3)	27 (9–165)	**100**	**34 (9–165)**	<.003
Breathing Amplitude Thoracic (μV)	95 (21–597)	1212 (356–2598)	**100**	**12.49 (2–123.7)**	<.001
Heart rate (Bpm)					
Increase	122.5 (117–155)	155 (139–173)	**100**	+24% (11–33%)	.001
Decrease	122.5 (117–155)	122 (81–130)	93	–8% (–0–50%)	.001
Saturation in oxygen (%)	97.5 (91–100)	94 (85–99)	93	–3% (0–7%)	.001

Note: The figures represent median and range values. Wilcoxon-Mann-Whitney tests were used to compare values before and after stimulation.

2. *Non-EEG signals*

- ECG: increases in heart rate, followed by a decrease in heart rate equal or more than 10% of basal values. The heart rate variation during basal period was in median 4% (range 1 to 7%).
- Breathing amplitude: increases in amplitude were seen mainly at the level of the thorax ($\geq 2 \times$ of basal values). There was no statistical difference in breathing frequency with a
  - median value of 34 breath/min in basal period and 32 breath/min after stimulation (range 25 to 50 breath/min) (NS). After stimulation,

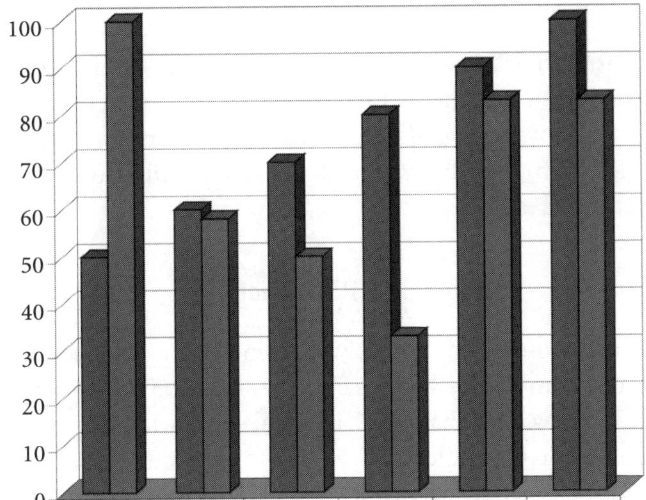

	1	2	3	4	5	6
■ Threshold (dB)	50	60	70	80	90	100
■ % Global response	0	58	50	33	83	83

Figure 4. Distribution of global reaction to increasing auditory stimuli intensities in REM sleep.

breathing was irregular in frequency and in amplitude in all cases. In 28% of cases, breathing irregularities were followed by a central apnea.

- Appearance of global body movements (trashing type) and/or increase in EMG tonus about 8 times of basal values.

The repetition of the auditory stimuli at increasing dB (A) during REM sleep lead to:

- An arousal response in 51/74 challenges (69%);
- An "U shape" arousal reaction curve, with increasing auditory intensities: arousal responses were seen initially following the first stimulation (50 dB) and again at high intensities (90–100 dB) (Fig. 4).

A global arousal was found before auditory stimulation in a median of 5 min 23 (range 4 to 12 min.). Comparing to basal situation, the frequency of occurrence of global arousal was increased when exposed to auditory stimulation ($p = .001$).

Following 16.6% of the stimuli, only a partial response was seen, that included:

- Drops in heart rates that were seen in all cases of partial responses.
- In addition to heart rate changes, changes were seen in one or two of the following signals: EEG, EMG, breathing movements (frequency, apnea, sigh). The types of changes were similar to those seen during global arousal responses.

Auditory arousals during NREM sleep

Auditory arousals challenges were done in 10 instances. The median time of auditory stimulation was 0:04 AM (range 22:53 PM to 2:02 AM). In 8 of 10 cases, there was no change in sleep stage following the arousal response; in two cases, the infants awoke.

Global reactions were obtained with auditory stimuli equal or greater than 70 dB in NREM sleep. The auditory arousal thresholds needed to induce an arousal were higher during NREM than during REM sleep. (Fig. 5).

The initial reactions were:

- A partial reaction (4 out of 10 challenges);

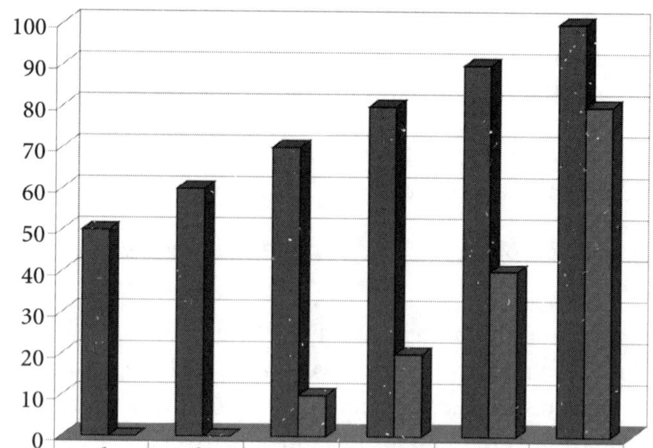

	1	2	3	4	5	6
■ Threshold (dB)	50	60	70	80	90	100
■ % Global response	0	0	10	20	40	80

Figure 5. Auditory challenges during NREM sleep.

Table 8. Quantitative data of global reaction during NREM sleep

REM sleep	Before	After	Frequency of changes %	Ratio after/ before(×)	P
EEG Frequency (Hz)					
Spectral					
Decrease all leads	3.10 (1.3–7)	1.25 (0.5–7.8)	89	0.39 (0.16–2.6)	.002
Decrease O1 lead			**100**	**0.35 (0.20–0.72)**	.018
Increase all leads	3.10 (1.3–7)	9.60 (1.2–22.5)	82	2.56 (0.24–11.23)	.001
Visual	3 (2–5)	2 (0–7)	78	0.5 (0.2–1.75)	.009
EEG Amplitude (μV) All leads	95.55 (60.5–180)	242.45 (111–596)	**100**	**2.65 (1.05–4.94)**	**<.001**
Increase T3 lead			**100**	**2.11 (1.07–4.94)**	**.018**
EOG Amplitude (μV)	18.5 (2–35)	121.5 (63–244)	**100**	**7.91 (2.37–122)**	.001
EMG Amplitude (μV)	5 (4–8)	27 (13–89)	**100**	**10.17 (2.63–32)**	.027
Breathing Amplitude **Thoracic** (μV)	275 (13–525)	1258 (326–2896)	**100**	**6.15 (2.81–75.77)**	.018
Heart rate (Bpm)					
Increase	121 (114–144)	155 (142–210)	**100**	**+29% (20–48%)**	.018
Decrease	121 (114–144)	118 (96–130)	85.7	–4% (–3–21%)	.042
Saturation in oxygen (%)	97 (94–99)	97 (95–98)	14	0% (1–4%)	NS

Note: The figures represent median and range values. Wilcoxon-Mann-Whitney tests were used to compare values before and after stimulation.

– A global reaction (6 out of 10 challenges, but 2/6 responded at 100 dB (A) only).

The median delay for partial and global arousals was 3 sec (range 0 to 9 sec), and the mean duration was respectively for partial reaction 4.5 sec (range 3 to 11 sec) and 36 sec (range 11–60 sec) for global reaction. The median auditory threshold was 80 dB (range 60 to 100 dB) for a partial reaction and 90 dB (range 70 to 100 dB) for a global reaction.

The changes seen during the arousal reactions in NREM type 2 sleep included:

- Changes similar to those seen in REM sleep;
- Less frequent changes in EEG frequencies (–25%), amplitude (× 1.5) and in EMG amplitude (× 2);
- The suppression of EEG spindles (in all cases);
- The appearance of EOG movements.

In the partial response:

- The presence of a sigh associated with an increase in heart rate was included in all cases.
- Changes in EEG or EMG can be associated. These changes were similar to those described during REM sleep.
- A global arousal was found before auditory stimulation in a median of 7 min 35 (range 4:28 to 14:48 min). Compared to the basal situation, the frequency of occurrence of global arousal was increased when exposed to auditory stimulation ($p = .011$).
- The repetition of the auditory stimuli at increasing intensities during a NREM period lead to progressive increases in the frequency of arousals, without the "U shape" response seen in REM sleep.

Comments

The evaluation of arousal thresholds contribute to a better understanding of the infant's reaction to environmental stress. The information is of particular value for a better understanding of some mechanisms associated with severe clinical conditions, such as the occurrence of the Sudden Infant Death Syndrome (SIDS). It can be shown that normal infants exposed to conditions known to increase the risk for SIDS develop a greater difficulty to arouse from sleep than when challenged in non-risk conditions. Such observations were reported in infants lying prone to sleep, for both spontaneously occuring (Groswasser et al., 2001) or induced arousals (Franco et al., 1998). Auditory arousal threshods were also increased in infants exposed to cigarette smoke during pregnancy (Franco et al., 1999), or sleeping in a warm environment (Franco et al., 2001).

Additional studies have also linked risk situations for SIDS to changes in heart rate autonomic controls with an increase in heart rate sympathico/vagal balance (Franco 1996, 2000a: 401). In infants, sleep apnea develop when exposed to cigarette smoking during gestation or to high environmental temperatures (Kahn et al., 1994) (Figure 6). These findings were reminiscents of the ob-

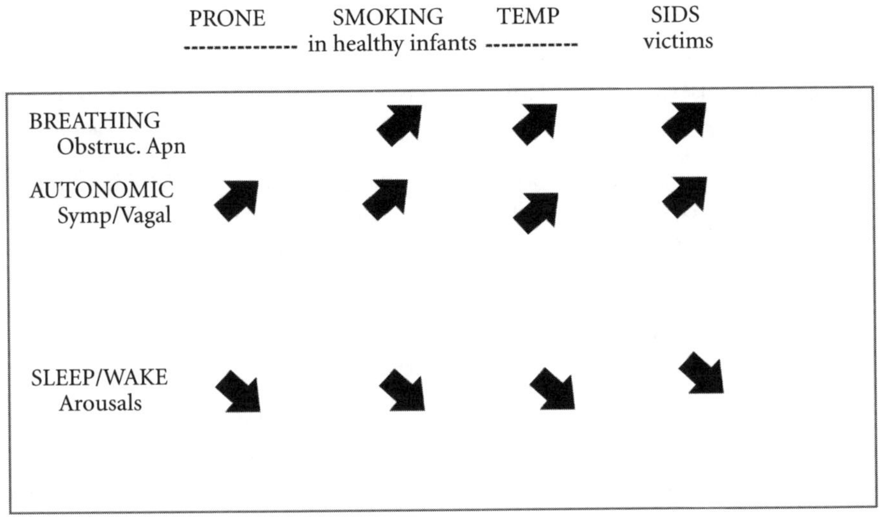

Figure 6. Environmental factors and SIDS.

servation of an increased frequency of arousals, an increase sympathico/vagal heart rate balance and an increase in obstructive sleep apneas in infants who became victims of SIDS (Franco et al., 1996; Kahn et al., 1992). Healthy infants exhibited more frequent spontaneous arousals and lower arousal thresholds when placed in situations associated with a lower risk for SIDS, such as breast feeding or the use of a pacifier during sleep (Franco et al., 2000b: 775).

These findings strongly support the possibility that arousal from sleep could play a crucial role in the occurrence of SIDS. It also emphasizes the complexity of the arousals, as breathing, cardiorespiratory and autonomic controls appear to be closely linked to the changes in brainstem and cortical status. Finally, the above studies further argue for a common definition of arousals. A consensus on the terminology and methodologies for the scoring of arousal in infants will benefit all those involved in research studies on infant sleep/wake behaviours in various clinical conditions.

Acknowledgments

We wish to thank Drs L. Curzi-Dascalova, M. Katz-Salamon, J. Milerad and S. Scholle who contributed to the selection of arousals in infants.

References

Franco, Patricia, José Groswasser, Martine Sottiaux, Emilie Broadfield & André Kahn (1996). Decreasesd cardiac responses to auditory stimulation during prone sleep. *Pediatrics, 97*: 174–178.

Franco, Patricia, Anne Pardou, Sergio Hassid, Pierre Lurquin & André Kahn (1998). Auditory arousal thresholds are higher when infants sleep in the prone position. *Journal of Pediatrics, 132*: 240–243.

Franco, Patricia, José Groswasser, Sergio Hassid, Jean Pierre Lanquart, Sonia Scaillet & André Kahn (1999). Prenatal exposure to cigarettes is associated with decreased arousal propensity in infants. *Journal of Pediatrics, 135*: 34–38.

Franco, Patricia, Henri Szliwowski, Michèle Dramaix & André Kahn (2000a). Influence of ambient temperature on sleep characteristics and autonomic nervous control in healthy infants. *Sleep, 23*: 401–407.

Franco, Patricia, Sonia Scaillet, Vanessa Wermenbol, Fiona Valente, José Groswasser & André Kahn (2000b). The influence fo a pacifier on infants' arousals from sleep. *Journal of Pediatrics, 136*: 775–779.

Franco, Patricia, Sonia Scaillet, Fiona Valente, Serge Chabanski, José Groswasser & André Kahn (2001). Ambient temperature is associated with changes in infants'arousability form sleep. *Sleep, 24*: 325–329.

Groswasser José, Tony Simon, Sonia Scaillet, Patricia Franco & André Kahn (2001). Reduced arousals following obstructive apneas in infants sleeping prone. *Pediatric Research, 49*: 402–406.

Guilleminault, Christian, & Michel Souquet (1979). Sleep states and related pathology. In: Korobkin R., Guilleminault C. (Eds), *Advances in Perinatal Neurology* (225–247). New-York: Spectrum Publications.

Kahn, André, José Groswasser, Elisabeth Rebuffat, Martine Sottiaux, Denise Blum, Martine Foerster, Patricia Franco, André Bochner, Marc Alexander, André Bachy, Patrick Richard, Michel Verghote, Daniel Le Polain & Jean-Louis Wyenberg (1992). Sleep and cardiorespiratory characteristics of infant victims of sudden death: a prospective case-control study. *Sleep, 15*: 287–292.

Kahn, André, José Groswasser, Martine Sottiaux, Igor Kelmanson, Elisabeth Rebuffat, Patricia Franco, Michèle Dramaix & Jean-Louis Wayenberg (1994). Prenatal exposure to cigarettes in infants with obstructive sleep apneas. *Pediatrics, 93*: 778–783.

Index of names

Index of terms

In the series ADVANCES IN CONSCIOUSNESS RESEARCH (AiCR) the following titles have been published thus far or are scheduled for publication:

1. GLOBUS, Gordon G.: *The Postmodern Brain.* 1995.
2. ELLIS, Ralph D.: *Questioning Consciousness. The interplay of imagery, cognition, and emotion in the human brain.* 1995.
3. JIBU, Mari and Kunio YASUE: *Quantum Brain Dynamics and Consciousness. An introduction.* 1995.
4. HARDCASTLE, Valerie Gray: *Locating Consciousness.* 1995.
5. STUBENBERG, Leopold: *Consciousness and Qualia.* 1998.
6. GENNARO, Rocco J.: *Consciousness and Self-Consciousness. A defense of the higher-order thought theory of consciousness.* 1996.
7. MAC CORMAC, Earl and Maxim I. STAMENOV (eds): *Fractals of Brain, Fractals of Mind. In search of a symmetry bond.* 1996.
8. GROSSENBACHER, Peter G. (ed.): *Finding Consciousness in the Brain. A neurocognitive approach.* 2001.
9. Ó NUALLÁIN, Seán, Paul MC KEVITT and Eoghan MAC AOGÁIN (eds): *Two Sciences of Mind. Readings in cognitive science and consciousness.* 1997.
10. NEWTON, Natika: *Foundations of Understanding.* 1996.
11. PYLKKÖ, Pauli: *The Aconceptual Mind. Heideggerian themes in holistic naturalism.* 1998.
12. STAMENOV, Maxim I. (ed.): *Language Structure, Discourse and the Access to Consciousness.* 1997.
13. VELMANS, Max (ed.): *Investigating Phenomenal Consciousness. Methodologies and Maps.* 2000.
14. SHEETS-JOHNSTONE, Maxine: *The Primacy of Movement.* 1999.
15. CHALLIS, Bradford H. and Boris M. VELICHKOVSKY (eds.): *Stratification in Cognition and Consciousness.* 1999.
16. ELLIS, Ralph D. and Natika NEWTON (eds.): *The Caldron of Consciousness. Motivation, affect and self-organization – An anthology.* 2000.
17. HUTTO, Daniel D.: *The Presence of Mind.* 1999.
18. PALMER, Gary B. and Debra J. OCCHI (eds.): *Languages of Sentiment. Cultural constructions of emotional substrates.* 1999.
19. DAUTENHAHN, Kerstin (ed.): *Human Cognition and Social Agent Technology.* 2000.
20. KUNZENDORF, Robert G. and Benjamin WALLACE (eds.): *Individual Differences in Conscious Experience.* 2000.
21. HUTTO, Daniel D.: *Beyond Physicalism.* 2000.
22. ROSSETTI, Yves and Antti REVONSUO (eds.): *Beyond Dissociation. Interaction between dissociated implicit and explicit processing.* 2000.
23. ZAHAVI, Dan (ed.): *Exploring the Self. Philosophical and psychopathological perspectives on self-experience.* 2000.
24. ROVEE-COLLIER, Carolyn, Harlene HAYNE and Michael COLOMBO: *The Development of Implicit and Explicit Memory.* 2000.
25. BACHMANN, Talis: *Microgenetic Approach to the Conscious Mind.* 2000.
26. Ó NUALLÁIN, Seán (ed.): *Spatial Cognition. Selected papers from Mind III, Annual Conference of the Cognitive Science Society of Ireland, 1998.* 2000.
27. McMILLAN, John and Grant R. GILLETT: *Consciousness and Intentionality.* 2001.

28. ZACHAR, Peter: *Psychological Concepts and Biological Psychiatry. A philosophical analysis.* 2000.
29. VAN LOOCKE, Philip (ed.): *The Physical Nature of Consciousness.* 2001.
30. BROOK, Andrew and Richard C. DeVIDI (eds.): *Self-reference and Self-awareness.* 2001.
31. RAKOVER, Sam S. and Baruch CAHLON: *Face Recognition. Cognitive and computational processes.* 2001.
32. VITIELLO, Giuseppe: *My Double Unveiled. The dissipative quantum model of the brain.* 2001.
33. YASUE, Kunio, Mari JIBU and Tarcisio DELLA SENTA (eds.): *No Matter, Never Mind. Proceedings of Toward a Science of Consciousness: Fundamental Approaches, Tokyo, 1999.* 2002.
34. FETZER, James H.(ed.): *Consciousness Evolving.* 2002.
35. Mc KEVITT, Paul, Seán Ó NUALLÁIN and Conn MULVIHILL (eds.): *Language, Vision, and Music. Selected papers from the 8th International Workshop on the Cognitive Science of Natural Language Processing, Galway, 1999.* n.y.p.
36. PERRY, Elaine, Heather ASHTON and Allan YOUNG (eds.): *Neurochemistry of Consciousness. Neurotransmitters in mind.* 2002.
37. PYLKKÄNEN, Paavo and Tere VADÉN (eds.): *Dimensions of Conscious Experience.* 2001.
38. SALZARULO, Piero and Gianluca FICCA (eds.): *Awakening and Sleep-Wake Cycle Across Development.* 2002.
39. BARTSCH, Renate: *Consciousness Emerging. The dynamics of perception, imagination, action, memory, thought, and language.* 2002.
40. MANDLER, George: *Consciousness Recovered. Psychological functions and origins of conscious thought.* 2002.
41. ALBERTAZZI, Liliana (ed.): *Unfolding Perceptual Continua.* n.y.p.
42. STAMENOV, Maxim I. and Vittorio GALLESE (eds.): *Mirror Neurons and the Evolution of Brain and Language.* n.y.p.
43. DEPRAZ, Natalie, Francisco VARELA and Pierre VERMERSCH.: *On Becoming Aware.* n.y.p.
44. MOORE, Simon and Mike OAKSFORD (eds.): *Emotional Cognition. From brain to behaviour.* n.y.p.
45. DOKIC, Jerome and Joelle PROUST: *Simulation and Knowledge of Action.* n.y.p.
46. MATHEAS, Michael and Phoebe SENGERS (ed.): *Narrative Intelligence.* n.y.p.
47. COOK, Norman D.: *Tone of Voice and Mind. The connections between intonation, emotion, cognition and consciousness.* n.y.p.